Praise for *Naturally Pain Free*

"I love Letha's writing style. *Naturally Pain Free* reads like she is talking to a good friend in a calm informative voice."

—Gerald D. Ginsberg, MD, Director, Plastic Surgery,
New York Downtown Hospital

"*Naturally Pain Free* is great! Just what is needed. It's loaded with good advice, and will fly off the shelves."

—Christopher Phillips, CCH, RSHom (NA), classical homeopath, New York

"Letha Hadady is informative…calming…sweet…reassuring…and most important…knowledgeable. *Naturally Pain Free* makes natural health practical…and not at all frightening and that's crucial."

—Kevin Harry, Network Television Executive, New York

"*Naturally Pain Free* is well-researched and charmingly written. A fine contribution."

—Dr. Alan Lazar, MD, FACS, Clinical Assistant Professor, College of
Osteopathic Medicine, Nova University

Naturally PAIN FREE

Prevent and Treat Chronic and Acute Pains—Naturally

LETHA HADADY, D.AC.

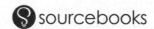

Published by Sourcebooks, Inc.
P.O. Box 4410, Naperville, Illinois 60567-4410
(630) 961-3900
Fax: (630) 961-2168
www.sourcebooks.com

Library of Congress Cataloging-in-Publication Data

Hadady, Letha.
  Naturally pain free : prevent and treat chronic and acute pains—naturally / by Letha Hadady.
    p. cm.
  Includes index.
  1. Chronic pain—Alternative treatment—Popular works. 2. Chronic pain—Prevention—Popular works.
  3. Chronic pain—Popular works. 4. Self-care, Health—Popular works. I. Title.
  RB127.H323 2012
  616'.0472—dc23

                                2012014791

            Printed and bound in the United States of America.
                    VP 10 9 8 7 6 5 4 3 2 1

Also By Letha Hadady

Asian Health Secrets
Personal Renewal
Healthy Beauty
Feed Your Tiger

*This book is dedicated to your inimitable spirit
that becomes wise by overcoming pain.*

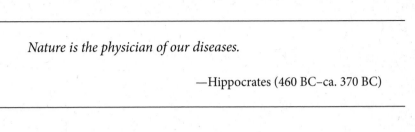

Nature is the physician of our diseases.

—Hippocrates (460 BC–ca. 370 BC)

Contents

Introduction

OUR LIVES BEGIN IN PAIN. JETTISONED FROM THE SAFE COMFORT OF OUR mother's womb, we are born into glaring light, noise, and challenges we must face alone. From the trauma of that separation we may eventually gain strength and wisdom or else seek reentry into darkness. This book is our journey of discovery and freedom from ignorance and slavery to that harmful lifestyle. Everywhere I go I meet people in pain who are bewildered, lacking an awareness of its cause and best remedy. Using a daily pain pill as commonly available as aspirin is a way of life for countless people. The illegal resale of prescription pain medicines has become black-market big business, while the public remains unaware of potential dangers associated with their use, especially in combination with medicines or certain foods. This book addresses a major international health problem, which is pain resulting from poor habits, aging, injury, environmental and political threats including terrorism, and a variety of everyday stress factors that too often lead to drug addiction, depression, and challenged immunity. Both personal and journalistic, *Naturally Pain Free* draws upon my own clinical experience as well as on research information from experts and treatment centers throughout the world. According to the American Pain Foundation:

> Chronic pain is a complex condition that affects forty-two to fifty million Americans. Despite decades of research, chronic pain remains poorly understood and notoriously hard to control. A survey by the American Academy of Pain Medicine found that even comprehensive treatment with painkilling prescription drugs helps, on average, only about 58 percent of people with chronic pain.

Despite the fact that tremendous scientific advances have been made around the world in naturally preventing and treating chronic and acute pain and injury with respected Asian herbs and advanced medical treatments, most people rely on their old favorites—denial, alcohol, addictive medical drugs, and over-the-counter pain pills—that fail to address the actual sources of pain and often result in harmful side effects. Do you use the same pain treatment for a toothache, headache, arthritis, menstrual cramps, or sciatica? Do you have chest pains from a heart health issue or an emotional heartache? They are all very different sorts of agony, stemming from different origins. Different pains require specific, individualized prevention and treatment in order to reduce reoccurrence and complications.

Naturally Pain Free presents safe, *pleasurable* ways to avoid common pains and long-term ailments that sap vitality and spirit. Comforting, preventative treatments detailed here include cleansing and slimming foods, calming herbal teas, revitalizing baths, energy-balancing massage, targeted use of LED-light therapy and cold-laser treatments, and pain-relief exercises done while sitting or lying in bed. Why suffer pain while trying to relieve it? You have suffered enough. You may think of this approach as hedonistic pain relief; I think of it as smart pain prevention and treatment.

Herbal tonics are nature's gems and address many health and beauty issues simultaneously. You can find Asian herbal capsules for sale at Walmart or in your local pharmacy, but you may not know how to use them. Shark cartilage, for example, gives us protein and minerals from the shark's backbone. It supports and lubricates your stressed joints, while it improves flexibility of blood vessels and helps prevent cancers. If you grew up in a traditional Chinese family, you probably ate it in soup during lunar New Year celebrations. Ashwagandha root, originally from India and now available in health-food store capsules, supports adrenal health and thereby improves physical endurance, memory, and sexual vitality, while it reduces lower back and leg aches and muscle fatigue. Aloe vera, the desert plant, is a supreme internal cleanser and a topical skin treatment for burns. If you were alone in the desert, it could keep you alive and pain-free. Drinking aloe juice reduces inflammatory pains, acid indigestion, menstrual cramps, and a wide variety of discomforts. These are among my favorite herbs.

All cultures value herbal traditions, whether as natural medicine or in cooking. With wise use, herbs are tools for prevention and treatment of pain and injury. To reduce confusion whenever possible, I avoid using traditional Asian medicine terms unless they are necessary to explain a specific treatment. For example, the Chinese word "qi" can refer to a measure of vitality, circulation, or organ functioning. However, I use the term to explain qi tonics or Chinese herbs such as panax ginseng that enhance our natural energy and support the health of internal organs. Most people do not realize that the *origin* of an herb is only part of its use. Many herbs and spices such as clove, cinnamon, and ginger are shared by many cultures. The difference comes in how they are used to affect our health. Students sometimes ask me whether people born in the West can use Asian herbs to treat pain or illness. My answer is, "Of course they can." Herbs do not have to originate in your backyard to be effective. Their best use depends upon a correct diagnosis, treatment, and follow-up.

How can you find an herbalist? Accredited herbal health professionals are listed by their associated organization such as the NCCAOM (National Certification Commission for Acupuncture and Oriental Medicine) located in Washington, D.C. and online. Ethnic communities throughout the world sell herbs that have been used with confidence for centuries, and a growing body of international research available online supports their use. Some people prefer to follow their nose by consulting an herbalist recommended by friends in order to get a sense of how he or she works and of whether the treatment may be effective. In that case, it is important to supply as much information as possible about your condition, ask questions, and give the treatment time to work. Herbs are not like daily vitamins that we use to supplement nutrition. They should be adjusted by an herbalist when necessary according to your energy, immunity, and even the seasonal changes. An Asian view of wellness is holistic in that it aims to enhance your individual vitality and mood in order to reduce pain. It ties everyday pains together with deeper issues such as circulation, inflammation, and digestion.

I have come to think of my physical pain as a life-saving warning to adjust my posture and nourish vitality with the right foods, herbs, and body treatments. Using nature's way to ease pain, I refresh my commitment to lasting good health. We grow into our bodies in a spiral of past and present habits and desires. Body shapes mind and mind shapes body. Pain also shapes us, allowing us to use our experiences to develop clarity, understanding, and personal growth. How we as individuals experience pain greatly determines our attitudes and expectations of it. The Lebanese-American poet Kahlil Gibran wrote, "Much of your pain is the bitter potion by which the physician within you heals your sick self."

Pain presents important communication about what is happening to us; some people accept it as normal, knowing more or less what to expect, while others feel threatened and deeply harmed by the same pain. Dr. Matthew Gammons, MD, specializes in sports medicine at Killington, Vermont, the largest, most active ski mountain in the northeastern United States. He says, "It is not a matter of courage or fortitude that allows some people to more easily bear pain. Emotional factors and nerve communication are involved as well as injury." A sensitive health professional can often identify physical injuries as well as the deeper harm pain does to the nervous system and emotional balance. However, few untrained people are able to recognize the nature of their pain, its origins, and natural treatment. This book brings together many approaches to prevent and ease some of your worst hurts and fears.

Is there such a thing as *good* pain? Many dancers, athletes, and bodybuilders believe there is. Building muscle mass stretches, sometimes tears connective tissue, and it hurts unless steps are taken to rid the body of acid waste by-products. A natural diet to alleviate workout pain includes alkaline green drinks and homeopathic natrum phosphate to reduce acidity. Drinking water to stay hydrated is helpful but not enough to ease muscle pain. Over-the-counter painkillers and steroids have bad side effects. There are better ways to deal with workout pain; you can find those ways in chapters covering injury and energy tonics.

Here is a different example of *good* pain. As I take the elevator to surgery on the fifth floor, I smile, anticipating a warm greeting from my longtime friend, Dr. Gerald Ginsberg, MD, FACS., Director of Plastic Surgery at New York Downtown Hospital. He has reshaped my Hungarian thighs using liposuction. His beauty treatments are a pleasure because they are my choice and I know the pain is both tolerable and temporary. They involve *good* pain. During our time together, we chat about family and vacations, which enhances a healing atmosphere. To support his expert treatments, I use a traditional Chinese herbal medicine to avoid excess bleeding, swelling, and bruising, and speed healing to a fraction of the usual time. In other words, I control my pain. The Chinese People's Army uses the same capsule of astringent and circulation-enhancing herbs to stop hemorrhage from gunshot wounds and help prevent infections. Office surgery avoids the usual risks and expense of general anesthesia and a hospital visit.

Dr. Gerry has often remarked upon my ability to stay calm and focused, while staying awake, during plastic surgery. He and I have the same goal, and I have total confidence in him. I am realistic about what to expect from treatments and I use natural pain-treatment methods during surgery. I breathe deeply, apply targeted acupressure point stimulation, and follow up with additional remedies to speed healing. After years of treating others' chronic pain issues, including female complaints, arthritis, computer-related pains, and everyday injuries, I know how to deal with pain. I have maintained a private health practice, and I presently write and answer health queries from around the world on my own and other websites. I can say with certainty that no over-the-counter or prescription pain medicine builds health. The more you know about *your* pain—its origins and effective, affordable treatments—the more calm, focused, safe, and content you can remain. The purpose of this book is to educate you about your pain in order to help prevent and eliminate it.

Sometimes, despite all our best efforts, pain conquers us because of injury, aging, and life's shocks. Maybe you jog or play tennis. Maybe you lifted the front room easy chair the wrong way and wrenched your back. Maybe you twisted your ankle, which is swollen and painful. Perhaps you have a chronic, debilitating illness that requires pain sedation. I am pleased to share my knowledge on natural and controversial pain therapies ranging from stem-cell injections to meditation and even marijuana. Luckily, a new frontier of regenerative medicine is slowly coming to light in America and is more advanced elsewhere. Once thought unimaginable, regenerative medicine accelerates the natural healing process to fully restore the health of damaged tissue and organs. Chapter 18, "The Future of Pain Medicine," features cutting-edge pain treatments, including my personal experience with platelet-rich plasma (PRP) and bone marrow stem-cell injections that use my own blood and stem cells to treat severe arthritic damage and pain.

This is truly an exciting direction in sports medicine and orthopedic surgery that hopefully will someday replace risky, expensive joint-replacement surgeries and enhance healing for all sorts of illness and injuries. I am thrilled to share my positive experience with this approach because it points the way to advanced treatment of acute and chronic pains. Great health research news is coming from China. Wujing General Hospital in Beijing specializes in autologous (taken from your own blood and bone marrow) stem-cell transfer treatments for heart disease, diabetes, and neurological illnesses, including Parkinson's disease and multiple sclerosis. We are at the dawn of a new day in medicine. This discovery, as important as the invention of surgery and antibiotics, brings up to date the ancient theories of qi and self-healing. We can heal the body with the body itself.

Chronic pain is exhausting, demoralizing, and aging. Acute, disfiguring injury is among our greatest fears. Pain depletes enthusiasm and life force. However, people since earliest times have treated pain with natural remedies from mud and bee stings to modern high-tech drugs and electrical stimulation. This book is your guide to treatments suited to your needs and budget. Chapters address different sorts of pain, ranging from superficial irritations affecting the skin's surface to heartaches. Scientists now know that the brain reacts to social rejection as though it were injury. Because body is connected to mind and emotions in a sensitive balance, wellness may be enhanced while treating either. For example, an essential oil can lift energy and mood, enabling positive thought and action. We strive to achieve total wellness, ease of movement, and comfort in order to achieve our best work and relate to others in positive, meaningful ways. The pleasure of beautiful music, loving touch, and pleasant natural aromas from cooking and flowers are no less important to well-being than a drug or surgical technique. They are the comforts of a loving home.

In modern Western society we stress aggressive action by using "painkillers." An Eastern approach, proven throughout the centuries, strives to ease discomforts and achieve balanced circulation and emotions in order to enhance vitality.

A healthy body is the perfect home of an open mind and generous spirit. An important source of our productivity is the confidence and enthusiasm resulting from the pain-free lifestyle described in this book. Why is a natural approach better? You may be able to temporarily ignore being overweight, having beauty problems, or having low energy, but no one can ignore a pain that stops you in your tracks. Try to sedate it, but sooner or later pain threatens vitality and shortens life. How we observe pain often points to the prescribed treatment approach. A research scientist might describe it like this: "Pain follows C-fiber activation, central sensitization, spinothalamic tract activation, insular cortex activation, and so on" in an inevitable chain of events. But chemical reactions do not express our experience. Pain hurts! It can be sharp, dull, deep, surface, hot, tingling, and all sorts of other feelings. Natural doctors, yogis, and parents have found ways to make pains stop. We need to pay attention to factors that aggravate our pain, such as age, excess weight, stress, diet, weather, emotional upset, and fatigue, and try to alleviate the underlying causes. This book will help. Good health provides comfort and well-being, and we are ill to the extent that we vary from this sensation.

A primary function of pain is communication. Political torture forces confessions. Pain always gets a reaction. Pain is a message from a specific area that something is wrong. You might tell me, "I have a headache." I would ask, "Where exactly does it hurt? Describe the pain." With my help, identifying and relieving your sources of pain may easily be done at home—without relying on clinics, expensive drugs, surgery, and machinery. Some people go to the dentist only after feeling a toothache. It is smarter to have regular checkups. Regular, natural pain prevention gives us the opportunity to enhance health and avoid discomforts of illness and aging.

Do men and women experience pain differently? It's hard to say. An April 2008 Clinical Update from the International Association for the Study of Pain entitled "Gender, Pain, and the Brain" finds many relevant factors such as hormonal fluctuation, differences in body size, skin thickness, blood pressure, social expectations, and differences in psychology such as anxiety and depression. It's not surprising that scientists find gender-related response to pain inexact. However, I think women react intuitively to pain. Some expect it monthly and for that reason are better prepared to handle it. We recognize its effects and are up for the challenge. We want a quick answer, not studies and diagrams, for injury and discomfort. This book is a tool to stop suffering.

Drugs have their place, which may be the hospital and battlefield more than the home. Prescription drugs should be monitored by medical professionals. Opiates are widely used in hospitals and following surgery to block pain, as are anticholinergic drugs that reduce spasm of smooth muscle in the lungs, gastrointestinal tract, and urinary tract. Many side effects are associated with these drugs, including hallucinations. One of my friends used a prescription drug for sciatica pain and cut up his bathroom towels with scissors in his sleep. Another client, using a drug for migraines, had the delusion that snakes were in her bed. Lawsuits are pending for people who were able to drive a car or commit crimes while under the influence of a popular sleep remedy. Morphine causes dizziness and headache, hampers digestion, and stops normal elimination. So can Oxycodone, or a combination of a narcotic and Tylenol, which is widely prescribed by doctors and sold illegally on the black market. It can be addictive to users and their unborn children.

One of the saddest and riskiest aspects of chemical pain-relief is drug withdrawal. We now have newborn junkies who must withdraw from painkillers their mothers took during pregnancy. An April 2011 *New York Times* article outlines the problem. A mother buys the prescription painkiller Oxycodone on the street. She takes it for the first twelve weeks of pregnancy and then tries to quit cold turkey. That results in her unborn baby having seizures, which could cause miscarriage. The mother takes methadone to reduce her drug cravings and withdrawal. But the baby nearly dies of withdrawal from methadone.

Taking a natural approach makes pain a tool for recovery. By recognizing the source of a chronic pain and preventing and eliminating it with foods, herbs, massage, movement, and a healthy outlook, we reinforce wellness. The body's subtle communication—the impulses that course through acupuncture meridians, chakras, and the surrounding ether, our network of wellness—remains intact as we gain resilience.

Your Comfort Zone

We each have a preferred location and climate that has nothing to do with our place of birth, work, or relationships. It is our comfort zone. Mine is a warm tropical beach. A light breeze from the south is blowing. It is late afternoon and I am in my solitary space singing a raga. Warmth, quiet, peace, and music are healing for me. Despite midsummer heat, if I eat too many cold, raw foods or iced beverages, if I linger in a cool swimming pool too long, I get deep chills that hurt muscles, joints, and bones. Usually a cup of cinnamon tea helps normalize my internal temperature and gets my blood moving to reduce pain. For me, internal or external cold retards circulation, causing stabbing pain.

Your pain may improve with cold treatments such as ice and anti-inflammatory aids; mine does not. You have to concede there is that difference among us: Some require warmth and others colder treatments in order to reduce chronic pain and enhance comfort and general health. Treatments recommended for everyone may not work for you or me, which is why I've outlined a number of recommendations to each ailment discussed in this book.

You may be reading these words in book form, or on your computer or mobile phone on a train or plane. My herbal suggestions are easy to find in your kitchen, in your health shop, in large chain stores and supermarkets, and online. Throughout *Naturally Pain Free*, I have provided appropriate Internet links to sources for top-quality natural health products featured in the book and, in some cases, links for additional reading. Most chapters include sections called "Letha's Advice" in which I share practical tips or personal insights on methods described in the chapter. The healing practices covered in detail in the book have been applied in my teaching at various educational centers in the New York area, including Beth Israel School of Nursing and Columbia Presbyterian Medical Center.

All research and product information is updated regularly with health articles, videos, books, and my personal comments to inquiring readers at my interactive, multilingual website, www.asianhealthsecrets.com.

Part One

Pain Prevention and Care

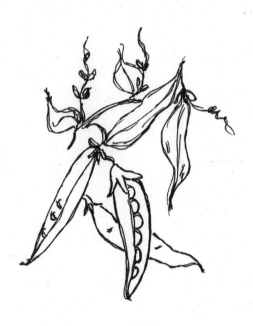

CHAPTER ONE

Five Ways to Beat Pain

I can stand anything but pain.

—Oscar Levant (composer, actor, 1906–1972)

OSCAR LEVANT, KNOWN FOR HIS ACERBIC WIT, SOPHISTICATED PATTER, AND perpetual cigarette-smoking while playing Gershwin on the piano, appeared in classic Hollywood movies with John Garfield, Gene Kelly, and the dance team of Fred Astaire and Ginger Rogers. The actor/composer had a famously bad temper, but Levant hit the right note when referring to pain. Perhaps his temper contributed to the problem, as mood affects our experience of pain. Depressed, agitated, and exhausted people often feel pain more acutely. How do you deal with nagging pain? According to psychologist Richard Stephens at Britain's Keele University, swearing increases pain tolerance for some people. However, I prefer increasing pleasure, not complaints. For that reason, we begin with five pleasing ways to recharge, regroup, and reverse everyday pains and annoyances with corrective diet, herbs, massage, meditation, and relaxing activities.

Letha's Advice: Two Rules of Thumb

Our needs and capacities vary considerably. You may feel gradually better by using my suggestions that affect metabolism, circulation, mood, or structural issues. Be kind to yourself by realizing that the discomforts you feel have evolved over the years and it will take time to improve.

- Start slowly with any new health regime and listen to your body and feelings while making changes to your routine. That can indicate the best dosage and frequency necessary for you.

- Add one new health idea at a time in order to clearly observe your progress. For example, change your diet for a week or more, and then add
  exercise or massage or other treatments recommended in this book.
  You may wish to keep a diary to record the most effective treatments.

Making any adjustment to long-term habits may result in temporary
pain while your body adjusts to new patterns of circulation, an enhanced
level of energy, and or other factors. Be patient and give yourself a
chance to observe and benefit from the progress you make.

1. Adjust Your Diet

Healthy blood circulation is key for pain management because blood supplies
oxygen and nutrients to stressed areas, beginning the healing process. The
circulation issue makes a low-fat, high-fiber diet most effective for reducing
pain as well as for lowering harmful cholesterol. Dr. Neal Barnard, MD, on the
advisory board of *Vegetarian Times* magazine, has written *Foods That Fight
Pain*. The doctor and I agree that "food and lifestyle changes can, over the long
run, rival the power of drugs or surgery in restoring circulation." He draws an
interesting connection between poor lumbar circulation (because of arteries
clogged with plaque) and chronic low back pain. Reducing plaque can improve
circulation and thereby reduce pain. Apparently, blocked blood vessels cause
problems anywhere in the body depending upon their location. The result may
be heart trouble, stroke, low back pain, or sexual dysfunction. One sign that
arteries may already be blocked somewhere, Barnard writes, is chest pain and
leg cramps in the calf.

The right sort of cleansing diet to unclog arteries, improve circulation,
and reduce stiff joints, backache, and inflammatory problems ranging from
migraines to PMS is simple, sparse, and vegetarian. It includes certain whole
grains, fruits, vegetables, and legumes. Barring allergies, I also recommend seaweeds, select mushrooms, moderate use of nuts, and tea as a daily refreshing
health beverage. However, I think few people are ready for a Spartan diet even if
testing proves its value. The problem with a medical testing approach to diet is
that findings are based on statistics and not upon your needs, desires, and tastes.
You might begin by adding healthy snacks that reduce inflammation and cholesterol—for example, rice cakes, dried nori seaweed, and green tea. Reducing
sugar and fried foods can make a major difference without totally revamping
your diet. Start slowly and increase foods that reduce pain.

Without a coherent energy theory of how the body works, such as that developed by the traditional Asian (Chinese medical or Ayurvedic) approach, we

are left to make choices among contradictory studies that may be funded by special interest groups. Scientists break down foods into ever smaller particles for study, often ignoring how foods influence the highly complex, coordinated actions of body and mind. Some of your favorite foods, such as coffee, chocolate, or garlic, which are beneficial for preventing disease, may also be your pain triggers. You have to observe their effects and decide to use or eliminate them for yourself. In some cases I will suggest treatments to overcome the pain they cause.

Pain Triggers

How do you find out what foods trigger your pain? Follow the elimination diet detailed below for two weeks. Observe the results. Then, each week, add one food to see if and how it triggers your pain. It is worth the time and effort to become pain-free. By eliminating congesting, fatty foods, we ease digestion and elimination of toxins that create pain. Observe how this diet affects your pain, complexion, digestion, breathing, energy, and mood. Diet always affects more than one aspect of vitality.

A Pain-Free Cleansing Diet

This elimination diet can improve migraines and other aches, itchy or red blemishes, certain allergies, and constipation for many people. This diet can also aid in weight loss, which improves arthritis by reducing stress placed on damaged joints. The diet features cleansing alkaline foods. Try to keep a 60/40 ratio of vegetables and select grains to fruits, with roughly six to nine servings of cooked and raw vegetables, more cooked than raw, and *barring diabetes* two fruits daily.

For two weeks, eat only foods from the following list:

- Brown rice, shirataki noodles, and unsweetened rice cakes
- Cooked or dried fruits (cherries, cranberry, figs, black grapes, pears, prunes, but no apples, citrus, bananas, peaches, or tomatoes)
- Cooked green, yellow, and orange vegetables: artichoke, asparagus, broccoli or broccoli cooking water, chard, collards, lettuce, spinach, string beans, squash, sweet potato, tapioca, and taro; fresh salad without dressing or with a little olive oil
- Water, plain or sweetened with black cherry concentrate; prunella tea, oregano leaf tea, ginger tea, or olive leaf tea; green tea, barley water with sliced ginger
- Modest amounts (one to two tablespoons daily) of kelp digitata, dulse, or nori seaweed
- Vanilla extract is optional; no honey, vinegar, or salt

Completely avoid these pain-trigger foods: dairy foods, chocolate, eggs, citrus, all meats (including turkey and fish as well as red meat and pork), wheat (including bread and pasta), nuts, tomatoes, onions, corn, apples, and bananas.

Other diet tips to keep in mind:

- Do not drink a raw juice first thing in the morning or else you certainly will develop a headache by three or four in the afternoon. Traditional Chinese doctors call that reaction "rising liver fire," the result of weak digestion.
- If you start to space out from hypoglycemia or weakness from the diet, try eating one boiled egg for protein. Be sure to pay attention to whether or not it gives you a headache.
- If you suffer from caffeine withdrawal while on this diet, have a cup of coffee or black tea to see if it takes away your migraine.

After losing daily headaches and joint pain with the elimination diet, you might try adding one pain-trigger food each week or two, to see if it actually gives you pain. Try other whole grains, not corn. Try different nuts, which provide healthy fats. Try a banana, a starch that is a source of potassium. You see what I mean.

Mulberry Leaf Tea: Erase the Carb Pain Trigger

Carbohydrates, especially bread, pasta, pastry, and potatoes, are a serious pain trigger for many people. One way to have your carb and eat it too is to drink warm mulberry leaf tea before a carbohydrate meal. An enzyme in mulberry leaf inhibits the absorption of carbohydrates in the intestine. That makes it an especially good tea for weight loss.

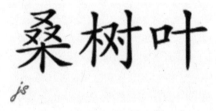

The Chinese character for mulberry shows a tree that is food for silkworms.

Letha's Advice: Mulberry for Blood Sugar Balance

I sometimes add a pinch of dried mulberry leaf to the teapot when making my breakfast Chinese gunpowder green tea. Mulberry leaf has a slight bittersweet flavor and nice aftertaste. If you have diabetes or are susceptible, have mulberry leaf tea before the big meal of the day to avoid a spike upward in blood sugar. Try boiling a few mulberry leaves for five minutes in water with pasta; then remove the leaves. Mulberry does not change the flavor of carbohydrates, but reduces their pain-trigger effects. In Chinese herb shops the bulk mulberry leaf called sang ye is sold in large bags. White mulberry leaf tea and extract are widely available and can be found online at major sources such as Amazon.com. On the main floor of Kam Man, New York's first Chinese supermarket, located at 200 Canal Street between Mott and Mulberry streets, and at most other Chinese supermarkets, a box of Ji Sheng Cha (mulberry leaf and twig tea) can be found with the medicinal herbs. It is very inexpensive.

Chinese herbalists have been using mulberry leaf and twig as herbal medicine for centuries. The leaf lowers blood sugar for type 2 diabetes. It is considered cooling and detoxifying for the lungs and liver. The twig and bark are used to reduce chronic joint pain and rheumatism. Chinese herbalists say it reduces nerve pain and water retention in legs and arms. It is perfect for improving your tennis game and dance steps.

Drinking the tea decreases pain in several ways. It adds water to lubricate muscles and joints. It reduces acid buildup and inflammation in the digestive tract and lets carbohydrates pass through the body without harm.

Simple Recipes

Shirataki Noodles with Hummus

You can find Japanese shirataki noodles for sale in the refrigerator section in many American supermarkets and most Chinese and Japanese food shops. It is the only refrigerated noodle packed in water. They are made with a no-calorie yam and are used to cleanse the digestive tract of harmful cholesterol. If you like Japanese sukiyaki, you have enjoyed these clear white noodles. They can be eaten cold or warmed with any sauce. Za'atar is a mixture of spices and sesame seeds. It usually contains cumin, coriander, and saffron and can be found in Middle Eastern food shops and online.

Serves 1

Ingredients:
1 8-ounce package of shirataki noodles
1 tablespoon hummus
1 teaspoon light sesame oil
Sesame seeds or za'atar
Fresh parsley, chopped

Rinse the noodles with plain water and place them in a bowl. Mix the hummus and oil with a few drops of water, and add sesame seeds or za'atar. Blend the mixture with the noodles and add parsley. Another variation: substitute a low-fat nut butter for the hummus and za'atar. You might add ½ teaspoon of low-fat nut butter whipped with 1 teaspoon of water until creamy. However, peanuts are a pain trigger for some people.

Barley Water

Easy to make, pleasant, digestive, and laxative, this beverage hits the spot. You have to use organic grains to make sprouts and fermented beverages such as this, or they will spoil. Discard a fermented liquid that stinks.

Ingredients:
1 quart purified or spring water
1 tablespoon raw organic barley
1 tablespoon raw ginger, peeled and sliced

Rinse off the barley and place it into a sterile, airtight glass jar. Add water and ginger and allow to ferment in a dark, dry place overnight. Taste the beverage during the following day or two. You can sweeten it with optional vanilla extract. The longer it stays undisturbed, the stronger the fermented taste will be. To stop fermentation, place the jar in the refrigerator. Each time you drink, add fresh water and allow it to ferment again.

The Power of Real Tea

There is something special about sitting and sipping warm tea. Real tea (*Camellia sinensis*) calms you and chases cares. According to research cited by the National Institutes of Health,

> "Tea is known to be a rich source of flavonoid antioxidants. However, tea also contains a unique amino acid, L-theanine, that may modulate aspects of brain function in humans. Evidence from human electroencephalograph (EEG) studies show that it has a

direct effect on the brain (Juneja et al. *Trends in Food & Science Tech* 1999; 10; 199–204). L-theanine significantly increases activity in the alpha frequency band, which indicates that it relaxes the mind without inducing drowsiness."

I cannot start the day without drinking a pot of hot caffeinated green tea. It clears the senses, lifts the spirit, cleanses the body, and speeds digestion. It is the primary health, beauty, and weight-loss beverage around the world. Drinking tea reduces absorption of dietary fats in the intestine. Whether or not tea may be considered a pain trigger, its benefits are enormous. They include reducing harmful cholesterol and enhancing our natural protection against heart disease, cancer, and depression. All styles and flavors of teas—white, green, oolong, or black teas—are made from the same tea leaf, *Camellia sinensis.* The difference comes in processing. Tea leaves are dried and toasted, and some are fermented to create the many flavors and health benefits of tea.

White tea has the least caffeine and a subtle flavor. Like all teas, it is full of antioxidants. Green tea is cooling, diuretic, and digestive. Oolong tea is semifermented and useful for slimming. There are many styles of oolong, depending on where and how it is grown and processed. For example, oolong teas grown on sunny hillsides in northern Thailand and sold from www.siamteas.com have a light and delicate aftertaste, whereas Chinese Ti Quan Yin oolong (also known as Tie Quan Yin or Ti Kuan Yin), named for the Iron Goddess of Mercy (iron in this case means "strong"), is perfumed with charcoal smoke and tastes pungently delightful.

Pu-erh, a richly flavored, earthy-tasting, red-colored fermented tea from Yunnan, warms digestion and reduces cholesterol and hangover. I ordered pu-erh tea on Amazon.com and sent it to my mother in New Mexico because recent research indicates that natural statins such as those in pu-erh can help prevent heart trouble and stroke. Black tea has a higher caffeine content than green tea and stimulates the nervous system.

All these teas are easily available in many supermarkets, herb shops, and online at major consumer websites. Choose your favorite tea according to your taste, health needs, and the degree of nervous stimulation you require. Some

Kitchen Herb and Spice Teas

Cleansing, cooling herbal teas include prunella tea, oregano leaf tea, or olive leaf tea. *Prunella vulgaris* is a broad-spectrum anti-biotic herb recommended to help clear swelling and lumps in the throat or breast, herpes, fevers, and hyperthyroid conditions. It is soothing and very mild. You may want to flavor it with vanilla. Oregano and olive leaf are pungent flavorful teas that improve energy and immunity. You can make a strong tea by adding one-half teaspoon to each cup of boiling water.

people are sensitive to caffeine. (If caffeine increases nerve pain, take a capsule of Siberian ginseng to reduce nervous irritation.) You can also splash cold tea on your face. The invigorating aroma is only part of the pleasure. Acids in tea protect skin cells against damage from sun exposure and kitchen burns.

2. Incorporate Herbs That Stop Pain

Some herbs used in cooking or household teas, such as ginger and mint, may reduce chronic pain because they enhance digestion, eliminate impurities and acid indigestion, and reduce fatigue. Mint tea relaxes smooth muscles in the abdomen, reducing cramps. Here are a few pain-relieving herbs for daily use. These are easily found in health-food stores and Asian food shops. We will revisit them again in detail in appropriate chapters.

Ginger

Researchers say ginger is anti-inflammatory because it shows anti-inflammatory effects in test-tube experiments. It blocks histamines and enzymes that would otherwise make inflammation-producing prostaglandins in the body. However, according to traditional Chinese medicine, ginger increases digestive qi and warms the stomach. Adding one-half teaspoon of dried ginger powder to a cup of water, for example, as recommended for reducing muscle and arthritis pain, feels warming in the throat and stomach. It warms the entire body and activates circulation. It is supposed to be cooling, but for me it is not. I look at my tongue after taking one-half teaspoon of ginger powder in water. I see dryness, red color, and many cracks in the tongue where the stomach line is. That shows dehydration. In other words, ginger powder is drying, stimulating, digestive, and anti-phlegmatic, and that action helps reduce joint pain. We are not aware of our prostaglandins—I have never met one—but we do feel digestive heat and improved circulation.

You should not use powdered ginger at all if you have stomach ulcers, chronic thirst or hunger (with or without diabetes), a hyperthyroid condition, bad breath, burning in the stomach, insomnia from hunger, or red irritated facial blemishes on the cheeks. Ginger may be too irritating if the digestive tract is already too acidic. Otherwise, if you can easily tolerate ginger, add one-half teaspoon to a cup of water once or twice daily to reduce stiffness and pain, especially in humid or cold weather. It works quickly. But to feel the full benefits of improved circulation may take one to three months.

Guggul (*Commiphora mukul*)

This famous cleansing, drying, stimulating, and rejuvenating herb, originally used by Ayurvedic herbal doctors in India and now available in American health-food stores, is a relative of myrrh. According to Ayurveda, the classical medicine of India, chronic pain may result from a variety of causes, including increased toxins and inflammation trapped in muscles and joints. Guggul is stimulating and detoxifying, and capsules have been recommended to reduce body fat and tumors. Guggul is often recommended for pain that is considered a result of "excess kapha" (phlegmy asthma and swollen joints). Ginger and guggul are detoxifying, aiding digestion and elimination. Guggul especially helps dissolve phlegmy congestion, which may improve asthma and fibroids. It speeds weight loss and lowers harmful cholesterol. It purifies like myrrh. For pain relief, it is often added to Ayurvedic formulas for arthritis and heart care. For general cleansing, to improve circulation and ease muscle and joint stiffness and pain, you might take one or two 375-milligram capsules once or twice daily.

Triphala

Triphala (also known as trifala) is a famous Ayurvedic remedy made from three fruits. Amla (*Emblica officinalis*) is high in rejuvenating tannins that protect the heart, hair, and complexion. Haritaki (*Terminalia chebula*) is a moistening laxative, blood cleanser, and antibiotic that clears complexion problems. Bibhitaki (*Terminalia bellirica*) is digestive and antispasmodic. I have mentioned triphala in several chapters because it does so many good things for body and mind. It improves diabetes, heart conditions, immunity, and vision. It stimulates bile secretion as it detoxifies the liver, helps digestion and assimilation, and significantly reduces serum cholesterol and lipid levels throughout the body. Triphala can be used along with guggul or used alone as an efficient cleanser that reduces inflammation, phlegmy congestion, and nerve pain. It helps protect against malabsorption illnesses including osteoporosis. Most people find triphala to be rather bitter, so the pills are easier to use than the powder. For inflammatory pain, PMS, and digestive complaints, take one or two pills with meals.

Skullcap

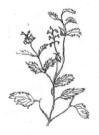

Skullcap

Skullcap (also known as *Scutellaria lateriflora*, helmet flower, blue pimpernel, Quaker bonnet, and mad dog weed) grows wild in the woods of eastern North America. Skullcap was originally used for rabies because of its tranquilizing effect on the central nervous system. Clinical studies have demonstrated skullcap's ability to improve blood flow in the brain, inhibit muscle spasms, and act as a sedative. Some alternative health practitioners use skullcap to treat symptoms of attention deficit hyperactivity disorder (ADHD). Skullcap is useful for a wide range of nervous conditions including insomnia, hysteria, anxiety, delirium tremens, and withdrawal from barbiturates and tranquilizers.

A medicinal infusion of the plant promotes menstruation and should not be given to pregnant women since it can induce a miscarriage. The infusion is usually given as a tea for nervous headaches, neuralgia, fever, atherosclerosis, cholesterol, anxiety, and insomnia. If you have never used skullcap or are very sensitive to herbs, start by adding three to five drops of the liquid extract to a cup of water and observe the results. You may feel more relaxed.

Skullcap's side effects may include increased body temperature and muscle aches that subside rapidly. Severe side effects occur as a result of extremely high dosages of the herb. Signs of allergic reaction include trouble breathing, skin rash or hives, swelling of the throat or the mouth, wheezing, and itching. Skullcap overdose may cause temporary giddiness, confusion, and twitching. Stop using skullcap if you develop shortness of breath, liver pain, or jaundice, a yellow color to skin or eyes. Do not mix skullcap with Tylenol, especially not the combination of Tylenol and alcohol because that combination has been shown to result in liver damage. Skullcap should not be used by anyone with epilepsy, any seizure-related disorders, liver disease (like cirrhosis, liver failure, or hepatitis), or kidney disease (like renal failure). You should not self-medicate with these disorders.

Aloe vera

I love aloe. It is clean, cool, and fresh, the scent of high desert filled with sunlight and sage. Smear the thick pulpy gel that lies under the crisp green peel on sunburn to ease burning pain. Drink pure organic aloe juice or gel in water to soothe an upset stomach; to reduce menstrual cramps, bad breath, and constipation; and to eliminate complexion blemishes and some food allergies. Aloe is an alkaline food that resembles the healthy tissue of internal organs, free from impurities and acids that age us and create pain. Many times, I have recommended aloe as a daily beverage for people who want to lose weight, control diabetes, and ease inflammatory pain or correct menstrual problems. See the chapter on women's issues beginning on page 89. A nice way to enjoy aloe is to add up to one-fourth cup daily of the juice or gel to mango, papaya, or prickly pear juice. Those juices are quite beneficial in themselves. Also see Nopalea on page 59. That beverage is a delicious blend of nopal cactus and fruit enzymes that is cooling and detoxifying to reduce inflammatory pain.

3. Massage: The Healing Power of Touch

Most people appreciate healing touch from a loved one or a professional therapist. While there are many products on the market to ease spasm, bruising, and pain, increase circulation, and relax nervous tension, nothing replaces touch. Moving stiff, painful areas where circulation is trapped frees us physically and emotionally. Where do you hold your stress? Neck, shoulders, back, arms, face, even hands and feet may feel the impact of overwork, poor habits, emotional upset, and chronic pain anywhere in the body. Massage frees the flow of vital energy so that painful areas of the body may benefit from healthy blood circulation. During or following a massage you may perspire or have chills, develop a temporary rash, or experience temporary pains as circulation shifts. Have you ever laughed or cried after a massage? That release of pent-up pain and emotions begins your healing. Beyond any massage technique, a subtle energy exchange between people is part of the treatment. That is why I always choose as massage therapists healthy, strong, nonsmokers who are dedicated to easing suffering. Reiki, Japanese shiatsu, Chinese tui na, Thai massage—there are many forms of Asian massage that help realign qi and nerves deranged by overwork, exhaustion, and emotional or physical trauma. They are all wonderful but appeal to varying tastes.

Reiki, healing touch, and Swedish massage are soft touch techniques that may gently improve long-term, deep problems. Reiki engages a healing flow of life force from universal wellness beyond the practitioner. Swedish massage strokes muscles to ease spasm and improve circulation. Thai massage uses stretches. The massage therapist may pull and twist your arms, legs, and back to free areas stuck, congested, and malfunctioning. In Bangkok, Thailand, the massage is done on the porch of a temple where it originated. The atmosphere is serene and quiet. Japanese shiatsu and Chinese tui na are deep, often painful, massage practices, manipulations, and stretches that originated to help martial arts practitioners and others recover from injuries as well as treat chronic disease. Acupuncture meridians may be addressed during the massage, and techniques using oils and ointments, cupping, and moxibustion may be used.

Cupping, not as popular in the West as in China, has been used by people in the Mediterranean and throughout Eastern Europe and Asia to draw congestion and pain away from areas buried deep within the body and bring pain closer to the skin surface and eliminate it. Special glass cups are heated inside and placed on the skin to form a vacuum that draws out impurities. One woman told me it was the only treatment that really helped her herniated disc back pain. The Chinese doctor moved the cups up along both sides of the spine to free the pinched nerves. Another soothing warming home treatment is a sweat bath. Adding up to one-fourth cup of ginger powder from the kitchen to warm bath water can draw out impurities in a similar way.

Moxibustion, a warming, energizing practice of burning mugwort herb over acupuncture points is used by traditional Chinese hospitals and is rarely done in the West. It smells like burning weeds and has been replaced by a myriad of massage balms available everywhere from Walmart to Walgreens and Rite-Aid and online, such as red (warming) Tiger Balm or white (cooling/warming) Tiger Balm. Blue emu massage cream is made with deeply penetrating emu oil and nutritional supplements such as glucosamine, which is recommended for joint pain. There are also cooling roll-ons that contain menthol.

Lymphatic Drainage Massage

This is a special sort of light stroking massage that guides energy flow in the body along the route to eliminate excess fluids, toxins, and other emotional stuff trapped in the lymph system, one of the body's major organs of detoxification. It can be used for weight loss, emotional trauma, and after surgery to help realign energy flow and rid the body of excess lymph fluid buildup. It is especially important to have this massage after breast cancer surgery in order to avoid pain and further problems. Here is a summary detailing how to do this massage at home for yourself.

Before my morning shower or during fifteen minutes of sunshine on the porch, I give my body a light lymphatic drainage massage, using fingertip strokes from the top of my head, down toward the face and neck and chest toward the heart, from the hands upward toward the underarms and heart, and from the feet toward the kidneys. Lymphatic drainage massage refers to the stimulation of the lymph system. It "suggests" to the body in a subtle way a healthy direction for energy circulation so that impurities and water retention may be eliminated. During cold weather, I sometimes I use light sesame oil, adding a few drops of lavender and geranium essential oils to enhance circulation during a massage. It's soothing and uplifting. If sesame feels too warming, you may prefer olive or coconut oil instead.

Posturology

Most people have some irregularity in their structure such as a slightly lowered shoulder from carrying heavy bags, or a slightly shorter leg or other postural problem. Over time the unevenness causes pain. We compensate for discomfort, developing a limp, a tic, or other inadequate means of self-protection, and pain becomes "frozen" in incorrect posture. Good posture is important for everyone because it helps prevent chronic pains resulting from poor circulation and emotional stress.

If you Google "posturology" you will find athletic coaches in the U.S., Canada, and Europe who are training athletes to reach their full potential. In Clearwater, Florida, where Paul St. John teaches this therapy, the aims are different. Paul St. John is a "neurosomatic educator" who works with body alignment and helps people in pain with their body structure. His view is that form and function are interdependent. His school of posturology gives seminars around the country. Many of the referrals to their pain clinic in Clearwater come from dentists, who need to find successful ways to reverse jawbone loss. Doctors, massage therapists, chiropractors, and others are coming to realize cures for specific ailments cannot take place unless posture is addressed.

Paul St. John analyzes and charts clients' dysfunctional postural patterns. Once these patterns are analyzed, a comprehensive program is designed to guide the client through the five stages of rehabilitation:

- Eliminate muscle spasm
- Restore flexibility
- Restore proper biomechanics
- Increase muscle strength
- Increase muscular endurance

The purpose is to not only to eliminate pain, but to educate the patient about ways to prevent recurrence of the injury. A stable body alignment that supports and maintains wellness should be the goal of body treatments. Otherwise, we fall into habits that create pain. For a list of qualified practitioners in your area, contact www.neurosomaticeducators.com.

I was fortunate to find someone in Vermont who had studied with St. John. At the Rutland farmer's market I met the husband-and-wife healing team of Bryan and Cheri Bush. They had set up a massage table near someone selling pastry and garden greens. I was having a tough day with hip and lower back pain from humid weather conditions and fatigue, so I decided to get a twenty-minute massage. It was amazing. As Bryan worked on my deep muscle spasms, my lower back felt warm. I asked Bryan if he was heating the massage table. He said, "That's your blood circulating freely where it could not go before." His massage was deep and somewhat painful at times. But his touch was very sensitive to my limited range of motion. Afterward, I felt new ease. As I slid off the table smiling I said, "My joints feel juicy!" My pain was mostly gone. Also very important, since Bryan works with structural alignment, he suggested ways to stand and stretch in order to maintain the treatment advantage. That sort of approach is a key component of Asian health practices such as yoga and tai chi movements because they improve posture and enhance circulation with alignment and breathing. Massage uses passive movement (stretching, pulling) and healing touch and is suitable for people who may be weak, elderly, exhausted, and in chronic pain.

4. Meditation: As Effective as Drugs for Easing Pain

"If a tree falls on you in the forest while you're meditating, does it still hurt? Well, yes. But maybe not quite as much as it would if you weren't meditating," reported researchers from Wake Forest University School of Medicine in Winston-Salem, North Carolina, and Wisconsin in the April 2011 *Journal of Neuroscience*. Individuals who practiced mindfulness meditation (also known as samatha or vipassana silent meditation) during a clinical observation reported much less discomfort than they did in earlier meditation-free sessions. Samatha, the research team wrote, "flipped switches on or off in diverse regions of the brain underlying attention, expectation, and even the awareness of thoughts themselves." The team published photos showing parts of the brain activated by pain that were much less stimulated during meditation. We are constantly bombarded with physical stimuli, and simple things like raindrops or a breeze blowing against our arms we often ignore. Meditation may help people to similarly let their "ouch!" reflexes go. Meditation can desensitize us to nagging pain. Try the following simple relaxation exercise.

To avoid extraneous stimulation, turn the lights out and your machines off. Sit quietly or lie flat in bed. Breathe slowly through your nose into the lower abdomen. Relax and exhale through the mouth. As you breathe, the abdomen rises and falls. Imagine a warm light such as a candle flame very slowly passing through your body from head to feet. As the light passes an area, it melts everything so that your pain dissolves. Repeat silently to yourself: "Hair relax… scalp relax…brain relax…face relax…" etc. Take all the time you need in order to melt your pain. If troubling thoughts or memories arise, put them aside for another day. Repeat breathing into a painful area as often as necessary before moving on to another area. Don't let yourself go to sleep because you will feel the effects better if you relax down to your feet.

5. Activities: Walking, Dancing, Sex

Like it or not, research from the 1990s in England and Norway shows that exercise helps reduce acute back pain. Our first impulse may be to rest, but doctors in England asked a group of back pain patients to rest in bed for forty-eight hours and another group to avoid bed rest between 9:00 a.m. and 9:00 p.m. Within seven days, more patients in the active group had fully recovered than in the bed-rest group. More recently, a 2004 article published by Ted Forcum, DC and Thomas Hyde, DC, states,

> People with low back pain often find some forms of exercise too painful to continue, and therefore don't get the exercise they need to maintain good health. Exercise walking is one way to benefit from regular exercise while not aggravating the structures in the lower back. For some back conditions, walking will aggravate or cause too much pain to be bearable. For these patients, other low-impact exercise may be advisable, especially water therapy (pool therapy such as aqua-jogging or deep water aerobics). The body's buoyancy reduces joint compression, allowing for more pain-free movement.

Benefits of Walking Daily

- ❏ Strengthens muscles in the feet, legs, hips, and torso—walking increases the stability of the spine and conditions the muscles that keep the body in the upright position.
- ❏ Nourishes the spinal structures—walking for exercise facilitates strong circulation, pumping nutrients into soft tissues and draining toxins.
- ❏ Improves flexibility and posture—exercise walking along with regular stretching allows greater range of motion and helps prevent awkward movements and susceptibility of future injury.
- ❏ Strengthens bones and reduces bone density loss—regular walking for exercise helps prevent osteoporosis and can aid in reducing osteoarthritis pain.
- ❏ Helps with controlling weight—any regular exercise routine helps maintain a healthy weight, especially as one ages and metabolism slows.

Most exercise experts recommend: Walk briskly, but maintain enough breath to be able to carry on a conversation. Start out with a five-minute walk and work up to walking for at least thirty minutes (roughly two miles) at least three or four times a week. Maintain good form while walking to get the optimum aerobic benefit with each step and help protect the back and avoid injury.

I have found the following walking practice useful for calming the mind while building leg muscles. Stand tall with your head centered between the shoulders. Focus your breath in the lower abdomen, inhaling and exhaling deeply a few times. As you move forward, engage the abdominal muscles by paying attention to your breath. Avoid leaning forward as you walk. Allow your arms to swing freely without effort. With each step, land gently on the heel and midfoot, rolling smoothly to push off with the toes. Be mindful about using the balls of the feet and toes to push forward with each step.

As you walk, take a step with each slow breath: Inhale to the count of two and exhale to the count of four. Eventually you can lengthen your breath by inhaling to the count of five and exhaling to the count of eight or ten. This sort of slow walking helps deepen breath, calm emotions, and reduce stress and encourages the body to release its natural pain remedies.

Movement encourages the body to release natural painkillers called endorphins. Endorphins are made in the pituitary gland at the base of the brain. Endorphins act like morphine in the brain, nerves, and bloodstream. Athletes and dancers may have a higher pain tolerance because they produce more endorphins. Acupuncture also works for pain because it releases endorphins.

If you can't move out of bed because of pain, try lying on a wooden back roller or place a rolled-up bath towel at your waistline while you lie flat in bed. That pressure brings blood circulation that helps release pain.

Dance and Sex

You might say, "Dance is exercise with heart and soul." Dance engages imagination as it enhances breathing and circulation. Whatever form of dance you choose, be sure to warm up adequately with stretches before beginning any exercise, avoid overstressing delicate joints, and stop when you are tired. I believe muscle and joint pain and injury may be due to inattention as much as to muscle weakness and fatigue. To ease exercise pain, apply a cream or ointment containing homeopathic arnica in order to enhance circulation and reduce inflammation.

Research has shown that a six-mile run stimulates endorphin release roughly equivalent to 10 milligrams of morphine. Though runners might agree, not very many of us can run six miles. Instead of sweating on a racetrack, I prefer a roll in the hay. Sex releases endorphins too. And you don't have to go the full six miles to reap the benefits. That warm flush of pleasure, a deepened breath, and slight sweating may be our best indications that those endorphins are doing their stuff. Herbal tonics discussed in Part Three can improve sexual vitality and circulation and therefore reduce pain. A look, a kiss, a touch are never wasted.

Chapter Two

Headaches

A great wind is blowing, and that gives you either imagination or a headache.

—Catherine the Great of Russia (1729–1796)

Sophie Augusta Fredericka von Anhalt-Zerbst-Dornburg, known as Catherine the Great—the empress who brought Russia into the modern world, expanded its territory, defeated the Ottoman Empire, and oversaw brutal reprisals during the largest peasant revolt in Russian history—had great imagination and frequent cause for headaches. It is interesting that traditional Chinese doctors describe a certain type of headache as the result of a "reckless wind" from weak digestion, liver inflammation, and excess digestive phlegm.

Does your headache feel as though heat is rushing to your head? Do your face and head feel stuffed with congestion or expanding as though your senses pound with pain? Is the pain on top of your head (excess phlegm) or behind the eyes (liver irritation)? When you think of something you ate or an argument you had and that memory makes the pain worse, it may be a cause of your headaches. Headaches stemming from poor digestion may also respond to emotions. We will see in a later chapter how our digestive center involves our emotional center.

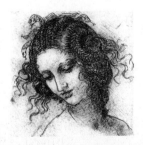

Ancient Chinese medical texts describe how, in a weakened condition, a "wind" (nerve irritation) can rise in our body to increase fever, dizziness, and headache. Accordingly phlegm may "obscure the senses." Everyone has experienced this. You feel dizziness, headache, or intense pressure in the head accompanied by a runny nose or mucus congestion in the face. It feels like a head cold but may be the result of rich eating and drinking. However, in traditional Chinese medicine, phlegm (*she* in Chinese) represents more than mucus. It is a *humor* that affects body and mind. The four humors of Hippocratic medicine were black bile (*melan chole* in Greek), yellow bile (*chole* in Greek), phlegm (*phlegma* in Greek), and blood (*sanguis* in Latin). They created, respectively, melancholic, choleric or angry, phlegmatic, or sanguine illnesses.

The causes of digestive phlegm include an indigestible diet of overly rich or cold raw foods, overweight, slow metabolism, a lethargic lifestyle, a cold damp climate, and medications or emotions that weaken digestion. These are some factors that often lead to a pounding, dizzy headache at the top of your head.

The *location* of head pain, such as the top of the head, behind the eyes, or on one side of the head, is a symptom used by Chinese doctors to help determine the cause and cure for the headache. Why not just take an aspirin for your headache? It may temporarily relieve discomfort, but does not touch the real cause of your chronic pain. With natural treatments, you can be more precise and prevent further damage. Have hours of staring at a computer screen made your eyes throb? Do you have pounding, dull pain accompanied by sinus congestion? Do you awaken mornings with a stiff neck and numb fingers? Is someone you know a pain in the neck? There are many reasons why your head, neck, and shoulders hurt. Most chapters dealing with a specific pain include a discussion of secondary discomforts. We start here with a common example that illustrates the role of diet in headache pain prevention.

Example: Nancy's Migraine

Nancy developed a migraine every afternoon at work around three o'clock. It wasn't her job. She loved working in a television studio. Her background was history, and she had an advanced degree from Harvard in Russian studies. But she found the light-hearted atmosphere, the pressing deadlines, and highly creative people at work refreshing. She was happy in her marriage and had two bright, young children. Her daily migraine, I found out, was the result of her breakfast. She drank a big glass of raw green juice every morning at 7:00 a.m., a time when digestion is particularly vulnerable.

Her cold, raw breakfast upset her digestion in a way that any trained Chinese herbalist would recognize: her "digestive qi" was weakened. It takes a stronger digestion to consume something cold and raw than something warm and cooked. People weakened from illness are often fed soups, not iced drinks, salads, and raw foods. Put another way, the raw juice detoxified her liver quickly and the result was fever, headache, a runny nose, and nausea—a sick headache—by midafternoon. I advised her to start the day with a meal that fortified digestion (digestive qi): for example, warm green tea with toast or a cooked cereal. If that was not warming enough, she could add sliced ginger to the warm tea. Within a day or two, her migraines disappeared.

The origin of Nancy's headaches was weak digestion. How did I know? The pain was intense, pounding, and located at the top of her head, and she had sinus congestion, a feverish feeling, a phlegm-coated tongue, a runny nose, and a slightly upset stomach. If Nancy's headache was a hangover resulting from overindulging in rich foods and alcoholic drinks, she would have felt intense pain throughout the head, especially at the temples and eyes, and experienced nausea, and her treatment would've been different. I would have given her acupuncture to reduce inflammation in the head and recommended a dose of homeopathic Nux vomica 30C, a liver cleanser. The result would be no head-ache and a healthier liver.

Practical Suggestions for Food, Herb, and Homeopathic Remedy Use

One of the worst mistakes the casual natural-remedy user makes is to take remedies according to convenience instead of at the optimum time. For example, lots of people have told me they take a handful of pills with coffee at breakfast because it suits their schedule or because they can remember to take them that way. Unfortunately, giving the body mixed messages weakens digestion, which can increase headaches. Natural remedies, like drugs, should be used when the body needs them most. Here are a few simple rules to follow:

1. If the problem results from digestion, such as cramps, burping, or phlegmy, nauseous migraine headaches, take digestive herbs such as ginger, mint, lemongrass, or others with or after meals. If the problem is not digestive, such as joint pain, back pain, skin rash, or insomnia, take the appropriate herbs between meals. That separates the remedy from digestive acids.

2. Never mix homeopathic remedies, which work on the cellular level, with foods, beverages, herbs, or toothpaste, in order to avoid making a mess of reactions in the cells. According to directions for specific use, we are usually told to wait one hour before eating or around two hours after eating before using a homeopathic remedy. A homeopathic remedy is made from an extremely dilute form of a plant, animal, or mineral product, but it is not digested like a food or an herb. Homeopathic pills or liquids are absorbed into the blood passing through the

blood vessels in the mouth. They work quickly and after being absorbed by the body leave no trace.

3. In general, during spring or allergy season, use green foods: bitter, cleansing raw and steamed green foods and herbs. In summer, enjoy the reds and blues—sweet ripe red and blue berries, cherries, and plums—because they are cleansing and blood-enhancing. In autumn and winter, enjoy earth-colored foods: cooked pumpkin and squash, cooked whole grains, and nuts and mushrooms for protein. In winter, or if you are especially weak and chilled, you can benefit from warming spices, energizing herbal tonics, and cooked foods.

How, When, and Why You Hurt

Pay attention to *when* you get headaches. Do they regularly occur about the same time of day or month? What conditions are present that may trigger a headache? Do you notice a connection to diet, hormones, or activities? Gradually, you will learn to recognize the characteristics of the pain that indicate the cause. The following are common examples to help you: pain from eye strain; tension and poor circulation pain, including neck and shoulder pain; digestion-related headaches; PMS and menopausal issues; and temporomandibular joint (TMJ) pain. Head, neck, and shoulder pains frequently occur together.

Eye Strain Headaches: Cucumbers and Chrysanthemum Flowers

Do you stare at a computer screen for hours, then watch television to relax? Rubbing your eyes is not the answer.

Characteristics of the pain:

- eyes hurt or burn
- vision is cloudy or there are floaters

Treatment

Increase blood and moisture circulation to the eyes:

- Take a five-minute break, lie down on your back or sit in a chair with your head back, place a slice of cucumber or wet tea bags on closed eyes, and relax. Black tea reduces under-eye swelling and is antiseptic.
- Steep a handful of dried Chinese chrysanthemum flowers (ju hua) in a ceramic, glass, or earthen teapot of hot water for five minutes.

Between meals, sip a glass of warm or cool Chinese chrysanthemum flower tea, recommended for cloudy vision, migraine, sunstroke, hot flashes, and stress headaches. It is naturally sweet and delicious.

Both white and yellow Chinese chrysanthemum flowers are used medicinally. Ju hua, as it is called in China, is a popular summer beverage. Chrysanthemum flower is anti-inflammatory, antipyretic (heat-reducing), and antihypertensive (reducing high blood pressure), as well as soothing to the liver. It is excellent for fevers with headache and for counteracting the effects of hot climates. The white chrysanthemum flower has been used to relieve hypertension and vertigo, and to improve vision and eye soreness, conjunctivitis, night blindness, and eye strain.

The yellow chrysanthemum flower is more effective for cold and flu symptoms of fever and sore throat. Research has demonstrated chrysanthemum's potential in treating angina (chest pain) by dilating coronary arteries. This flower is antibiotic against a wide range of pathogens. Out of fifteen compounds isolated from this edible flower, all showed potent inhibitory effects against abnormal cells.

Tension and Poor Circulation–Related Aches

Tension headaches are often aggravated by neck and shoulder pain, after sitting for hours without moving and from poor posture. Aching neck and shoulder muscles may occur in response to overexertion, prolonged physical stress, or emotional tension. Muscles may also develop hard knots that are sore to the touch, sometimes called trigger points.

Characteristics of the pain:

- dull
- nagging
- deep
- immovable
- worse with fatigue or emotional upset

Treatment

For simple tension headaches and a stiff neck, increase blood circulation to the painful area with massage in order to nourish tense muscles with blood and oxygen. Apply heat or cold to increase comfort. A pleasantly fragrant Chinese analgesic liquid called White Flower, recommended for muscle and joint pains from simple headaches, arthritis, sprains, and bruises, contains oil of wintergreen, menthol, camphor, eucalyptus, peppermint, and lavender. Apply it to the back of the neck at the hairline and temples as needed. Avoid the eye area. Another useful remedy is homeopathic arnica ointment. Increasing local circulation relieves tightness and tension headaches.

Stop your usual activities that aggravate neck tension and pain. You may notice muscle or nerve pains in your neck upon waking or after using your computer. If neck pain involves nerves, for example muscle spasm from pinching a nerve or a cervical disc pressing a nerve, you may also feel numbness, tingling, or weakness in your arm or hand. Here are natural approaches for easing neck pains and secondary discomforts.

Morning Stiff Neck

When you wake up with a painful stiff neck, that's likely a muscle spasm—a sudden, powerful contraction of neck muscles, which some people call a "crick" in your neck. Muscle spasm can result from a muscle injury or a disc or nerve problem, so that the muscles tense in order to stabilize the neck and prevent you from moving in a way that will cause pain or further damage. Neck muscle spasms sometimes accompany emotional stress, but often there is no identifiable reason for muscle spasm. If you often wake up with a stiff neck or headache, you may also be using the wrong pillow. Many people sleep on their side. If the pillow is too large, it puts the neck at an extreme angle that may aggravate existing circulation problems.

Characteristics of the pain:

- neck stiffness and a cracking or grinding sound
- tight neck muscles, knotted or impossible to move
- finger numbness or tingling

Treatment

Try to use a pillow that conforms to the shape of your neck and head. When lying on your back, use a cylindrical pillow that supports the back of your neck. If the pain continues and/or includes numb extremities, have a neck X-ray to check whether whiplash or a vertebrae problem may be impairing circulation. See page 30, on "When to Consult a Health Practitioner."

Chronic Computer-Related Neck and Shoulder Pain

An orthopedic surgeon once told me he had devised a cure for all sorts of neck pain. "Throw your computer out the window," he said. How often do you take a break from work to walk around, drink water, or stretch? Neck-related headache (cervical headache) is most often felt in the back of the head and upper neck, where muscles extending along the skull are contiguous with neck muscles that become tense or spasm. It is aggravated by neck movement and often accompanied by stiffness and tenderness of neck muscles.

Characteristics of the pain:

- not noticed until you stop working
- dull, aching, fixed (not moving), and persistent
- worse with fatigue, stress, and emotional upset
- may coincide with chest tightness, wrist pain, and numbness in the hands

Treatment

Muscle pain, stiffness, and numbness from overwork often can be relieved with massage using a warming, soothing oil or ointment. For example, Tiger Balm ointment comes in two forms: red is warming and white feels cooling. White Flower Chinese analgesic oil contains lavender, menthol, and other stimulating scents and feels simultaneously warming and cooling. That switch from warm to cool to warm enhances circulation, which relieves pain. Tiger Balm can be dotted at painful points at the hairline, on the neck, on the top of the shoulders, at the elbow, and at the wrist in order to relieve stiff neck, shoulders, and arms resulting from hours spent at the computer. Additional treatments for computer pains are in a later chapter. It is important to stretch muscles to make them supple, and strengthen and build them to make them more resistant to sprains and injury.

Digestion- and Nerve-Related Headaches

Does your headache feel worse from noise, light, irritating people, and stress? Does it improve with quiet music or a nap? (See chapter 16.) Do cold or hot room temperatures or certain foods make your pain worse? We have seen how weak digestion can cause headaches. Nerve injury may also be at the root of your problem. Pinching the roots of spinal nerves causes pain. Depending on the nerves involved, the pain may shoot down the arm or even into the hand.

Characteristics of nerve pain:

- sharp
- moving or fleeting
- severe
- pins and needles

- hot or electric
- PMS headaches and shoulder pain with digestive troubles or food allergies
- emotional upset makes it worse

Treatment

Harmonize digestion to relieve belching, gastrointestinal disorders, and body aches. Herbs useful for tension headaches that occur with digestive problems include a combination of bupleurum, pueraria, pinellia, cinnamon, white peony, ginseng, skullcap, ginger, and licorice. One example of a remedy that uses these herbs is Ease 2 pills by Health Concerns, a company located in Oakland, California.

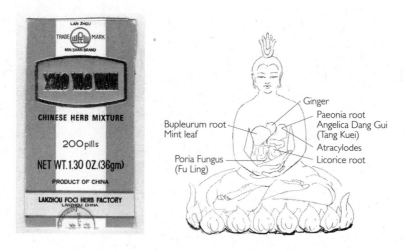

Xiao Yao Wan (also known as Relaxed Wanderer or Relaxx Extract) is a Chinese patent remedy pill sold in Chinese herb shops for a few dollars per bottle and online for a high price. It contains digestive herbs—ginger, bupleurum, mint, atractylodes, tang kuei, peony, and poria—to regulate digestion and reduce bloating, nervous stomach, chest and rib pains, irregular menstruation, depression, and anxiety. It improves digestion and therefore reduces food allergies and allergic headaches. I often recommend Xiao Yao Wan for nervous headaches accompanied by bloating and cloudy thinking from excess phlegm. Supporting digestive energy can also help regulate emotional upset. Even if you are too busy to eat or have irregular dietary habits, use this or another digestive remedy daily to help support digestion, blood sugar balance, and emotional equilibrium.

PMS and Menopausal Stress Headaches

Please see the entire chapter relating to women's issues beginning on page 89. Is there a single herb remedy for women's perimenopausal and menopausal headaches? I think so. Imagine a soothing cap placed over your head that removes heat, stress, insomnia, and spasms: skullcap.

Characteristics of the pain:

- sudden, hot throbbing or accompanying hot flashes
- temper
- anxiety
- hypertension
- insomnia

Treatment

Skullcap (also known as *Scutellaria lateriflora*, helmet flower, blue pimpernel, and Quaker bonnet) was used in colonial America to treat rabies. This plant produces a flower that resembles a hat, or "skullcap," worn by American colonists. Skullcap has a tranquilizing effect on the central nervous system. Clinical studies have demonstrated skullcap's ability to improve blood flow in the brain, inhibit muscle spasms, and act as a sedative. Some alternative health practitioners use skullcap to treat symptoms of attention deficit hyperactivity disorder (ADHD).

Skullcap supplements are often used for the following conditions: allergies, anxiety, epilepsy, fever, hardening of the arteries, high cholesterol, inflammation, insomnia, muscle spasm, nervous tension, stroke prevention, and paralysis caused by stroke. In China, one species of skullcap, *S. baicalensis*, is used to treat high blood pressure and insomnia. *S. baicalensis* is also believed to have antioxidant effects as well as antihistamine and anti-inflammatory effects, and is used to treat allergies, tumors, and, combined with other herbs, prostate cancer. The chemicals in skullcap are thought to work by preventing swelling and inflammation and by sedating pain. No recommended dose for skullcap has been established. The results vary.

Skullcap comes in different forms, such as liquid extracts or teas. The recommended doses for these products differ, due to differing potencies or other factors. Be sure to follow the specific directions for your particular skullcap product. Certain people, including heart patients and others, should not use sedatives of any kind. See my warnings against using sedative herbs in chapters dealing with heart health.

Trigger Points for Head, Neck, and Shoulder Pain

Trigger points are painful points and areas of referred pain resulting from poor blood circulation. The name "trigger point" may be misleading because it would seem that massaging them could trigger pain. In fact, massaging or stimulating trigger points can help eliminate pains. Here is a website indicating the trigger point locations for the head, neck, and shoulders according to muscle location: www.painclinic.org/musclepain-headneck shoulderarm.htm.

Trigger points are located at some distance from the referred pain. When applying pressure to them, use steady movement downward along the path of referred pain, not jerky harsh movement. Most often pain is removed from the area of most pressure—the center of pain—towards the extremities. For example, massage that applies pressure downward from neck to arms and hands often helps relieve inflammation (a hot throbbing pain) in the head and neck. You might also apply Tiger Balm or a sports rub ointment to areas of referred pain to enhance circulation.

A Spice Tea for Chronic or Computer-Related Neck and Shoulder Pain

Deep, aching shoulder pain that results from overwork, fatigue, or poor posture can be improved with a warm tea made by adding one-fourth teaspoon turmeric powder and one-fourth teaspoon cinnamon powder to a cup of hot water. Consume this without food between meals and you can feel the warming blood circulation soften your stiff shoulders and neck.

Letha's Advice: A Simple Treatment for Stiff Neck and Shoulder Pain

Apply a dot of red Tiger Balm or White Flower analgesic ointment along the back of the neck at the hairline and also along the top of the shoulders. That allows blood circulation to flow and relaxes muscles so that the cervical (neck) vertebrae can more easily find their correct position. Take a few deep breaths into the painful area and allow the exhalation to melt your shoulders down to your toes.

TMJ

Trigeminal neuralgia, a terrible pain affecting the trigeminal nerve, makes your face and jaw feel on fire. It can result from an incorrect bite that can be fixed by a dentist. It may also be tension-and-diet-related. See the article and video entitled "Headache and TMJ" at www.asianhealthsecrets.com. You may be able to improve TMJ pain at home by applying Tiger Balm and with massage.

Percussion Massager for Chronic Muscle Pain

A percussion massager, such as one made by HoMedics that has one or two massage heads, can be used to deeply increase circulation in the neck and shoulders. Massage at the back of the neck from the hairline down toward the top of each shoulder. Be careful to use a gentle setting at first and avoid the jugular vein located deep at each side of the neck. Always avoid using a massager or other stimulating device over the heart area.

My HoMedics percussion massager is my third arm. I use it to enhance circulation, reducing congestion pain made worse from sitting for hours writing. Other massagers are made as massaging pads you can add to your chair or place in the driver's seat of your car. A lively *zizzz* provides a good break from work when you don't feel like walking around the room. It eases tight painful muscles and spasms, and gets your circulation singing.

Daily Prevention of Head and Neck Pains

- Use relaxation techniques and regular exercise to prevent unwanted stress and tension to the neck muscles.
- Stretch every day, especially before and after exercise. A massage therapist can help you use stretches specifically for your neck and shoulders. For example, whiplash requires lying on a cylindrical pillow to help maintain the proper neck curve.
- If you tend to get neck pain from exercise, apply White Flower analgesic liquid to your neck for ten minutes after physical activity. Ice reduces inflammation but may increase nerve pains.
- Use good posture, especially if you sit at a desk all day. Keep your back supported. Adjust your computer monitor to eye level. This prevents you from continually looking up or down.

- At the computer, stretch your neck every hour or so. Don't forcefully twist your neck around but press with the palms of your hands against the tops of your shoulders and gently lean in the opposite direction.
- Use a headset for the telephone.
- When reading or typing from documents, place them in a holder at eye level.
- Make sure your sleep pillow is properly and comfortably supporting your head and neck. (A person who needs three or four pillows in order to breathe and is short of breath may have a heart or energy problem. Do not neglect to get that tested.)
- Make sure your mattress is firm enough.
- Use seat belts and bike helmets to prevent injuries.

When to Consult a Health Professional

Most chronic neck pain is not medically serious. Try self-care strategies before seeking medical help. However, if your neck pain is so severe you can't sit still, or if it is accompanied by any of the following symptoms, contact a medical professional.

- Fever, headache, and neck stiffness. This triad of symptoms might indicate bacterial meningitis, an infection of the spinal cord and brain covering that requires prompt treatment with antibiotics.
- Pain traveling down one arm, especially if the arm or hand is weak, numb, or tingling. Your symptoms might indicate that a herniated cervical disk is pressing on a nerve.
- Loss of bowel or bladder control. This might indicate pressure on the spinal cord or spinal nerve roots, needing immediate attention.
- Extreme physical instability. If you can suddenly flex or extend your neck much farther than usual, it might indicate a fracture or torn ligaments. This occurs only after significant injury, and is more likely to be detected by your doctor or an X-ray than by you.
- Persistent swollen glands in the neck. Infection or tumor can result in swollen glands and neck pain.
- Chest pain or pressure. A heart attack or inflamed heart muscle can cause neck pain along with more classic heart symptoms.

A Hit on the Head

If you fall or hit your head, there may be a concussion or possible neurological damage. Check for these warning signs: dizziness, weakness and fainting, fever, dilated pupils of the eyes, and lack of coordination when walking. Here is a simple test for neurological damage to the brain or nervous system that my chiropractor brother, Eric Hadady, DC, taught me.

Stand in an empty corner of your home. In the chiropractor's office, the doctor will stand behind you to catch you if you fall, so you have to protect yourself from injury by standing close to the walls. Put your feet together pointing forward. Put your hands together palms upward as though carrying something in the palms. Raise the arms to shoulder level with the upturned palms outstretched. Close your eyes and tilt your head slightly backward. You will waver somewhat but may soon find your balance. Count to ten slowly, then open your eyes and check your posture.

Are you tilting to one side, to the front or back? If so, there may be neurological damage resulting from your traumatic injury. If you cannot hold your balance at all, your self-regulating mechanism may be impaired by your injury. Check with your chiropractor, who will repeat this sort of test and others to determine the location and severity of your problem. He/she may be able to alleviate certain symptoms, such as dizziness, with an adjustment. Further testing may also be necessary.

If there is no serious damage from the injury, rest quietly and apply ice for twenty minutes daily or White Tiger Balm as needed to reduce swelling. Homeopathic arnica 30C is recommended for injuries resulting in superficial pain, swelling, and bruising. You will find many natural pain treatments for injuries in Chapters 8 through 10.

CHAPTER THREE

Backaches

Great ideas originate in the muscles...I never did a day's work in my life. It was all fun.

—Thomas A. Edison (1847–1931)

THOMAS ALVA EDISON, THE LAST OF SEVEN CHILDREN IN HIS FAMILY, DID NOT speak until he was four. By the time he was twelve, he had read Gibbon's *Decline and Fall of the Roman Empire*, Sears' *History of the World*, and Burton's *Anatomy of Melancholy*. He devoured *World Dictionary of Science* and books on practical chemistry. Whether or not your great ideas originate in your muscles or your brain and how back and brain are connected remains to be seen. Can you think better without back pain? Certainly! Does chronic backache squash your vitality and enthusiasm? Of course!

In the spirit of "the wizard of Menlo Park," the inventor of the light bulb, phonograph, and motion picture camera, this chapter contains several *fun* treatments for simple backache resulting from fatigue, weakness, and overwork. The following baths, massage oil, and mineral milk fortify muscles, ligaments, and bones and reduce nerve pain to help prevent injury and pain. I get my best writing ideas while floating in a swimming pool, when pressure is taken off muscles and joints. This chapter will help you to experience that healing pleasure at home.

背中の痛み
腰痛
גב כאבי
боль в спине
mal au dos
Rückenschmerzen
dolor de espalda
hátfájás
rugpijn
backache

Everyday Fatigue and Stress Back Pain

Does your back feel tight, stiff, or pinched? Is the pain dull or sharp? Is the pain worse with fatigue, emotional stress, caffeine, smoking, or alcohol?

- Fatigue-related back pain feels dull, deep, and heavy. You may also have difficulty breathing, heart palpitations, or numbness in the limbs.
- Disc injury or muscle spasm feels sharp, sudden, and very severe. Disc injury requires a visit to the chiropractor and possibly X-rays.
- Dehydration back pain feels worse from stress, aging, and chronic diarrhea, and from consuming drying spicy foods, drinking alcohol, and smoking. Dehydration dries the discs and increases likelihood of injury and chronic pain.

Back Injury Risk Factors

Although anyone can have back pain, a number of factors greatly increase your risk. They include age, level of fitness, diet, race, occupational hazards, disease, and smoking. The person most at risk of back injury and chronic pain would be:

- thirty or older
- an out-of-shape weekend warrior with weak muscles, eating a high-calorie, high-fat diet
- a non-Caucasian (African American women, for example, are two to three times more likely than white women to develop spondylolisthesis, a condition in which a vertebra of the lower spine slips out of place)
- a person who may have inherited a tendency toward disc problems
- a smoker
- a person who works in a job that requires lifting, pushing and pulling, or twisting or vibrating the spine

Treatments for a Simple Backache

Tired, aching muscles need to breathe and expand. Many health professionals advise drinking lots of water, as muscles, bone, and flesh are mostly made of water. I would add: eat seaweed daily for vital minerals that muscles and bones need. Naturally salty-flavored, delicious, and crisp nori, dulse, and kelp (soaked until soft and consumed along with the soaking water) make excellent snack foods. We also absorb water and beneficial nutrients from a bath.

A Detoxifying Seaweed Bath

*This refreshing soak feels great after exercise or overwork, and to help correct long-term dietary overindulgence. Separate your bath from a meal by at least two hours. Imagine you are at the seashore, breathing the healing peace of the ocean. Kelp seaweed (*Laminaria longicruris*) encourages relaxation, tones and tightens the skin, and promotes blood circulation and lymphatic drainage (an anticellulite treatment!). It improves aching muscles and arthritic joint pains. Kelp digitata (*Laminaria digitata*) has also been suggested as an antiradiation treatment.*

Ingredients for the bath:
1 cup sea salt
1 cup baking soda
2 cups Epsom salts
2 or more tablespoons powdered kelp
2 tablespoons dried ginger powder
1 cup apple cider vinegar

Draw a warm bath. Mix the dry ingredients (sea salt, baking soda, Epsom salts, kelp powder, and ginger powder) in a bowl. Add water and combine well to make a paste. Pour the vinegar into the bathwater and add the seaweed mixture. Soak for 20–30 minutes. Brush the skin with a towel or take a 30-second cool shower as you prefer. Wrap in a dry towel and lie down for another 15 minutes to enjoy the benefits of improved circulation.

Kelp Massage Oil Rub

A massage oil should invigorate as well as relieve tension and reduce pain. Steep two tablespoons of kelp powder in eight ounces of oil for two weeks or more. Use an oil according to your energy needs. Coconut, olive, or soy oil are cooling for warm weather or inflammatory conditions. Sesame oil is warming and rejuvenating for cold weather, chronic chills, and weakness, and useful for the elderly or persons with arthritic stiffness that feels better with application of warmth. Almond oil has a neutral temperature and is beautifying for the complexion. Keep the oil in an airtight container, away from sunlight and heat.

The oil absorbs kelp's abundant sea minerals. The primary known constituents of kelp include algin, carrageenan, iodine, potassium, bromine, mucopolysaccharides, mannitol, alginic acid, kainic acid, laminine, histamine, zeaxanthin, protein, and Vitamins B2 and C. It is especially high in natural iodine, plus the cell salts so important for the proper functioning of the body and especially the thyroid. Kelp oil is useful for everyone because of its strengthening effects. It's especially useful for ailing and convalescent persons and during pregnancy. It improves weight loss and chronic depression from low vitality. If you hate the smell of seaweed, add a few drops of an essential oil such as lavender, lemon, or mint.

A Simple Back Rub

Before or after your seaweed bath, apply a few drops of kelp oil to face and dry skin areas. For weight loss, detoxification, or after surgery to release toxins from the body, a light-touch lymphatic drainage massage works best. Massage gently with your fingertips using a pressure no heavier than the weight of a dime, stroking from the head toward the heart and from the feet toward the kidneys. That encourages lymphatic cleansing.

To soothe an aching tired back and muscle spasms, a heavier touch works better. Some people prefer a strong steady pressure, not light stroking, to sedate pain. If you are massaging the back, start from the waist or buttocks and place the sides of your fists on each side of the spine. Inhale with the person you are massaging. With the exhalation, press firmly but with a touch sensitive to that person's needs, moving your fists upward toward the center of the shoulder blades. I recommend using the fists, not the flat of the hands, because that stresses your wrists less. You might also try using the side of your forearm on each side of the spine. Moving upward on the back for massage reverses the direction of gravity and can sometimes remove stress from the discs that tend to collapse from sitting.

A Rejuvenating Mineral Bath

The more your muscles, joints, and ligaments are nourished with blood, necessary fluids, and oxygen, the easier it will be to increase movement and sustain comfort. Your back muscles support your standing and sitting. The lumbar area is particularly stressed by hours of sitting under the pressure of overwork, sugar, caffeine or tobacco, and worries. Foods and exercise are not enough to stop the pain. Nourishing tonics that rejuvenate muscles improve comfort and mobility. Here are two ways to insure muscle strength and flexibility: bioplasma and shilajit.

Bioplasma is the name given to a combination of twelve essential minerals (also known as cell salts or Schuessler Tissue Salts). They are not table salt but support healthy cell tissue and cell function. The formula includes forms of calcium, potassium, magnesium, iron, and silica. Add ten to twenty small white pills to a bath of warm water and soak for twenty minutes. During your mineral bath, turn out the lights and imagine yourself in a cozy dark cave. Reconnect with your inner strength. (Growing up in New Mexico, I might connect with my inner Gila monster.)

Shilajit

For thousands of years in India, China, Tibet, Pakistan, and Russia, people have enjoyed the benefits of shilajit (also known as mineral pitch, bitumen, or fulvic acid), the thick black liquid minerals that drip from cracks in Himalayan rocks during hot weather. Shilajit is made of decomposed, centuries-old plants and rocks formed under pressure. It is a coal by-product on its way to becoming diamonds. The black semisweet liquid is extruded from rocks with geothermal pressure and then purified, and is thought to prevent and cure nearly every discomfort and disease known to man. Shilajit's highly condensed minerals and amino acids fortify core energy responsible for physical, sexual, and spiritual power.

One of the most potent rejuvenating substances used in Ayurveda (the classical medicine of India), shilajit is used as a general tonic that improves libido, helps stabilize

When a Backache Is Not a Backache

Unexplained, persistent back pain can be an early sign of cancer. Pain in the lowest part of the back, upper thigh, and hips can be a sign of prostate cancer, while pain in the upper back can signal lung cancer. A pain in the upper abdomen and back is one of the few early signs of pancreatic cancer. Men with testicular cancer report a heavy, aching feeling low in the belly or abdomen, or in the scrotum or testicles. They sometimes describe it as a feeling of downward pulling or as a generalized ache throughout the groin area. Prostate cancer that has spread to the lymph nodes often makes itself known as discomfort in the pelvis or swelling in the legs. Other signs of possible prostate cancer include blood in the urine or semen, and difficulty with urination, which may be difficulty starting or stopping urination. There may also be swollen lymph glands in the neck, underarm, or groin. If any of these problems arise, you should check with your doctor for further analysis and, if necessary, take steps to eliminate prostate problems. Anti-inflammatory herbs, such as the Chinese patent remedy Kai Kit (also known as prostate gland pills) are useful for simple benign prostate discomforts.

blood sugar, heals injury and broken bones, and improves immune function, arthritis, hypertension, and obesity, among other things. Shilajit helps move vital nutrients and moisturizing relief to aching muscles and bones to stop back pain. It relaxes ordinary daily tensions and improves sleep patterns essential to healing pain and injury. It improves stamina for overworked, overstressed people. Everyday wear and tear to the spine from standing and sitting, poor nutritional habits, and age naturally increase dehydration of muscles and joints that directly affect lower back pain. Shilajit can help reverse dehydration and therefore slow signs of degeneration, including muscle and bone loss and chronic pain.

As a general tonic, swallow one capsule of shilajit with a few sips of milk (or water), either during the mineral bath or before bed. The only contraindications for using shilajit are high uric acid levels, gout, or kidney stones made of uric acid. To reduce uric acid stones and gout I recommend adding one tablespoon of black cherry concentrate to a glass of water daily. Another treatment is a course of homeopathic formic acid 6X (homeopathic ant) prior to using shilajit. Consult with your homeopathic health specialist for specific individualized recommendations.

Enhanced Sexual Vitality and Less Back Pain for Men and Women

A backache can seriously slow your game. Traditional Asian medicine acknowledges the intimate connection between back and leg muscles, lower back comfort and flexibility, hormone balance, and sexual wellness. Many Asian energy and sexual herbal tonics combine remedies that reduce tight aching muscles in back and legs as they fortify sexual hormones. For enhanced muscle strength and male potency, combine shilajit with an equal amount of ashwagandha, sometimes called "Indian ginseng," known to fortify muscles and nerves. If added testosterone is required for sexuality, add an equal amount of gokshura (*Tribulus terrestris*) to the above herbs.

For female hormones and sexual rejuvenation, combine shilajit with an equal amount of shatavari, wild East Indian asparagus, which nourishes fragile vaginal tissue to increase sexual comfort for postmenopausal women and fertility for younger women. This combination is not digestive and increases phlegm and sexual fluids. Therefore, take it between meals. See more tonic herbs in Chapter 17.

Back Pain Caused by Your Shoes

Joint injury happens when the hip rotates forward and becomes stuck in an abnormally painful position. Forward rotation of the hip and/or pelvis is often the result of wearing high-heeled shoes. Pain comes from twisting, pulling, and stretching many tendons, ligaments, muscles, and pinching the sciatic nerve. You may have sciatica and/or muscle strain due to a sacroiliac (SI) joint problem. If you continue to wear high heels, stretch out the back of your legs and thighs by standing with your toes on top of a book or door frame in order to raise your toes an inch or two higher than your heels. Then, standing straight, bend forward with your entire body, not just the waist, to stretch the back leg muscles. Hold that position for the count of ten and repeat several times. Massage the feet and entire leg, hip, and groin to improve circulation and alignment.

Smoker's Chronic Back Pain

Smoking is dehydrating and blocks the body's ability to deliver nutrients to the back muscles and discs. Repeated coughing from smoking may also cause back pain. Smokers are less physically fit and healthy than nonsmokers, which increases their likelihood of pain. And smoking impairs circulation and breathing, which slows healing, prolonging pain for people who have had injuries, back surgery, or broken bones.

Letha's Advice for Smokers

Quit! Try chewing a spicy cinnamon stick instead of continuing a stinky habit. Cinnamon enhances circulation to reduce pain, helps normalize body temperature, improves pancreas function in diabetes, and, some say, reduces our chances of developing brain fatigue (even Alzheimer's). Not a bad trade-off. Acupuncture has helped many people to stop smoking. Points for the lungs, nervous system, and common addiction are located on our ears.

Lower Back, Leg, and Groin Pain

It has been estimated that 80 percent of chronic low back pain involves the sacroiliac (SI) joint, located at the very bottom of the back on either side of the spine. The sacroiliac joints at the rear part of the pelvic girdle sit between the sacrum (vertebrae S1-S5) and the ilia (hip bones). The SI joint allows torsional or twisting movements when we move our legs. Without the sacroiliac joints, the pelvis would be at higher risk of a fracture. SI joint dysfunction can happen if the SI joint either becomes "locked" or too mobile. Many women, because we can give birth, are very flexible (too flexible) in the SI joint. Certain yoga positions can also increase this flexibility. Do you waddle from side to side with each step? Other people, because of hip joint damage, feel stuck in the lower back and walk with a stiff leg. Either walk leads to problems with surrounding ligaments and muscles and therefore causes a wide range of discomforts throughout the lower back and buttocks, or even the thigh or groin.

Symptoms of SI Joint Injury

- Pain is located either to the left or right of your lower back or tail bone. The pain can range from an ache to a sharp pain that restricts movement.
- Pain may radiate into your buttocks and low back and will often radiate to the front into the groin. Occasionally for men it is responsible for pain in the testicles.
- There may be referred pain into the lower leg, mistaken for sciatica. (See chapter 4 for sciatica.)
- Classic symptoms of SI dysfunction are difficulty turning over in bed, struggling to put on shoes and socks, and pain getting your legs in and out of the car.
- There may be stiffness in the lower back when getting up after sitting for long periods and when getting up from bed in the morning.
- One side of your lower back may ache when driving long distances. There may be tenderness on palpating the ligaments that surround the joint.

Injury to the sacroiliac joint can result from trauma; biomechanical problems such as leg-length discrepancy, a twisted pelvis, or muscle imbalances; hormonal changes during pregnancy; or inflammatory joint disease. To avoid pain and further injury, doctors recommend rest, applying a warming pack, or using an anti-inflammatory. They may inject corticosteroids or use electrotherapy. However, most over-the-counter painkillers, especially aspirin and acetaminophen, increase the risk of bleeding ulcers and liver damage, and steroids thin bone mass. Plus, they offer only temporary relief. A leg-length discrepancy (when one leg is shorter than the other) should be corrected with a shoe insert or other means, or else injury will continue.

The SI Joint Roll

You can feel some relief from muscle tension and painful ligaments and nerves surrounding the SI joint if you do this simple movement a few times a day. Other movements for people who cannot get out of bed are detailed in chapter 9 on Sports Injuries. For example, the hip rolls can be done in bed or the bath tub.

Lie on your back. Put your knees together and bring them toward your chest. Do not strain or push. It should be comfortable. Gently and slowly lean your knees first to the left then to the right. If that hurts too much, lean them against a wall or chair or other immovable object, then release them. You should be able to get into the position easily, with no effort. The aim is to relax tension and pain. Breathe slowly and deeply and repeat this movement several times.

Backache and the Weather

If you have chronic back and leg pain, or have had a previous injury to the area, try to avoid temperature extremes, especially the effects of cold, wet weather. Dress in rain gear and a neck scarf to protect your muscles from spasm. A spasm is the body's warning that a muscle is not comfortable, often because it lacks circulation and nourishment from blood and oxygen. Protecting against spasm pain will save you lots of trouble and help prevent injury. After being outside in nasty weather, enjoy a cup of warm cinnamon tea to prevent hypothermia and enhance circulation for the entire body.

SI Joint Quiz

1. **Is my pain worse when I get out of bed?**
2. **Does my pain get worse after prolonged sitting?**
3. **Is my pain worse after prolonged standing or walking?**
4. **Is my pain better for a while after I change my position or activity?**

If you answered yes to at least three questions, you likely have sacroiliac joint dysfunction as your most basic pain problem. Disc dislocation or herniation usually accounts for only 5 percent of back pain.

Herbal Pills for Back Pain

A natural herbal remedy for back and leg pain should free stuck circulation, strengthen sinews, bones, back, and knees, and fortify adrenal health. One easy-to-remember herbal remedy that combines herbs to fortify testosterone and, therefore, muscle strength is called Backbone.

Backbone is a Chinese herbal pill for low back pain made by Health Concerns in Oakland, California. It combines warming, stimulating herbs that feel like a deeply soothing yet invigorating massage. Along with treating back pain, it is used for urinary incontinence, spermatorrhea (loss of sperm), impotence, weak back and knees, and reduced hearing and vision stemming from low adrenal vitality. It is not recommended for people with fever, night sweats, chronic thirst, a red tongue, rapid pulse, painful urination, insomnia, red eyes, or constipation with hard stools or blood in excretions.

Backbone pills are a warming, invigorating tonic for people who more often feel chills, weak muscle strength, and fatigue from work, sexual excess, or aging. They may be pale with cold limbs and have watery diarrhea or excess urination. Chinese doctors call these internal cold symptoms "kidney yang deficiency." Do you wear extra clothing in cool weather, sleep with lots of covers, feel weak after being in cold weather, or develop diarrhea after eating salad? If so, you need a warming tonic such as this. Its use may be temporary, just until you feel stronger and warmer; for example, two to three pills three times daily, up to a week or two. Stop taking a warming remedy if you begin to feel hot, flushed, and insomniac or have dark urine.

> **Important Note**
>
> Always avoid all warming herbs and energy tonics such as Chinese ginseng if you have a fever or cold/flu symptoms. The tonic drives the cold/flu symptoms deeper beyond your natural defense system.

Backbone pills contain herbal precursors to testosterone: eucommia bark, cistanche, and cuscuta seed; a source of calcium from tortoise shell; herbs to enhance circulation such as tang kuei; myrrh; and herbs to fortify adrenal health including cornus fruit (a wild cherry), rehmannia, and others. Eucommia, woodwardia, acanthopanax, dipsacus, and tortoise shell (from *Chinemys reevesii*, a farmed pond turtle) strengthen bones, muscles, and sinews (tendons).

If you prefer an all-vegetarian herbal pain-relieving formula for lower back and nerves, take one-half teaspoon of ashwagandha powder and a pinch of clove (the kitchen spice) powder in a cup of warm water along with two capsules of shilajit twice daily for at least two weeks and give yourself a gentle kidney and lower back massage with seaweed oil. If you develop thirst and other heat symptoms, omit the clove powder. You might use instead one-fourth teaspoon ashwagandha powder and one-fourth teaspoon shatavari powder (or two 300-milligram capsules of each) with a little milk or warm water twice daily.

Discs, Sprains, Curves, and Back Injury

If your pain is severe, sudden, long-lasting, or is accompanied by fever, dizziness, or other changes in consciousness you should see a specialist. **It is essential to get a correct diagnosis, whether you choose medical or natural treatments**. The herbal baths, oil, and pill treatments that I recommend may be combined with medical treatments to speed healing as they reduce discomforts. However, allow adequate time for them to work, even if they alleviate pain. Using soothing natural treatments for preventing and treating back pain, you can eventually feel increased energy, strength in lower back muscles, better flexibility, and ease of movement. However, eliminating back pain is not enough to solve your problem. Since the back muscles are vital for movement and balance, they may affect your gait, your senses, and your mood. Continue with regular daily natural treatments in order to prevent discomfort and further damage.

If you experience severe pain, the problem may be mechanical: a problem with the way your spine moves or the way you feel when you move your spine in certain ways. The most common mechanical cause of back pain is intervertebral disc degeneration. It occurs when the discs located between the vertebrae of the spine break down with age and wear and tear. The problem leads to pain if the back is stressed. Other mechanical causes of back pain include spasms, muscle tension, and ruptured discs, also called herniated discs.

Spine injuries such as sprains and fractures can cause either short-lived or chronic pain. Sprains are tears in the ligaments that support the spine, and they can occur from twisting or lifting improperly. Fractured vertebrae are often the result of osteoporosis, a condition that causes weak, porous bones. Less commonly, back pain may be caused by severe injuries that result from accidents and falls.

Many medical problems can cause or contribute to back pain. They include scoliosis, which causes curvature of the spine and does not usually cause pain until midlife; spondylolisthesis; various forms of arthritis, including osteoarthritis, rheumatoid arthritis, and ankylosing spondylitis; and spinal stenosis, a narrowing of the spinal column that puts pressure on the spinal cord and nerves. While osteoporosis itself is not painful, it can lead to painful fractures of the vertebrae.

Other causes of back pain include pregnancy; kidney stones or infections; endometriosis, which is the buildup of uterine tissue in places outside the uterus; and fibromyalgia, which causes fatigue and widespread muscle pain. Problems could also arise from infections or tumors. Although the causes of back pain are usually physical, it is important to know that emotional stress and use of nerve stimulants such as caffeine also play a role in how severe the pain is and how long it lasts.

Prevent Back Pain

One of the best things you can do to prevent back pain is regular, gentle exercise to keep your back muscles strong. If you walk or run, get fitted for shoes that are right for your stride, including lifts as needed. Swimming is excellent because it places no weight on joints. If you can't swim, walk in the water. Another good exercise is, while facing the center of the swimming pool, rest your arms against the rim of the pool to create a stable support and ride an imaginary bicycle in the water in order to tighten abdominal muscles and release leg pain. Exercises such as tai chi and qigong or any weight-bearing exercise that strengthens your balance are good ones to try.

My friend Sharon Smith is a qigong master, who for many years has taught people how to move gracefully and pain-free through life. Her Asian movement practice has shaped her personality. She is an attractive, audacious traveler who spends summers in Thailand and China refining her skills and teaching workshops. The grounded center of her vitality is qi developed from breath, concentration, and slow movement, freeing meridians that enhance life force. One summer she visited sacred Buddhist sites in China and sent me an email from the Yak Hotel in Lhasa, Tibet! Her physical and mental freedom gained from qigong enables a wider expression of body, mind, and spirit. Consider that when you exercise. What is the ultimate goal of your exercise—to build muscles or to free your body and expand your mind?

A healthy diet is a very important step to prevent back pain. For one thing, eating to maintain a healthy weight helps avoid putting unnecessary, injury-causing stress on your back and legs. To keep your spine and all bones strong, you need to get up to 2 grams of calcium and 2,000 IU of vitamin D3 every day. These nutrients help prevent osteoporosis, which is responsible for many bone fractures that lead to back pain. Your skin makes vitamin D when you are in the sun. Try to spend fifteen minutes in the sun or with a sun lamp daily.

When to See a Health Specialist

A trip to the doctor, chiropractor, osteopath, or other specialist is a good idea if your pain is severe and doesn't improve with natural treatments and rest, or if you have pain or dizziness after a fall or an injury. It is also important to see your doctor if you have pain with any of the following problems: trouble urinating; weakness, pain, or numbness in your legs; fever; or unintentional weight loss. Such symptoms could signal a serious problem that requires treatment. You may need to have X-rays, an MRI, a CT scan, or blood tests for the final diagnosis. Many times, the precise cause of back pain is never known, but it may be comforting to know that back pain can get better whether or not you find out what is causing it.

Sample Diagnostic Tests for Back Pain

X-rays: Traditional X-rays use low levels of radiation to project a picture onto a piece of film (some newer X-rays use electronic imaging techniques). They are often used to view the bones and bony structures in the body. Your doctor may order an X-ray if he or she suspects that you have a fracture or osteoarthritis, or that your spine is not aligned properly. The best modern X-ray equipment uses less radiation; however, to protect yourself after being exposed to X-rays, take at least 1,000 milligrams of easily absorbable vitamin C for several days.

Magnetic Resonance Imaging (MRI): MRI uses a strong magnetic force instead of radiation to create an image. Unlike an X-ray, which shows only bony structures, an MRI scan produces clear pictures of soft tissues, too, such as ligaments, tendons, and blood vessels. Your doctor may order an MRI scan if he or she suspects a problem such as an infection, tumor, inflammation, or pressure on a nerve. An MRI scan is needed if the pain persists more than three to six weeks, or if your doctor feels there may be a need for surgical consultation. An MRI machine is a noisy tunnel. If possible, you may request an open MRI if you feel claustrophobic. Practice slow, deep breathing during the test unless instructed to do otherwise.

Computed Tomography (CT) scan: A CT scan allows your doctor to see spinal structures that cannot be seen on traditional X-rays. It is a three-dimensional image that a computer creates from a series of two-dimensional pictures that it takes of your back. Your doctor may order a CT scan to look for problems including herniated discs, tumors, or spinal stenosis. A CT scan exposes you to many times more radiation than X-rays. Experts advise to have no more than one scan a year. Before and after you have a CT scan, if not contraindicated for your condition, use tonics to enhance immunity such as vitamin C, zinc, and astragalus. Continue for at least one month following the scan.

Blood tests: Although blood tests are not used generally in diagnosing the cause of back pain, your doctor may order them in some cases. Blood tests that might be used include the following:

- **Complete blood count (CBC)**: CBC can point to problems such as infection or inflammation.
- **Erythrocyte sedimentation rate (also called sed rate)**: A measure of inflammation that may suggest infection. The presence of inflammation may also suggest some forms of arthritis or, in rare cases, a tumor.

Many useful natural anti-inflammatory herbs can ease pain depending upon its type and location. Remember, your comfort level is a vital part of diagnosis and treatment of back pain. As with other injuries, continue using natural treatments even after pain has stopped, because the back is vulnerable. In the womb we swam and did not walk or sit. Experts say that up to 90 percent of all MRI scans of the spine show some type of abnormality, and sometimes the X-rays and CT scans of people without pain show problems. Similarly, even some healthy pain-free people can have elevated sed rates.

Rules of Thumb for Treating Back Pain

Rest and Avoid Excess or Jarring Movements

Acute back pain, from spasm or other causes, may improve without medical treatment. But a relaxing bath and gentle massage often feels great. Also, get enough sleep. Pain aggravates insomnia and vice versa. Homeopathic Coffea cruda 6X is recommended to improve sleep and eliminate caffeine from the body. Take a recommended dose under the tongue without food one half hour before bed. Exercise is not advisable for acute back pain, nor is surgery. According to medical sources, chronic back pain, in the vast majority of cases, does not require surgery. Rest and home treatments are often enough to ease pain. However, when back pain is caused by a tumor, an infection, or a nerve root problem, prompt surgery is necessary to ease pain and prevent complications.

Hot and Cold Packs

In most cases, hot or cold packs, or sometimes a combination of the two, can be soothing to chronically sore, stiff backs. Heat dilates the blood vessels, improving the supply of oxygen that the blood takes to the back and reducing muscle spasms. Heat also alters the sensation of pain. Cold may reduce inflammation by decreasing the size of blood vessels and the flow of blood to the area. Although cold may feel painful against the skin, it numbs deep pain. Applying hot or cold packs for fifteen minutes or alternating every fifteen minutes may relieve pain, but it does not cure the cause of chronic back pain.

Gentle Exercise

The following four types of exercise are important to general physical fitness and may be helpful for certain specific causes of back pain: flexion (bending forward), extension (bending backward), stretching, and aerobics. The first three are easily and gracefully accomplished by doing the yoga salute to the sun. Or, if that is too difficult, try the cat posture. A cat loves to stretch. Kneeling on all fours, place your weight evenly on to your palms and knees. Inhale, curve the spine upward toward the ceiling, and then exhale as you reverse. Curve your back downward toward the floor. Inhale up and exhale down. Gently repeat to create a comfortable rhythm.

For back problems, always avoid exercise that requires twisting or vigorous forward flexion, such as aerobic dancing and rowing, because these actions raise pressure in the discs and actually do more harm than good. Always avoid high-impact activities if you have disc disease. Try three ten-minute sessions to start with and work up to your goal, no more than thirty minutes at a time. But first, speak with your doctor or physical therapist about the safest aerobic exercise for you.

Acupuncture

In Shanghai's teaching hospital, I witnessed and gave successful acupuncture treatments for low back pain, incontinence, "incomplete urination," a complication of prostate inflammation, paralysis, stroke, thyroid conditions, breast fibroids, and depression. Acupuncture works like turning on a light switch, moving circulation to dissolve stiffness and pain. It can reduce inflammation, affect the functioning of internal organs, and improve certain disease conditions. This ancient Chinese practice has finally gained popularity in the United States.

Inserting thin needles or using laser stimulation at precise locations along acupuncture channels by practitioners can unblock the flow of stuck qi circulation to relieve pain and restore health. This works partly by increasing the body's natural pain-numbing chemicals, such as endorphins, serotonin, and acetylcholine. Doctors have reluctantly agreed that acupuncture can be effective when used as part of a comprehensive treatment plan for low back pain, fibromyalgia, and several other conditions. Results will vary among patients and for the same patient at various times because the available level of qi will vary according to health condition. The very weak, elderly, or pregnant women should not receive acupuncture but should instead use energy tonics.

I believe the great advantage of using traditional Asian therapies such as acupuncture or acupressure comes with the diagnosis and careful, comprehensive follow-up. Western scanning is extremely precise in pinpointing a mechanical or structural problem or finding a tumor. However, acupuncture, which engages the body's subtle energy fields and herbs that support internal organs and blood quality, can be used to simultaneously improve vitality, mood, and circulation, and speed the healing process without side effects. Here is an all-too-common example that illustrates my point about traditional Asian diagnosis that is specific to the *person*, not to the disease.

Donna has chronic low back pain that is worse from fatigue or rainy weather. Her tongue is pale, swollen, and scalloped at the edges with marks left by impressions from her teeth. From the color, shape, and markings on her tongue I sense her metabolism and digestive energy are in trouble. Her pulses are slow, deep, soggy, and hesitant, indicating what acupuncturists call "stagnant qi." In other words, her energy is inadequate to support healthy circulation and heart action. Her complexion is slightly pale and ashen, her voice is breathy, and she is listless. She is pooped. An over-the-counter painkiller will not help her much. My diagnosis indicates she has edema with a puffy face, dark circles under the eyes, and waterlogged legs. She has slow, difficult digestion and low blood sugar. Her inadequate digestion and low vitality will more than likely lead to depression, irregular menstruation, and down the line, possibly a fibroid. I don't even have to ask: her radial pulses show she has low sexual vitality and no libido. Applying ice or heat to her back will certainly not treat her underlying problems, nor will a steroid injection. She needs better vitality to lift her spirits and ease pain. She needs stimulating, hormone-balancing herbs, nourishing foods, and energizing treatments with acupuncture or massage in order to build up her weak condition and improve her feeling of hopelessness.

Preventing back pain is not a one-shot treatment, but a lifestyle change that can help you to look and feel better, younger, and more positive. Hopefully Eastern and Western medicines will work more often in tandem to alleviate pain and treat the entire person. That requires precise testing and surgical or medical treatments coordinated with a natural approach to address the nutritive, energetic, and emotional aspects of pain. Note: medical treatments, including platelet-rich plasma (PRP) and stem-cell injections, are covered in chapter 18.

CHAPTER FOUR

Sciatica

Your pain is the breaking of the shell that encloses your understanding.

—Kahlil Gibran (poet, 1883–1931)

THE SCIATIC NERVE IS THE LARGEST, THICKEST NERVE IN THE BODY, FORMED BY the joining of lumbar (L4, L5) and sacrum (S1, S2, and S3) spinal nerve roots. It runs from the lower back down to the heel.

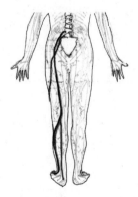

The sciatic nerve.

Characteristics of the pain:

- sharp, piercing, hot, electric pain that runs along the sciatic nerve
- pain may begin in the lower back, but travels down the buttocks, along the side or back of the leg, around the knee to the ankle

Causes of Sciatica

The actual cause of sciatica depends upon whom you ask. It is a pinched nerve that can drive you up the wall with pain or make you jump from the electric shock. It may be the result of a compression such as bulging disc fluid pressing against the nerve. Some people think sciatica is caused by a spasm of the piriformis muscle located deep inside the buttocks.

I have heard from orthopedic surgeon friends that sciatica stemming from the piriformis syndrome is rare. Usually it involves a back disc problem. In that case, X-rays and longer treatment may be necessary. Several spinal disorders can cause nerve compression and sciatica or lumbar radiculopathy. According to medical sources, the six most common in descending order are (most common) a bulging or herniated disc; lumbar spinal stenosis (the opening in the vertebrae is not wide enough to comfortably allow for the spinal cord); spondylolisthesis (a vertebra in the lower part of the spine slips forward onto a bone below it); trauma, piriformis syndrome, and (least common) spinal tumors.

It is commonly accepted that nerve pain reacts to stimulants, stress, and fatigue. After all, nervous energy drives our work and active social life. We cannot separate one nerve from the whole to examine our pain because the nervous system, brain chemicals, and our habits work together as a communication network. Here is an example to help us understand how that works.

A man I'll call Albert usually wrote several books simultaneously. However, he told me one biography stumped him, and he asked his ex-wife, a librarian, for help in obtaining rare original sources. She scribbled illegible notes on loose sheets of used paper at the library. Her sloppy disorganization was irritating, but her library connections provided access to books otherwise impossible to obtain. He generously gave her credit as a co-author. While promoting the book on television and radio, she assumed center stage, and was generally rude. Albert vowed to never work with her again. Then came the dawn: He needed her cooperation to write the sequel. He agonized for a few weeks whether or not to contact her. One morning, turning over in bed, Albert yelped in pain, unable to move. A searing sharp pain stabbed his right buttock and along a line that ran down the back of his right thigh and from the knee to the outside of his right ankle. Tears came to his eyes. He felt physically and emotionally stuck.

Was it a disc injury or emotional conflict causing the pain? Albert did not care. He wanted relief! Albert took three twenty-minute warm baths daily, adding Epsom salts to relax his back muscles. It helped somewhat, and he conceived new books while soaking in the tub. After consulting a medical doctor, Albert stopped taking the prescribed narcotic painkiller after it gave him hallucinations that he was slicing his ex-wife into pieces. He got manipulation treatments from both his chiropractor and osteopathic physician and laser treatments from me. He said they all helped a great deal. After nearly two weeks of agony, his sciatica became latent. It shows up when he fails to exercise, does not drink enough water to hydrate his muscles or works under pressure sitting many hours at his desk or driving a car. Most likely a locked SI joint is a problem for him, along with other individual factors including mental fatigue, caffeine, adrenal weakness, and overweight. Luckily, Albert has become conversant with the Internet and no longer depends on his ex-wife.

Albert's ongoing "pain in the butt" sciatica is rather easily treated with acupuncture. Here is how you can give yourself a massage treatment for sciatica based on acupuncture principles at home. Lie on the pain-free side. Allow the painful leg to rest on top of or in front of the other leg With your palm push downward from the most painful area of your hip toward the thigh. You can easily find painful points along that line of stuck energy. Use pressure strong enough to feel a release of tension and continue for ten minutes. Massage around the top, bottom, and side of the knee. Apply strong pressure along the lower leg to the ankle and massage the foot down to the little toe. You are bringing pain, stuck energy circulation, and inflammation away from the source of pain toward the body's extremity. That is how acupuncture and massage help to relieve inflammatory pain. Take the pain away from its source along an energy pathway and out of the body. You might also use a massage cream or ointment containing menthol or homeopathic arnica to enhance the cooling, relaxing treatment.

For such a case of simple sciatica, I use a painless cold laser, and it requires one to three treatments to bring inflammation down along the gallbladder meridian to the feet until pain is eliminated. Using a laser for this or for tennis elbow (see the treatment in chapter 9), never point the laser light toward the eyes, Adam's apple, or heart. Avoid laser or electrical stimulation if you have a pacemaker. You may be able to ease the pain considerably at home by lying on a tennis ball placed at the painful area in the buttocks or by doing the piriformis stretch shown in the illustration. Make sure to check with your chiropractor first to make sure that stretch will be beneficial in your case. Your sciatica may stem from another cause. Seated, bend the painful leg at the knee and place it on top of the nonpainful leg. That stretches the buttocks to relieve muscle tension.

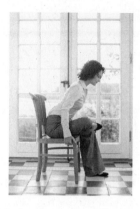

Sit with the ankle of the painful leg on top of the opposite thigh. Lean gently forward to stretch the lower back. If that hurts your groin, the problem may stem from your hip joint, not the sciatic nerve. Otherwise, if the stretch gives relief, continue with it gently several times a day.

Daily Prevention and Treatment of Sciatica

Stay Hydrated

At the swimming pool of a Vermont spa, I met Dr. Richard J. Nasca, MD, from North Carolina. He is a noted orthopedic surgeon who has written articles such as "Biomechanics of Existing and New Spine Implants" and worked with an international team of researchers to invent a plastic disc used to replace damaged discs and reduce spinal injury pain. Retired, fit, and active, he and his wife are avid golfers who travel to spend time with their children. He also stays in touch with research. To prevent injuries to bones, joints, and discs, he recommends staying hydrated with a drink such as Gatorade cut in half with water to reduce the sugar content. Gatorade is made of 94 percent water plus 6 percent high-fructose corn syrup, citric acid, salt, modified food starch, mono-potassium sulfate, sodium citrate, emulsifiers, and natural flavorings. Water and sodium puff the muscles and ease connective tissues so that you can stay limber. Gatorade provides carbohydrates and electrolytes lost during physical activity and a source of energy that's more dependable than caffeine drinks. Because of the sugar content, I recommend drinking water with added bioplasma, sold in health-food stores, instead of Gatorade-type drinks. Bioplasma, a homeopathic remedy made of twelve essential minerals including potassium, sodium, calcium, iron, and silica, provides support for the cells and eliminates workout odors.

Letha's Advice: Stretch Upside Down

Short of surgery, traction, or painkillers, I recommend a slant board for daily use to increase a healthy stretch. Lying with your head lower than your feet reverses the flow of gravity to help lubricate drying, aging spinal discs. I ordered a slant board online. When I lie on it, blood rushes to my head and refreshes my complexion. It stretches the spine, allowing for more space between vertebrae. Women with a tilted pelvis should lie face downward on the slant board to realign the pelvis. People with hypertension should use caution or avoid the slant board. Otherwise, most people find that lying on it fifteen minutes daily, avoiding mealtime, is a refreshing and relaxing experience.

Is your lower back and leg pain reduced by stretching in the opposite direction, for example, by allowing your leg to hang over the side of the bed? If so, the origin of your sciatic pain may be a jammed SI joint or even reduced cartilage at the hip joint. Try standing on the pain-free leg and bending the painful leg in half at the knee. Let it hang. Does that stretch feel better after about ten minutes? If so, that is the form of traction you should use. It may work better for you than a slant board.

A Lemon Foot Soak to Reduce Inflammation

Another way to reduce inflammation in the body is to soak your feet in warm water, adding the juice of one organic lemon. Recommended for fevers, a twenty-minute lemon foot soak also works nicely to relax tense muscles. Breathe deeply and gently into the lower abdomen, and as you exhale, relax from the waist down to the toes. After the soak, firmly massage your heels, especially along the outside edge at the bottom of the heel, where acupressure points relieve sciatica pain.

Correct Posture

Ayurvedic doctors in India believe sciatica is common for most people after age thirty who overeat richly and do not exercise. The doctors recommend sleeping on a firm surface or placing a mattress on the floor to support the sciatic nerves. Sleep flat on your back with support under the knees, not in the fetal position on your side. When sitting, avoid twisting or taking an unusual position that stresses the lower back. When you work, take breaks often and massage your lower back with the palms of your hands. Apply a pain patch to your lower back. Wear a magnet belt over the area of pain to support lower back muscles and reduce sciatica pain. Magnets enhance blood circulation and relax muscle tension.

A Cleansing Diet

Sciatica pain is compounded by constipation. Straining or indigestion exerts pressure on the sciatic nerve. Ayurvedic doctors recommend a light diet of fruits, vegetables, and complex carbohydrates, which provide roughage. Steamed and fresh green leafy vegetables are very useful. Bananas and peeled apples or applesauce are recommended. Avoid heavy meals, because they take a long time to digest and can aggravate constipation. Add turmeric powder and aloe vera gel to beverages when possible. Turmeric is antibiotic and anti-inflammatory, eases joint and ligament pain, and improves digestion and absorption. Add one-fourth teaspoon of turmeric powder per pot of green tea or juice. Aloe is cooling, alkaline, and slightly laxative, with a recommended dosage of up to one-fourth cup per day. Other useful Indian herbs include boswellia cream applied externally.

Supplements for Reducing Inflammatory Nerve Pain

Victorian ladies added nerve sedatives such as valerian root extract in their bath. The earthy-smelling herb may have sedated their senses more than the pain. Chinese doctors believe the underlying causes of arthritis, sciatica, and lumbago include poor circulation, accumulation of moisture and swelling in the joints, and inflammation from "blood stagnation," that is, poor circulation of blood and vital energy (qi). They recommend herbs that enhance blood flow specifically to painful areas and that rid the body of edema. One such American-made herbal combination is called Mobility 2. It is based on a traditional formula, Shu Jing Huo Xue Tang. It is worth studying this formula to see how it works. That will help you to select the right diet and herbs for yourself.

Mobility 2 pills contain red peony, persica, tang kuei, and ligusticum to invigorate blood circulation. Atractylodes, poria (a diuretic), and vitex reduce edema in the abdomen and lower body. Ligusticum, chiang huo, clematis, and angelica have analgesic effects. Citrus invigorates energy circulation. Tang kuei and rehmannia (Chinese foxglove) nourish blood. Ginger improves rheumatism, and siler, which reduces discomfort from windy, cold, and damp weather, is also used for rheumatic pain. Achyranthes relieves aching knees and back, and gentiana reduces inflammatory pain.

You can see that traditional Asian herbal formulas are complex. Mobility 2 contains seventeen herbs that work together in tandem to reduce pain and swelling and normalize circulation. The action of the herbs is much deeper and longer-lasting than applying hot and cold compresses. In addition, using an herbal formula instead of dulling sedatives supports the production of healthy blood, digestion, and energy flow. Mobility 2 is recommended for chronic arthritis or rheumatism characterized by inflammation, redness, and swelling in the joints; gout; sciatica; lumbago; and edema that aggravates pain.

Letha's Advice: Put Out the Fire

How else can you avoid inflammatory pain in the body? Avoid consuming chili peppers, tomatoes, sugar, red meat, cheese, alcohol, and cigarettes; protect yourself against inclement weather, and avoid arguments with persons who are a pain in the butt. You will find more foods and supplements for reducing joint, muscle, and nerve pains in the following chapter covering arthritis. Whether or not you have arthritis, if you have any sort of chronic inflammatory pain, develop a healing relationship with Nopalea, a miracle cleansing/healing food from the Arizona desert. See page 59 for details.

When to Consult a Health Specialist

In some cases, if sciatica stems from disc and back muscle issues, the hydrating foods and baths from chapter 3 will be helpful. Avoiding caffeine, stimulants, and stress can also generally improve nerve pains. However, you may need X-rays and medical treatments if home treatments fail to bring relief after a few days, if pain persists, or if pain becomes worse. Some sports medicine doctors now give natural nonsteroid injections for relieving pain. See chapter 18, "The Future of Pain Medicine."

CHAPTER FIVE

Arthritis

The aim of the wise is not to secure pleasure, but to avoid pain.

—Aristotle (philosopher, 384 BC–322 BC)

STRICTLY SPEAKING, OSTEOARTHRITIS MEANS JOINT INFLAMMATION, BUT IT HAS come to be experienced by many as that icky, achy, stiff feeling we equate with growing older. Actually, joint pain often results from repeated stress injury, such as jogging or typing. Pain may involve loss of protective cartilage that cushions the joints or from bone spurs (osteophytes), bony growth formed on normal bone in response to pressure, rubbing, or stress that continues over a long period of time. Stiffness and swelling from repeated injury make movement difficult. Is getting out of bed each morning a challenge? Do you avoid moving around? Chronic conditions experienced as pain arise from many factors. There may be physical trauma—a discrepancy in leg length provoking a limp, a slouched posture when seated, an injury to the SI joint in the lower back, or daily wear and tear in a joint—or poor circulation resulting from a poor diet and bad habits. Misery communicated throughout the body is hard to locate. We seem to hurt all over because joints, tendons, ligaments, muscles, and nerves are involved. That sort of pain is especially aggravated by age, overuse of stimulants, and emotional problems.

Joint Pain and the Mind

I vaguely remember a time when we wrote letters instead of emails, when lights were out at midnight, and when stock market crashes, tsunamis, and terrorist attacks were far from the tranquility of my home. Today we are a plugged-in, turned-on, networked society, and global anxiety is the result. For many, living knowledgeably and responsibly requires instant communication, but staying open has disadvantages. Stress increases acid conditions, and the result is joint pain. We need to regularly withdraw from the world to a soothing herbal bath or a cushioned chair for quiet, deep breathing, to enjoy a cup of healing herbal tea, and to get a massage or acupuncture treatment to remain pain-free.

Homeopathic gelsemium, made from the yellow jasmine, is recommended for free-floating anxiety and fear of future events. I have recommended it for performance anxiety, weakness and muscle aches during the early stages of a cold, and for mental and physical exhaustion. With guidance from a trained homeopathic specialist, it may be helpful for depression from overwork and worries.

Negative emotions such as anger and frustration harm vitality and circulation. Isolate your pain in order to find its cause. Is your pain in the neck and shoulders; in large joints at the shoulder, elbow, hip, or knee; at the groin; in the lower back; or in the entire leg? Is it muscle stiffness with lassitude? Or is the pain sharp and electric like sciatica? Essential oils act on the subtle energy of body and mind. Used in a healing bath or as an addition to tea, they are a daily pleasure.

Enjoyable Home Treatments

A soothing herbal or mineral bath does wonders, as we absorb nutrients through the skin. See the seaweed bath on page 35. Try soaking in a warm bath of mineral salts and pleasant essential oils in order to give up your pain to the water. If you prefer, add five drops of an essential oil to one teaspoon of cooking oil such as canola or olive oil and use it to massage painful areas. Essential oils of lavender, balsam pine, fennel, and rosemary are especially refreshing. Cooling essential oils for inflammatory pains include sandalwood, rose, and chamomile.

Warming and Cooling Foods and Spices

It is encouraging to know you can reduce chronic joint pains with kitchen spices. They are potent energy medicines used as teas. You might use up to one-fourth teaspoon of a recommended spice per cup of hot water as a tea. You need to recognize the type or nature of your pain, even if you do not know its cause. Joint and muscle pain may feel worse in cold, damp weather. That is often the case with early arthritis. Chinese doctors call it "wind damp disease." In this case, "wind" refers to nerve pain and dampness refers to swelling. This sort of pain may be improved with a cup of hot cinnamon tea to help avoid or treat hypothermia. Cinnamon gently increases sweating and, therefore, eliminates a chilled, heavy, logy feeling, while it enhances circulation to remove stiffness.

Warming herbs and spices, such as cinnamon, clove, and rosemary, correct pale tongue and chills which are signs of "internal cold."

On the contrary, inflammatory arthritis often causes burning pain; red, swollen joints; and joint damage resulting from loss of cartilage. In that case, cooling foods, herbs, and spices are comforting. Many people have reported improvement from chronic inflammatory pain by drinking Nopalea. TriVita, the Arizona company that makes this detoxifying beverage, recommends starting with three to six ounces daily for one month and then reducing the dose. That may be too strong for someone with a weak digestion or a history of bleeding ulcers or colitis. In that case, I recommend adding one to three ounces daily of Nopalea to a glass of water. Nopalea is made from nopal cactus and contains many fruit enzymes that detoxify the body and reduce inflammatory pain and swelling. Cooling nutritional treatments and herbs help correct a red, dry tongue; fast, erratic or tense pulse; chronic thirst and/or hunger; and other inflammatory discomforts.

Your pain symptoms and signs such as tongue color and pulse will change as you use a healing food or beverage. You have to monitor your comfort level carefully. If you continue to use a food or herbal treatment beyond its time of effectiveness, you will create an imbalance. Here is an obvious rule to follow.

Prevention Is Key

Now is the best time to take steps to prevent joint and bone damage before it becomes hard to get out of bed. Much discomfort can be prevented or greatly improved with a corrective diet and gentle, targeted exercise. Feeling better, you shall develop the willpower to continue. That process offers many rewards: among them are improved vitality, mental clarity, and emotional balance.

Be Flexible and Sensitive to Changes in Your Pain

- Your internal temperature may change with the weather but also from your habits.
- When chilled and weak, use a warming treatment until you feel stronger.
- When inflammatory symptoms burn, use a cooling treatment until you feel comfortable and calm.

You may feel numbness that is worse in bad weather. Humidity slows circulation and digestion. It dampens enthusiasm and drive. A cinnamon or ginger tea may lift your spirits and reduce a logy feeling. You may be able to predict an approaching storm when swollen joints lock in place, aggravated by a sudden drop in barometric pressure. That is rheumatism. Homeopathic dulcamara is recommended for joint pain that feels worse with damp weather. Always use homeopathic remedies according to directions, separated from meals, beverages, and toothpaste. It is always better to treat annoying, weakening joint and muscle pain with a supportive approach suited to your needs, instead of a general painkiller such as aspirin, because so many different sorts of physical and emotional discomforts come together simultaneously.

Cleansing and Building

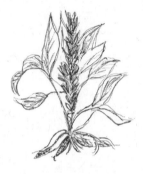

Turmeric herb.

What are the keys to bone, muscle, and joint health? Two things—cleansing and building. This chapter introduces a number of helpful dietary treatments for pain reduction and ease of movement. Healthy tissue and freedom of movement require adequate absorption of nutrients, especially protein and minerals. Vital nutrients cannot be absorbed if the digestive tract is clogged with phlegmy wastes and lacks adequate probiotics and digestive enzymes. For that reason, cleansing foods and herbs ensure proper nutrition. They may be bitter greens such as alfalfa and digestive herbs and spices such as turmeric, ginger, pepper, cinnamon, cumin, coriander, cardamom, or others. See the following chart. Nutritional herbs, such as alfalfa, and seaweeds are full of essential minerals for cleansing and building. To improve digestion and absorption, some nutritionists recommend chewing several alfalfa tablets with each meal. Maca powder, made from a Peruvian root vegetable, is a sexual hormone–balancing nutritional supplement that naturally enhances our own estrogen or testosterone as needed. It is useful to enhance digestive absorption, energy, and reduce stress-related pain for anyone over age thirty. Choose from the following tasty herbs and spices. Add them to cooking and use them to make teas between meals.

Daily Herbs and Spices for Digestion, Circulation, and Joint Pain Reduction

Herb/Spice	Detoxifying	Warming/ stimulating	Cooling	Function
Alfalfa	✓		✓	Minerals
Cardamom		✓		Digestive
Cinnamon	✓	✓		Circulation
Coriander	✓		✓	Diuretic
Cumin	✓		✓	Alkaline
Ginger	✓	✓		Digestive
Pepper		✓		Digestive
Turmeric	✓		✓	Circulation
Maca powder				Hormone Balance

To build muscle, bone, and joint health, you need two things: the building materials found in minerals, foods, and herbs that ensure hormone balance; and adequate circulation to bring the building materials where they are needed. Aside from everyday foods, several unusual Asian herbs are stressed—arjuna, triphala, and shilajit to name a few—because they accomplish those tasks so well. You will find them in Ayurvedic herb shops and online. You will read about arjuna and guggul in a later chapter covering pain in relation to heart health and circulation. This chapter stresses treatments for osteoarthritis, the most common form, but the recommendations will improve many rheumatic discomforts. Because health does not give itself to illness, this chapter offers an elegantly simple program to organize your treatments in order to leave time for wellness.

Causes and Holistic Treatment

The causes of rheumatoid conditions are many, including trauma, fatigue, genetic disposition, sodium deficiency, metabolic disorders, poor food habits and allergies, junk food, high stress, drug side effects, chemicalized drinking water, excessive perspiration increasing sodium loss, glandular imbalance, climate, and others. Improving digestion is key to eliminating unassimilated minerals and acid wastes that end up as bone spurs and joint pains. According to nutritionist Dr. Bernard Jensen, PhD, most arthritis patients are deficient in hydrochloric acid (stomach acid) and digestive enzymes needed to properly digest proteins. He suggests that people over age forty take a digestive enzyme tablet with meals.

Pain relief from drugs is not the answer. Drugs may mask the symptoms—like painting a car with a broken engine—but real relief comes from prevention through improving digestion, assimilation, circulation, and hormone balance.

Why Diet Fads Don't Work

Have you given up meat in order to detoxify the body? Or do you eat more protein to lose weight? Diet fads throw the body into abrupt biological changes. Many people feel great temporarily while fasting because the body is getting rid of excess acids. The joints feel better. But unless we go on a proper maintenance and buildup diet afterward, we start accumulating pain and trouble in the future. Diets need thought, analysis, and often supervision. For one thing, your energy type and addictions should be addressed. No permanent improvement is possible otherwise.

After age fifty, when rheumatic conditions surface, there is a 20–40 percent lowered function in all body parts due to aging. Men develop curves from lack of testosterone. Women more often have aches and irritability, and may develop facial hair, cellulite, and arthritis (poor calcium assimilation) from reduced estrogen. Fortunately, a lot of beauty issues can be covered over, tucked up, sucked out, etc. But we still need plenty of minerals throughout life to keep us going.

A holistic approach to preventing and treating arthritic pain maintains the health of the entire body in order to avoid problems. In the case of rheumatoid conditions, we need iodine from kelp seaweeds for the thyroid, exercise to enable mineral absorption, hawthorn berry and Asian herbs that support heart tissue and function to keep circulation strong, sufficient liquid intake, diuretic cleansing herbs to support the kidneys, fresh vegetables and fruits to provide fiber, foods high in calcium, sodium, and potassium to neutralize excess body acids, vitamin D3 to improve calcium assimilation, and a proper alkaline diet to meet nutritional needs. Reading the list of foods and supplements required blurs the senses. We need to start with an organized approach, or reaching a cure will never happen. A simple, wise, supportive diet suggested below is the way to start.

A Diet for Weight Maintenance and Joint Comfort

Often joint pain can be reduced with a cleansing slimming diet. This is especially true for painful knees and hips because they must carry our weight. A light diet that avoids pain triggers is most useful. A practical and highly effective baseline diet, suitable for achieving a healthy weight, while eliminating bad dietary habits, is described in *Feed Your Tiger: The Asian Diet Secret for Permanent Weight Loss and Vibrant Health*. The baseline diet, recommended for all readers, stresses alkaline, detoxifying foods. It includes daily two fruits, six to nine vegetables (raw or cooked), one source of protein, and one starch. It's easy. Increasing vegetables is in itself alkalinizing for the blood and tissues. Vegetables increase cleansing. Too many proteins eaten all at once confuse the body. Mixing fruit with protein and starch slows digestion and creates acids.

Bone Minerals: Food Sources

Arthritis requires particular minerals used as building blocks, including properly balanced potassium, calcium, sodium, and magnesium, to ensure strong bones and pain-free movement. Bone meal and mixed minerals may be the best way to go for people who have no time for juggling nutrients. Bone meal is a whole food made of joint material we have to replace in the body. The pills and powder are easily available in health shops and online. Dr. Bernard Jensen, who brought countless people back to health with diet, recommends four bone meal calcium tablets two times daily along with a high-sodium food, which is one tablespoon of powdered goat whey in a cup of warm water, along with a tablespoon of lecithin granules. He found that it takes at least five years to bring on rheumatism, arthritis, or osteoporosis in the body, and it takes at the very least one year to bring about improvement with a careful diet and lifestyle. The program of bone nutrients he describes in his book, *Arthritis, Rheumatism, and Osteoporosis: An Effective Program for Correction through Nutrition*, can compensate for dietary wrongs of the past. It speeds up the healing process by supplementing extra nutrients you should have had all through the years.

In every case of arthritis or rheumatic damage you can assume you are not getting enough potassium, natural vegetable sodium (not table salt), and absorbable calcium. Here are good sources for each of them.

Potassium Foods		
Almonds	Beef	Brussels sprouts
Apricots	Beets	Carrots
Artichokes	Beet greens	Cauliflower
Bananas	Blackberries	Chayote
Barley	Blueberries	Cherries, black
Beans, lima	Broccoli	Chervil

Potassium Foods

Chicken	Honey	Parsley
Chicory	Horseradish	Peaches
Chives	Kale	Peanuts
Coconut meat	Kohlrabi	Pecans
Corn	Lemon	Potato, baked
Cucumbers	Lentils	Prunes
Currents, black	Lettuce	Radish, black
Dandelion greens	Limes	Radish, red
Duck	Mangoes	Raisins
Eggplant	Mushrooms	Spinach
Endive	Mustard greens	Turnips
Figs, black	Olives	Watercress
Grapes	Parsnips	Zucchini
Halibut, smoked		

Sodium Foods

Butter, cow	Pears	Strawberries
Cheese, swiss	Pineapple	Swiss chard
Chinese cabbage	Pomegranate	Veal joint broth
Milk, cow	Pumpkin	Watermelon
Milk, goat	Raspberries	Whey
Okra	Rice, natural brown	Leeks
Papaya	Squash	

Calcium Foods

Asparagus	Cheese, swiss	Lettuce, Romaine
Banana	Chinese cabbage	Limes
Beans, lima	Chives	Mangoes
Blueberries	Cream, cow	Milk, cow
Bread, whole grain	Cucumbers	Milk, goat
Butter, cow	Dandelion greens	Mustard greens
Buttermilk	Endive	Oranges
Brussels sprouts	Grapefruit, fresh	Parsnips
Carrots	Honey	Parsley
Cauliflower	Kale	Peaches
Cheese, cow, cottage	Kohlrabi	Peas, fresh
Cheese, goat, cottage	Leeks	Pecans
Cheese, Roquefort	Lemons	Persimmons

Calcium Foods		
Pineapple	Turnips	Watermelon
Strawberries	Turnip leaves	Whey
Swiss chard	Watercress	

Barring individual food allergies, you can easily fit the above foods into the baseline diet: two fruits, six to nine vegetables, one source of protein, and one starch. Have your fruit for breakfast with tea, vegetables as a big lunchtime salad, and a protein with additional vegetables at dinner. I always advise my students to sun-ripen fruits from the supermarket in the window for several days until they become soft and extra-ripe. Commercially grown fruit is famously rock hard and, therefore, low in natural sodium. It is the sweet flavor of overripe citrus, plums, bananas, and juicy fruits that heals weak bones through improved calcium absorption.

To save time and trouble, in this chapter you'll find a handy daily schedule with recommended doses and additional Asian herbs that I will explain. Certain supplements are best absorbed with acidic foods such as fruit and tea. In general, take water-soluble B vitamins and vitamin C with water and oily supplements such as fish oils, flaxseed oil, and others with meals. I don't mix fish and dairy because they are each fat and increase phlegm. Phlegmy congestion, we will see later in this chapter, is an underlying factor in arthritic pain, swelling, and stiffness. Do not try to add all these new supplements at once. Give yourself a chance to gradually feel the difference. If your joint pain issues concern digestive problems, add digestion/absorption remedies. If circulation is your problem, add the heart herbs to improve circulation. If weak, thin bones are a problem, add digestive and nutritional supplements such as vitamin D3 and sources of minerals. Gradually, as you add necessary nutrients, your energy and mood can improve.

Daily Supplements for Joints, Muscles, and Bones

Why is it better to use an herbal combination for arthritis or other severe chronic illness over prescribed drugs? Because the discomforts are complex, involving so many aspects of our energy and well-being. The herbal combinations are "built" like a house in order to serve many purposes and avoid side effects. A good example of how common prescription medicines may deplete nutrition is a category of drugs used to reduce stomach acid. These drugs, called proton pump inhibitors (PPI) and histamine (H-2) blockers, reduce the uncomfortable symptom of excess acid. Also, both classes of medication inhibit vitamin B12, leaving you with a foggy head, no energy, and a poor mood. PPIs and H-2 blockers deplete folic acid, leaving you at risk for developing heart trouble, anemia, neural-tube birth defects, and poor detoxification. They deplete calcium and beta-carotene, leaving you prone to osteoporosis and loss of night vision.

A friend commented at my website that she relied on a combination of apple cider vinegar in water for two weeks and lost her gout pain for the first time in years. However, she was upset because she had gained unwanted weight with uncomfortable abdominal bloating, and she suspected that she now had a yeast infection. Merely changing our acid/alkaline balance is risky. And it does not always specifically address a problem.

Always use supplements that treat joint and muscle discomforts between meals or separated from food by at least two hours, because their aim is to enhance circulation at the joints and reduce joint swelling and pain. They are, therefore, not digestive. Asian supplements containing a variety of synergistic nutritional and painkilling herbs make caring for arthritis simple. They include Ayurvedic combination remedies originating in India such as JointCare made by Himalaya Company (see the main ingredients on the following pages), recommended for reducing arthritis pain, and several Chinese patent remedies, among them Vine Essence Pill, made with a secret formula which is said to increase blood circulation and reduce swelling and pain. The listed indications for Vine Essence Pill include rheumatic arthritis, sciatica, hypertrophic or productive spinitis, cervical spinitis, dorsal spinitis, lumbar spinitis, etc. I have used them and over time they reduce pain, swelling, and stiffness. However, a portion of their ingredients are labeled "proprietary herbal extract blend."

An American herbal medicine manufacturer located in Oakland, California, makes pills using purified, tested Chinese herbal ingredients, and they list all ingredients. Among pills useful for arthritis and sciatica is Mobility 2, which is anti-inflammatory and laxative for joint and nerve pains including sciatica, gout, lumbago, and edema (water retention). Another is Mobility 3, which combines warming, stimulating herbs useful for persons over age thirty who feel joint discomforts more when exposed to wind or cold, damp weather. It treats headache, numbness, and fatigue as well. The ingredients for these popular Asian and American-made Asian herbal pills are listed on the following pages. Many times the Asian-made products are less expensive when purchased in Asian groceries and herb shops. All are available online.

How to Use JointCare, Vine Essence Pills, Mobility 2, and Mobility 3

An herbalist can help you decide which of these combinations to ease joint pain and reduce joint damage would work best for you, depending upon your degree of joint damage and your usual health habits, but here are some pointers that will help you to chose the best approach. All the supplements that I suggest for joint health and comfort include herbs that enhance joint moisture and flexibility such as licorice, mallow, and Chinese foxglove. Joint moisture is an important issues for people over age thirty, for athletes and dancers who repeatedly stress joints, and for people who smoke. Other herbs contained in most Asian joint health pills include adrenal-support herbs or those that increase testosterone such as tribulus or morinda. Adrenal health is important because it maintains basic vitality necessary for movement. Bone and joint health building materials such as sources of calcium may also be included. Finally, Asian herbal combinations for joint health normally contain herbs such as boswellia that increase circulation and ease pain. Any of the herbal supplements that I recommend for joint comfort and health can prove helpful in most cases.

However, if you feel joint discomforts worse in cold damp weather, you require the warming tonic herbs found in Mobility 3 and Vine Essence Pills. If your joint pain is accompanied by sciatica, inflammatory joint pain and constipation, you require the cooling, moistening herbs in Mobility 2. If you want a general supportive supplement to delay joint damage and the effects of aging such as muscle and joint weakness, JointCare by Himalaya may be the best answer. You can combine the herbal combinations that best suit your needs.

In addition, you will need to adjust your herbal combination as your illness, your age, your level of pain, and the weather dictate. Using supportive herbs is more complex than taking an aspirin, but it ensures that you will be building healthy bones and joints, as you increase flexibility and reduce the source of pain.

I recommend taking herbs that affect joint comfort between meals, separated by at least two hours from meals or snacks. That way the herbs will not weaken digestion. The dosage of pain herbs, whether for joints or other areas, depends upon your needs. In general, Asian herbal pills made in China or India require a somewhat larger dose. For example, many Chinese patent remedies such as Vine Essence pill may recommend four pills three times daily. Health Concerns (Mobility 2 and 3) usually recommends three pills three times daily. However, you are the best judge of the dose you require. The body accepts herbs as it does foods, and the same rules apply for both. If you have a fever, avoid heating herbs. If you have chills, weakness, and diarrhea, avoid laxative herbs. Use common sense. Start with a lower dose—for example, two pills twice daily—if you are particularly sensitive, and increase the dose so that you feel the effects. Continue with the herbal regime as long as it feels comfortable for you. For joint health and comfort, that may mean for the rest of your life, since we stress and damage joints daily with movement and sitting.

The main listed ingredients in JointCare (made in India by Himalaya and sold in U.S. health stores and on Amazon.com):

- **Boswellia** (*Boswellia serrata*) is used for joint support and to provide an overall sense of well-being. The immunomodulating benefits of boswellia are the key to supporting healthy joints. Boswellia also has many cholesterol- and triglyceride-lowering properties.
- **Guggul** (*Commiphora mukul*) is a resin known to increase white blood cell counts and possess strong disinfecting properties. Guggul has been shown to promote bone mineralization and support all connective tissues like joints and nails. It is a famous broad-spectrum herb that strengthens the body's general defense mechanism through increased white blood cell production. Guggul has also long been known to normalize lipid metabolism and lower cholesterol and triglycerides, while maintaining or improving the HDL-to-LDL ratio.
- **Licorice** (*Glycyrrhiza glabra*) is primarily used to promote gastrointestinal health. It is a mild laxative, which soothes and tones the mucous membranes and relieves muscle spasms. Licorice is rich in flavonoids and is currently under intense investigation as an antioxidant and as a cancer-protecting botanical, boosting certain immune functions such as interferon production. Its mode of action is as an antimutagen, which prevents damage to genetic material.
- **Musk mallow** (*Hibiscus abelmoschus*) has been shown effective for nervous debility and in helping maintain healthy joints. An emulsion made from the seeds is regarded as antispasmodic and used as an aphrodisiac.
- **Indian madder** (*Rubia cordifolia*) is considered the best Ayurvedic blood-purifying herb and an immune regulator. Its antioxidant properties are also being investigated. Indian madder supports heart health because it regulates blood pressure, blood vessel constriction, and the tendency of blood to form clots.
- **Small caltrops** (*Tribulus terrestris*, also known as gokshura) is a mild diuretic, contains saponins that help maintain healthy coronary arteries and circulation, and improves the overall heart function by

dilating coronary arteries, thereby boosting circulation to the heart. It promotes the flow of urine, cools and soothes the membranes of the urinary tract, and inhibits the production of oxalate, a substance that causes microcrystals.

- **Guduchi** (*Tinospora cordifolia*) is effective in inhibiting the growth of bacteria and for enhancing immunity and strength.
- **Horseradish tree** (*Moringa pterygosperma*) contains a physiologically active constituent effective for a broad range of health needs. For example, it contains pterygospermin, an antibiotic-like substance.

Ingredients and Actions for Chinese Vine Essence Pills

- **Futokadsura stem** (*Caulis piperis futokadsurae*) reduces dampness (water retention and swelling) and promotes circulation to reduce pain.
- **Fo-ti** (*Radix polygoni multiflori* or he shou wu) is a blood tonic that supports kidney and liver tissue and function.
- **Gastrodia tuber** (*Rhizoma gastrodiae* or tien ma) is a nerve stabilizer used to ease spasm pain, headaches, and tremors.
- **Morinda root** (*Radix morindae*) is an adrenal and energy tonic, and precursor to testosterone, that indirectly improves circulation
- **Licorice root** (*Radix glycyrrhizae uralensis*) eases spasm pain and improves absorption of other herbs.
- **Chinese angelica root** (*Radix angelicae sinensis* or dong quai/tang kuei) is a blood tonic that supports healthy circulation and reduces pain. It is estrogenic. (Avoid using it for active estrogen-dependent cancers.)
- **Chuanxiong** (*Radix ligustici wallichii*) is a blood tonic that supports liver and kidney health.

Mobility 2 and Mobility 3 Made by Health Concerns

Ingredients and Actions for Mobility 2

Red peony (chi shao), persica (tao ren), tang kuei, and ligusticum are included to invigorate blood circulation. Atractylodes (bai zhu), poria (fu ling), and vitex (man jing zi) reduce water retention and swelling (known as dampness in traditional Chinese medicine). Ligusticum, chiang huo, clematis, and angelica have analgesic effect. Citrus peel and clematis enhance circulation. Ginger treats rheumatism and reduces phlegm. Siler resolves wind, and cold, damp conditions and achyranthes relieves aching knees and back. Gentiana eliminates inflammatory pain.

Ingredients and Actions for Mobility 3

Kirin ginseng, cinnamon, tang kuei, tienchi ginseng, ginger, spatholobus, and *Ardisia gigantifolia* enhance circulation; rehmannia or he shou wu enhances blood production; loranthus tones kidney and liver.

Other useful American-made combinations for joint pain and damage include Avoca ASU, a vegetarian combination of glucosamine HCI (nonshellfish), avocado and soybean unsaponifiables (ASU), and methylsulfonylmethane (MSM), all of which have been proven effective in reducing joint pain and the formation of bone spurs. Hyaluronic acid pills are used to irritate joints in order to provoke production of cartilage. Many people have noted improvement using such supplements, although they do not prevent or totally reverse symptoms.

LED Lights, Arthritis, and Chronic Pain

New work is being done by some innovative chiropractors and physical therapists who use LED lights for pain reduction and complexion beauty. The lights promote the natural production of collagen, which is similar in structure to cartilage. It is worth a good try and does no harm in the process. Here is current information on it from a variety of health sources.

Light-emitting diode (LED) light therapy is used to treat muscle pain and joint stiffness, symptoms typically associated with arthritis, through holistic, nonmedicinal, noninvasive means. NASA research has inspired the use of LED lights, which penetrate deep into muscle tissue, for treatment of chronic pain and stiffness and improving circulation. LED therapy is used on the Space Station and by the United States submarine fleet for pain relief and wound healing.

The Food and Drug Administration (FDA) has approved LED light therapy for the treatment of minor pain and stiffness and specifically for use by arthritis sufferers, which is why the system was created. The LED system transmits light waves at a speed of 880 nm into the deep muscle tissue, stimulating DNA production and normal cell growth and function, which can be altered by the effects of arthritis. Currently the LED Technologies infrared system, the only FDA-approved system, consists of two nine- by fourteen-inch panels containing

154 infrared and twenty red LEDs. Accessories include a stand to position the panels for use on the face and a strap to position them on the body. LED Technologies lists its LED therapy system at between $350 and $450 per unit.

How to Organize Bone, Muscle, and Ligament Health Treatments Throughout the Day

Most often supplement manufacturers combine vitamins and minerals in ways to insure their proper synergy. For example, minerals are mixed with trace minerals such as zinc, gold, or manganese that improve absorption. Try to find time-release and organic supplements when possible. The following program suggests the sorts of supplements to be taken during the day; however, you should make adjustments according to your needs. In general, cleansing herbs are used during the morning, as are herbs that support the heart. Tonics and energizing herbs are recommended during the afternoon hours between meals. Soothing nerve tonics are useful during evening hours. You do not have to take all the following herbs daily to feel good results. You will naturally require some more than others. Try to choose the ones best suited to your needs from each section: Morning, Between Meals, and Bedtime.

Morning Supplements with Water, Tea, Juice, and/or Light Breakfast

- Calcium, magnesium, mixed minerals, trace minerals (with acidic fruit or tea): Try to take a mixed supplement that has at least 1,000 milligrams of calcium and half as much magnesium.
- 2,000 IU vitamin D3; 400–800 milligram SAMe, as needed. SAMe improves depression while reducing joint pain.
- Two capsules guggul, 500 milligrams each (reduce joint swelling, pain, cholesterol, fat, fibroids).
- One-fourth teaspoon arjuna in tea; or two or three capsules HeartCare; or two capsules hawthorn (circulation, heart health, cholesterol reducing)
- Two or three triphala (a.k.a. trifala) pills, 475 milligrams each, once or twice daily with meals. It is an herbal blend of three fruits and provides cleansing for blood, acts as a laxative, and improves complexion and nutritional absorption.

- Super Enzyme Caps (Twinlab): pancreatin, papain, betaine hydrochloride, pepsin, bromelain (dissolves impurities, improves absorption) or equivalent
- Avoca ASU (soy and avocado oil and veggie glucosamine, chondroitin, MSM): Take as directed. This vegetarian formula of glucosamine/chondroitin is easier for digestion than the usual one made from shellfish shells. It is said to reduce arthritis pain, joint damage, and swelling and improve mobility.
- Others: 5-HTP if needed. Various forms of 5-HTP (a.k.a. L-5HTP 5-hydroxytryptophan) are useful for people who are depressed or addicted to breads and sweets, and who wish to lose weight. One source is griffonia seeds used to make Griffonex 5-HTP pills by Health Concerns. 5-HTP is not recommended to be taken with anti-depressant drugs or anti-Parkinson's drugs.

Breakfast

- Fruit, tea with optional powdered goat whey (minerals), cooked grain cereal, seaweed, nuts, seeds, and maca powder (iodine, hormones)
- One tablespoon tahini (it is fattening but a good source of natural calcium as needed), one tablespoon bone meal powder with goat whey and lecithin. These can be added to yogurt or cooked cereal.

Snacks Between Meals

- Figs and goat's milk or powdered goat whey in water or yogurt and four bone meal pills to provide minerals necessary for bone health and absorption
- Five to ten papaya enzyme pills (anti-inflammatory, heals wounds and broken bones) or one Super Enzyme Cap
- One packet unflavored gelatin in water to rebuild cartilage
- Raw celery (high fiber and necessary sodium; reduces cholesterol and cellulite)
- Okra, raw, steamed, or dried chips (high in sodium, which improves calcium absorption)
- Dried nori and dulse seaweed (minerals)

External Treatments (See Chapter 1)

- A seaweed bath with one cup of sea salt, baking soda, Epsom salts, one tablespoon ginger powder, one tablespoon kelp powder, and one cup apple cider vinegar
- Seaweed massage oil for lymphatic drainage massage (lymph carries calcium to muscles and joints and eliminates toxins)

Bedtime

- One cup of low-fat milk, almond milk, or oat milk with one or two shilajit capsules (bone health, arthritis, immunity, rejuvenation)

Asian Herbs for Joint and Bone Health Also Improve Circulation

The following herbs are mentioned in the above schedule and serve to support vitality in many ways because circulation, energy, and digestion are as important as nutrients that build bones and joints. For example, arjuna, hawthorn berry, and HeartCare, an herbal combination made by Himalaya that is called Abana when sold in India, strengthen the heart muscles and help regulate heart action. That is important for arthritis because blood brings vital nutrients and oxygen to all muscles and joints. Such herbs help to regulate the heartbeat and therefore circulation, while eliminating impurities including harmful cholesterol.

This is important: a strong, healthy heart protects against chronic fatigue, chronic pain from poor circulation, and depression. These factors underlie all joint discomforts and circulation problems.

The Joint Pain–Heart Health Connection

Normally, health experts treat heart and joint issues separately because they are medical specialties. However, the body does not work compartmentally. In a holistic view, circulation (stemming from heart health and adrenal strength) vitally affects joints, chronic pain, mood, digestion, and absorption of nutrients. For that reason, I have included a section treating circulation and indirectly blood pressure in this chapter for arthritis.

Arjuna: A Warrior in Your Cup

For enhanced circulation, I add a warrior (one-fourth teaspoon of arjuna herbal powder, a heart tonic) to my morning tea. Arjuna tree bark powder and capsules are considered the most important Ayurvedic herbal tonic for a healthy heart. It protects against heart weakness, chronic heart failure, and reduces harmful cholesterol. Arjuna bark is astringent and strengthens muscle. That means that, although it is not per se a digestive herb, it may nevertheless improve joint pain and flexibility during damp weather or overindulgence of rich foods. Read about arjuna beginning on page 233. A popular Ayurvedic heart remedy that contains arjuna and many other herbs in a capsule that I often recommend for people who "give from the heart" is called HeartCare. You will read about it in the heart health chapter beginning on page 225. Find the capsules online, made by Himalaya herb company.

Triphala

A major part of preventing and treating rheumatic aches is eliminating wastes, including acids, phlegm, and undigested minerals that have formed bone spurs. If you have effective absorption in the gut, you stand a much better chance of getting the calcium you need. Triphala (also known as trifala) is an herbal pill or powder made of dried powdered fruits of amla (*Emblica officinalis*), myrobalan (*Terminalia chebula*), and belleric myrobalan (*Terminalia belerica*), all of which are medicinal plants. Considered a gentle laxative and blood cleanser, triphala is often used to stimulate digestive health, improve liver and gallbladder function, boost immunity, ease inflammation, and manage chronic congestive conditions like asthma and overweight. It is also commonly found in many Ayurvedic supplements for joint and bone health, skin care, and other formulas that detoxify and cleanse the body and blood.

Test-tube studies have suggested that triphala offers antioxidant, bacteria-killing, and immune-enhancing benefits. And in animal-based research, scientists have shown that the herbal blend may help keep cholesterol in check. In other studies on animals, triphala has demonstrated anticancer effects. One study published in 2008, for instance, found that feeding triphala to mice helped suppress the growth of pancreatic cancer cells.

Choose triphala capsules (available at health-food stores) or pills available in East Indian groceries instead of the powdered form, because it is bitter and sour. It is generally safe to take triphala as a mild laxative on a longer-term basis unlike other, harsher laxatives. However, in some cases, triphala may trigger temporary gastrointestinal side effects such as gas, stomach upset, and diarrhea.

Shilajit

Shilajit, which is also covered on page 37, is a major Ayurvedic rejuvenation tonic. The active principle of shilajit is fulvic acid. Shilajit contains useful mineral and organic constituents taken to help digestion and the assimilation of foods. Shilajit is often used in combination with other specific plant decoctions to, for example, support respiratory and genitourinary functions. You will read more about the wonderful, rejuvenating benefits of shilajit in the following chapter on osteoporosis. Also see Part Three for information on tonic herbs, insomnia, PRP, and new or controversial approaches for reducing pain.

The Pain/Mood Connection: S-Adenosylmethionine (SAMe)

Though expensive, the supplement SAMe has become popular for osteoarthritis. It is a synthetic form of a naturally formed compound in the body made from the amino acid methionine and adenosine triphosphate (ATP), the energy-producing compound found in all cells in the body. The supplement is expensive, but interesting to me as an herbalist because it is also recommended for depression and liver disease. Pain, depression, and liver are linked. SAMe is stimulating in order to treat what Chinese herbal doctors might call stagnant qi from deficient liver function. Imagine wanting something badly and being told you can't have it, do it, or want it: that increases pain, frustration, and depression.

Studies on the effectiveness of SAMe for osteoarthritis find it to be as effective as nonsteroidal anti-inflammatory medications. SAMe increases the availability of mood neurotransmitters serotonin and dopamine, and evidence suggests that SAMe improves liver disease by helping to normalize liver enzyme levels and cholestasis, a condition in which bile cannot flow from the liver to the duodenum. In other words, it improves the flow of liver qi and thus aids in reducing pain and frustration. Note: people with psychiatric conditions should only use SAMe under the supervision of their health-care provider. SAMe has been associated with hypomania and mania.

The most common side effects are digestive complaints, skin rash, lowered blood sugar, dry mouth, headache, hyperactivity, anxiety, and insomnia. People with Parkinson's disease should avoid SAMe. Most practitioners recommend starting with 400 milligrams per day taken on an empty stomach and then increasing the dose depending on the results. See Part Three for more information on the pain/mood connection.

Letha's Advice: Simplicity and Courage

It is impossible to recommend only a few treatments for arthritis when there are so many wonderful remedies easily available to us. Your choice will depend on your needs and convenience of use. You might begin simply with three energy tonics: sunshine, seaweed, and shilajit. They each cleanse and build. There is something else important: our bodies hold memories even if movement is painful and limited. While writing this chapter, I watched dancers in a flamenco performance on YouTube. It made me weep. I felt their pride and the beauty of their movement. Our dances and walks leave a trace as a lover does inside us and in the ether surrounding us. I want to regain that feeling of graceful movement again. It may be with the tango, which requires less stamping. I have to grow stronger before I decide which dance to choose.

My advice to you is: prevent joint damage and pain early with the recommended remedies in this chapter. Make them part of your preparation for menopause and graceful aging. Use them after injury to ensure comfort and healthy qi circulation. They will speed healing. In later chapters you will find ointments for sports injuries. Apply them regularly to the areas of your hip joints, lower back, and knees to increase circulation and protect your cartilage. Do the simple stretches for hips and knees in chapter 9. We were not meant to sit in chairs. The foods and herbs I have recommended here will get you moving, dancing, loving, and living your life again.

CHAPTER SIX

Digestion

Laughter is the tonic, the relief, the surcease for pain.

—Charlie Chaplin (actor, 1889–1977)

OUR DIGESTIVE CENTER IS ALSO OUR EMOTIONAL CENTER. WE *DIGEST* FOODS, thoughts, and feelings or else suffer pain.

Aikima, dressed in corporate navy blue, her long jet black hair tied in a severe knot, nervously twisted her diamond ring. She appeared as though she could lift off straight up into the air. She smiled and spoke with carefully slow English and no trace of a Japanese accent. Three weeks after the earthquake and tsunami that took some twenty thousand lives in her native country, her job as hostess at a large Japanese company located in midtown Manhattan included reassuring customers that business would be conducted as usual.

"I cannot eat," she said shyly. "I have no appetite and when I eat my stomach hurts."

Her official bearing did not allow a show of emotions. Her coloring was slightly jaundiced. She complained of bad breath and burping, signs that tight rib muscles troubled digestion. Her tongue was red and had a thick yellow coating, indicating difficult slow digestion and excess acidity. Her radial pulses for liver and gallbladder were thin and tight, indicating extreme muscle tension from emotional stress. Powerful emotions reduced healthy bile flow. In an earlier time, her condition might have been called "bilious." The symptoms were digestive distress, although the origin was emotional. Both had to be addressed. A mere sedative drug would weaken digestive qi and trap poorly digested foods like poisons, making her feel even more miserable. A drug for reducing stomach acid could not improve her emotions.

A holistic approach aims to reestablish wellness on many levels by addressing underlying sources of physical and emotional vitality. Traditional Asian doctors work primarily with foods, herbs, and energy-enhancing methods in order to balance the driving forces that underlie wellness.

In practice, when a sick person sits in front of you suffering from symptoms, what you really want to know is: Where does this person hurt? How does she hurt, and why, and when did it start? How can I help her to feel at ease in her body, mind, and spirit? Very often, under extreme stress the patient feels separated from her center of gravity, from her source of vitality and emotional comfort. She may feel helpless, depressed, and confused. For problems that cut across many aspects of well-being, I suggest remedies that support healthy, comfortable digestion.

Our digestive center is also our emotional center. Aikima's rebellious digestive qi made her feel sick and stuck in the middle. Her jaundiced appearance from bile spilling into her blood, her halitosis, and her nervousness all pointed to stuck digestive qi rising up into her chest. It was not just acid reflux, but tension that stops normal digestion, blood production, and unglues emotions. Unless her digestive qi was regulated and comfort assured, she might later develop heartburn, chronic hiccups, headaches, a flushed appearance, or a skin rash. Down the line if digestive symptoms were not improved, she might develop irregular menstruation and a host of other digestion-related illnesses.

For Aikima, I recommended an herbal brew formulated for her, containing ginger and bitter digestive, laxative herbs to help normalize the flow of bile, support digestive organs, free stuck circulation in the chest, and thus regulate digestion and support emotional balance. I treated acupuncture points in her left ear, one called *shen men* ("spirit gate" in English) to ease nervous tension. (Sometimes massaging both your ears with your hands is enough to help release tension and reduce painful symptoms resulting from stuck emotions.) I showed her how to massage her lower abdomen to free energy flow from the small to large intestine. She gently pushed with her palms from the solar plexus, located under her ribs, toward her naval. Then she continued with circular movements around the navel from her right to left, following the ascending colon and across to the descending colon. She took a deep breath and began to cry. Soon her coloring became normal and she heaved a sign of relief.

By reaffirming the normal digestive process, we initiate healing. A strong digestion allows us to absorb nutrients necessary for survival. Then stable blood sugar ensures emotional comfort, and our food can be used for creating energy and immunity, not waste. Our digestive/emotional center is the origin of our belly laugh and optimism. Strong digestion underlies mental clarity and concentration. If balance brings health, than laughter is frosting on the cake. Laughter comforts: we feel happy in our center of gravity. Maintaining adequate digestive enzymes and a smooth circulation of qi for digestive organs also facilitates mental and emotional balance. American author Max Eastman (1883–1969) wrote, "Laughter puts your brain, your central nervous system, and your whole being into a state of free play." He also said, "Laughter is, after speech, the chief thing that holds society together." However, when life becomes too painful to laugh, then crying that frees digestion and breathing may bring relief. Digestion and emotions are intimately linked, and enjoying and sharing meals are fundamental to our communication in our family and society. Here are suggestions to enhance the many health benefits of our foods.

Mind, Body, and Digestion

For many years I have led walking tours for medical professionals and the public through New York's Asian neighborhoods in order to discuss and show Asia's medicinal herbs. I never let anyone talk about illness during our dinner that follows class. It's much better for digestion to have flowers, a lovely cheerful table setting, friendly chatter, and music. Do you burp or have cramps or indigestion in a stressful situation? Do you rely on nuts as a pleasant snack and sweets and coffee for energy? They are pain triggers. You need herbs to overcome their side effects. Choose either a physical or psychological approach, either a nutritive, energetic, or talking therapy, and healing can begin. A natural approach encourages healing on all levels.

Acupuncture meridians associated with digestive organs, especially the stomach meridian, pass through the auditory center of the brain. Certain aspects of the digestive process affect mentality in ways we do not expect. Have you been troubled by gnawing thoughts that replay like a broken record? Our digestion affects mental clarity as well as energy. Have fasting or dietary upset brought about spacey feelings? Some people even develop hallucinations from long-term stress and dietary abuse. We will deal with the impact of digestion on the nervous system, mind, and emotions in Part Three. For now, we are concerned with digestive pain, bloating, yeast problems, and acid reflux. To understand their origin, we must look inside.

What's the Dosage?

I have already advised you to take an herbal digestive pill along with meals so that it can work as needed. A question I always get when teaching and writing is, "What is the proper dose used for a given remedy?" Take the dose that works for you. You might start with the dose recommended on the bottle. But observe your tongue and other symptoms and change the dose accordingly. An herbal digestive remedy may increase cleansing (laxative or diuretic), cause temporary digestive upset, or change cravings. You can balance discomforts by adding herbs and spices according to your tongue observations. Observing the tongue ensures you will use the proper remedy as long as needed.

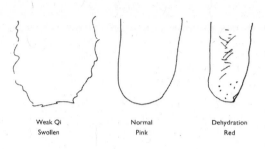

| Weak Qi | Normal | Dehydration |
| Swollen | Pink | Red |

Observe your tongue

Your Tongue

Traditional Asian medicine employs tongue diagnosis because it is an easy-to-see internal organ that tells us a lot about digestion, energy, and general health. As the illness or discomfort improves with natural therapies, our tongue's appearance will also change for the better.

The Shape of the Tongue

First thing in the morning or before a meal, look at your tongue with a mirror. A normal, healthy tongue fits neatly into the mouth and is neither too large and bloated with water nor too small and wrinkled. The teeth do not leave scallops at the edges of the tongue. The tip of the tongue corresponds to qi affecting the thyroid, chest, and heart. The center line from the tongue root to tip corresponds to the stomach qi. The fat areas on both sides of the center line correspond to the stomach/spleen qi. The edges of the tongue along the sides show liver qi. If there is liver congestion, that area may appear red and bloated with impurities. The root of the tongue shows the lower part of the body, especially the kidneys and adrenal energy. If an area of the tongue is puffy, bloated, or marked with dents, bumps, or spots, it indicates trouble in the corresponding area of the body and internal organs.

The Color of the Tongue

The color and markings on the tongue will vary somewhat with your diet. But there is an overall tendency of coloring you can observe from day to day. A healthy tongue is pink and moist with only a thin white coating. The tongue itself is not mauve, white, brown, or any other extreme color. The coating, if any, is not thick, which indicates excess phlegm. The coating color is not yellow, green, or brown, indicating excess acid conditions and toxins.

Pale Tongue

An overly pale tongue shows underfunctioning of internal organs or a tendency for body chills, weakness, water retention, chronic depression, and possibly low adrenal energy and potential heart failure. Stimulating, warming, and drying foods and herbs, such as ginger and clove tea, may help bring about balance. Often an herbal digestive remedy will contain warming herbs, such as ginger, to stimulate digestive acids, along with cooling or bitter herbs, such as mint or vervain, to regulate the liver and soothe muscle tension. (Vervain tea is recommended for nervous conditions and arthritis pain, but should be avoided by pregnant women.)

Red Tongue

A red tongue shows inflammation, dehydration, and excess acid in the body. It may correspond to anxiety or insomnia or fever conditions. There may also be chronic thirst and hunger, diabetes, or hormone irregularities. In this case, an appropriate digestive remedy would also balance blood sugar, reduce sweet cravings, and curb salt addictions. The Asian herbs used would be moistening, rejuvenating, and supportive of blood production and liver health. Some antiacid herbs and foods are also recommended. Below I recommend various digestive combinations for specific problems.

Common Digestive Problems, Uncommon Remedies

Since the digestive process is complex, encompassing several organs, their respective qi, and acupuncture meridians, the following remedies address numerous wellness issues beyond what are normally considered digestive problems.

Indigestion

Let's start simply: for bloating and gas, be careful about your food combinations. Trying to digest fruit with grains or protein can be problematic. Fruit sugar digests quickly and forms gas bubbles when combined with slow-digesting foods like proteins and starch. If you have weak digestion, eat fruits with tea or coffee, and wait for an hour before eating other foods. Ginger tea works well for indigestion with a pale tongue. Other useful herbs and spices for indigestion bloating include cardamom, fennel seed, and bay leaf.

Letha's Advice: Aloe Vera for Acid Reflux

To correct an underlying excess acid and tight rib muscles that cause reflux and GERD, drink up to one-fourth cup of aloe vera juice or gel added to warm water or juice. Aloe is alkaline, soothing to delicate digestive tissue, and relaxes muscle tension. Used over time, aloe corrects bad breath, menstrual cramps, skin blemishes and itchy rashes, and constipation. Do not use your garden aloe plant, but buy a quality, organic, health-food store bottle of aloe vera for internal use. Otherwise, you would have to destroy too much of the plant to get at the pulp, the part you need to correct acidity.

You may wonder, "Why bother to use a plant when over-the-counter tablets for heartburn are sold in every supermarket?" Here is the short list of side effects for the most popular heartburn tablet ingredient, famotidine: headache; dizziness; constipation; diarrhea; fussiness (especially for babies given the drug); hives and skin rash; itching; swelling of the face, throat, tongue, lips, eyes, hands, feet, ankles or legs (look for heart involvement if swollen ankles); hoarseness; and difficulty breathing or swallowing.

Burping

Burping can occur from stuck liver qi, from swallowed air, or from an unwise food combination. Making a baby burp after drinking milk is useful because babies swallow lots of air. However, burping is not a good sign in adults. It may indicate emotional tension that makes digestive energy feel stuck and painful. Try eating food that is less rich and drink a digestive tea such as ginger, mint, and lemongrass.

Hiccups and Hiatal Hernia

Hiccups and nervous hiatal hernia are painful conditions that occurs when, because of muscle tension, the stomach pushes upward against the diaphragm to cause a spasm. No structural problem is involved with nervous hiatal hernia. Relaxing rib muscles is key to solving this dilemma. I once had a client, Anna, who was a judge, and sitting on the bench daily listening to couples fight over their divorces made her nervous and gave her a hiatal hernia. She also drank five cups of coffee daily to stay awake.

At my suggestion, Anna switched to green tea, and her hiatal hernia slowly disappeared. I also stimulated a point with my laser on the top of her foot that brought her stuck stomach qi energy downward to relieve the stuck digestive qi. You might massage firmly the entire foot, top and bottom, and if the hernia is accompanied by fever, inflammation, and/or anger, soak your feet in warm water, adding the juice of one organic lemon.

Food Addictions and Pain

What is the first thing you think of when trying to cure your upset feelings and worries? It probably isn't yoga or an herb. Lots of people indulge in comfort foods to soothe emotions. Some crave "mother's milk" in the form of soft cheeses, sweets, cakes, ice cream, and sweet liquors. Others crave stimulating salty foods, hot spices, alcohol, bitter coffee, and tea to lift spirits. Many use caffeine to support mental focus. All those foods are pain triggers. You may be especially sensitive, as many people are, to aged cheese and caffeine. Balancing mental/emotional food cravings requires a digestive remedy that reestablishes a healthy digestive function and emotional comfort. One such remedy is a Chinese herbal pill called Xiao Yao Wan.

Chinese Xiao Yao Wan patent remedy (also known as Hsiao Yao San, Free and Easy Wanderer, Relaxed Wanderer, or Relaxx Extract) is such a balanced digestive remedy that it is recommended for everything from bloating to hiatal hernia and chest pains to depression and anxiety. Chinese herbalists can claim such broad-ranging results because Xiao Yao Wan regulates the digestive organs and their qi, which supports their proper function. It eases the flow of qi throughout the digestive and emotional center. Xiao Yao Wan works well for a pale tongue or a coated tongue. If the tongue is red and acidity is a problem, ginger in Xiao Yao Wan may be irritating. In that case, combine the pills with aloe vera juice.

An American-made product which contains some Chinese herbs is Quiet Digestion, made by Health Concerns. It is used for irregular digestion, occasional constipation or diarrhea, bloating, and spasms. According to TCM (traditional Chinese medicine), it is said to "disperse wind and dampness," which means it helps reduces bloating, water retention, and nervous digestion. Quiet Digestion combines barley with bitter magnolia bark in order to stimulate bile production. It contains some of the same ingredients as Xiao Yao Wan, such as atractylodes and poria, and adds other herbs to treat vomiting, regurgitation, gastric hyperactivity, bacterial or viral gastroenteritis, motion sickness, hangover, and jet lag. It improves digestive absorption.

Kick the Coffee Habit

Coffee brightens mood and improves short-term memory, and its antioxidants are known to prevent certain cancers. But for many, coffee causes digestive problems. If you love java but want to avoid jitters and cramps, splash strong cold coffee on your face and awaken your senses. Recent research suggests that coffee's caffeine may retard or prevent skin cancers. Not a bad trade-off. Awaken your senses. Use leftover brewed fine-grind organic coffee grounds to exfoliate rough, dry skin. Rinse with cold water or coffee to make your complexion fresh and tingling.

Two Health-Food Store Remedies for Sweet Tooth

5-HTP: A modern Western remedy to reduce sweet cravings, overweight, and depression is 5-HTP (L-5-HTP or 5-hydroxytryptophan), extracted from griffonia seeds. You can find it in one form or another in many health-food stores. It comes in pill form, called Griffonex 5-HTP, made by Health Concerns.

Gymnema: In gardens throughout India, a potted plant is placed within easy reach. Its leaves are used as an Ayurvedic herb to curb sweet tooth and support the pancreas. In India you chew the leaves to eliminate a sweet flavor from foods. But in America you can buy capsules labeled with its Latin name, *Gymnema sylvestre*. Take the capsules as directed for diabetes and weight loss. It is covered in detail in *Feed Your Tiger*.

You can reduce a sweet craving with meshashringi and use stevia as a sugar substitute. A holistic naturopath friend in New York recommends putting a drop of stevia liquid extract on your tongue daily to stop addictive cravings for sugar, drugs, and alcohol. She is Dr. Diane Gioia-Bargonetti, ND, CTN, also known as Dr. Di, who has served as the resident naturopath at the Association for Research and Enlightenment in New York City.

Ulcers

Depending upon the location, ulcers may hurt worse as a result of hunger or after eating. Sometimes eating under stress causes pain from hiatal hernia and excess dumping of stomach acid, and the result is ulcers. I like to recommend drinking aloe vera juice or gel (the kind for internal use and not sold in tubes for sunburn) to correct many digestive upsets, because aloe heals wounds, burns, acid reflux, and spasm. Try to eat meals at regular times. Add more green alkaline vegetables to the diet, and add some cooling spices such as cumin and coriander to reduce digestive acids. Others useful foods for treating ulcers are cabbage and homemade pickled vegetables. Digestive enzymes from pickled cabbage (made without salt and sugar) can help prevent yeast, indigestion, and pain. For bleeding ulcers or chronic gastritis, the Chinese patent remedy Yunnan Paiyao is recommended. You will read much more about that herbal capsule in later chapters covering bleeding and injury.

Dietary Infections

Dietary microbial and viral infections are alarmingly common and in many cases drug resistant because of poor dietary habits and ignorance of basic hygiene. Supergerms, including antibiotic-resistant bacteria and viruses are easily passed from person to person because of unclean habits while preparing and serving foods.

Infection is a large important topic for another book, but here are the basics.

Germs want to live like everything else, and they mutate in order to survive. Staph infections, originally skin infections that may become internal diseases causing pneumonia and heart failure, used to be confined to hospitals but are now passed on the street by coughing, sneezing, and touching foods that others consume. Staph germs live inside the body, and an estimated 30 percent of the world carries this bacteria that colonizes the sinus cavities, groin, vagina, anus, and deep folds in the skin. According to experts, about 58 percent of hospital workers have been exposed to and carry the germ. However, anyone who prepares and serves food or shares a meal at home or in a restaurant should also be careful to avoid passing germs by touching foods, coughing, or sneezing on foods. Instruct children to blow their nose away from the table and wash their hands before eating or touching food. Natural antibacterial agents include oregano oil capsules or tea. Oregano leaf is a powerful germ fighter that can be added to teas in order to build a line of defense against dietary bacteria. When using an antibiotic medicine or herb, it is advisable to increase your intake of yogurt or acidophilus in order to protect healthy digestive bacteria. Follow directions on the label and buy a nondairy acidophilus if you are allergic to milk or wheat.

Norovirus, sometimes called stomach flu or food poisoning, develops when foods that should be refrigerated are left to spoil or when an infected person touches foods we consume. Shellfish may be particularly vulnerable. Often an entire conference, school, meeting, or other large group that eats the same meal can become infected. The symptoms are sudden, violent vomiting and diarrhea and headache that may resolve by itself in a day or two. Hospitalization to prevent dehydration is often necessary for the elderly or very young or people with a compromised immune system. There is little protection against these germs except to enhance our natural immunity by washing our hands with an alcohol based soap and tea tree oil before and after food preparation and eating. The recommended treatment for norovirus is rest and drinking plenty of liquids.

Candida fungus causes a yeast infection that affects men and women causing a complex of unpleasant symptoms, including digestive bloating and discomfort, depression, and cloudy thinking, that are hard to eliminate. Often the result of using antibiotic drugs, surgery, or pregnancy, it is aggravated by consuming yeasty foods like bread, pastries, beer, and wine, oral contraceptives and contraceptive devices, high estrogen levels, or having sex with someone infected. candida is a complex of unpleasant symptoms that are hard to eliminate. *Candida albicans*, a common form, can cause infections (candidiasis or thrush) in humans and animals, especially in immunocompromised patients with diabetes or HIV. It frequently colonizes the oropharynx, skin, mucous membranes, lower respiratory system, and gastrointestinal and genitourinary tracts. Candida infections cause painful sores internally for women and unsightly rash and fungal infections externally on the skin and nails for either sex. "Systemic infections of the bloodstream and major organs affect over ninety thousand people a year in the United States, with a 40–50 percent mortality rate," according to Tarlan Hedayati, MD, author of *Candidiasis in Emergency Medicine.*

Letha's Advice for Candida

To kill the candida yeast, add one drop of Australian tea tree oil to a cup of warm water in a porcelain cup, not plastic or foam (tea tree oil melts foam). Drink this in water or coffee or use a drop on your toothbrush once daily. Do not put tea tree oil directly in your mouth or other sensitive areas—it burns. While the yeast is dying off, you will crave all sorts of yeast-increasing foods such as candy, sweets, sugar, pastry, soy, and breads. Avoid them. But do take acidophilus or eat plain yogurt daily to replenish necessary digestive bacteria. Vitamin Shoppe and other major health-food stores and supermarkets sell homeopathic products formulated to treat nagging candida yeast symptoms including digestive bloating, burping, abdominal cramps, uncomfortable itching and burn- ing pain in the sexual area, and discharge, as well as to help prevent reoccurrence. They include YeastGard and Candida Yeast, a combina- tion homeopathic remedy made by NatraBio. (See my advice for curing vaginal candida infections in the following chapter.)

Dizziness/Ménière's Syndrome

Are you dizzy with spinning vertigo (when the room seems to spin) if you turn your head around? Do you have ringing in your ears or hearing loss? It may be related to your diet. Not all causes of Ménière's syndrome are as obvious as the following. My friend Sam, an overweight heart patient, ate three cheese blin- tzes, a poppy seed hamantash pastry, and some grapes and nuts, and wondered why he awoke in the middle of the night so dizzy he could not stand. Digestive phlegm muddled his senses. In the past, he has had Ménière's syndrome, diz- ziness that becomes worse when turning your head around. It often happens for him during times when stress, rich foods, and damp weather have caused digestive trouble.

Some people develop Ménière's syndrome after using an antibiotic that has left behind phlegm, which troubles circulation in the inner ear. The best, fastest treatment for such dizziness is acupuncture to points in the head, arm, and leg to treat dizziness, headache, and digestive phlegm. But that is not always practical, especially when a friend calls in the middle of the night. So it is a good idea to keep digestive aids such as Xiao Yao Wan in your pocket if you eat richly and end up dizzy or spacey, or get a pounding dull phlegm-related headache at your crown that makes you feel as though your head is expanding. A homeopathic medicine recommended for motion sickness, Cocculus indicus, may help as well. Medical treatment of Ménière's syndrome is only palliative, usually involving Valium for anxiety and possibly diuretic medicines. Unless dietary and circulation issues are cleared, excess dietary phlegm will continue to "obscure the senses."

When to Consult a Health Specialist

Check to see if you have blood sugar problems, especially if there is diabetes in the family, if you feel weak and faint after eating certain foods, if you have chronic thirst and/or hunger, or if you cannot get through the day without snacks. Check with a health specialist if digestive pain, indigestion, or a skin rash do not improve after simplifying your diet, or if you see blood in urine, stool, or other digestive sputum. Watch your diet for sweets and fats in order to avoid problems with cholesterol and candida. Your doctor may not be able to spot a problem until it turns into a serious disease. Simple everyday health and beauty issues such as skin rashes, bad breath, menstrual cramps, and headaches can easily be improved with dietary changes and a few simple herbs such as aloe vera. If pain is severe and continues or if stress relief treatments do not help, you should have medical testing to help determine whether or not the problem may be ulcers, irritable bowel syndrome (IBS), or a cancer.

Unexplained recurrent stomachaches may be early signs of colon cancer. People with pancreatic cancer often describe a dull ache that feels like it's pressing inward. Many liver cancer patients say they had stomach cramps and upset stomachs so frequently that their doctors thought they had ulcers. Liver cancer patients and those with leukemia may experience abdominal pain resulting from an enlarged spleen, which may feel like an ache on the lower left side. Your doctor may order an ultrasound test. Finding a liver or pancreatic tumor early can make all the difference in treatment.

The most common early sign of stomach cancer is pain in the upper or middle abdomen that feels like gas or heartburn. It may be aggravated by eating so that you feel full without eating. The pain can sometimes be relieved by antacids. An unexplained pain or ache in lower right side can be the first sign of liver cancer. Feeling full after a small meal is a common sign of liver cancer as well. Other signs include a jaundiced (yellowish/orange) complexion, unexplained weight loss, and weakness or frequent infections.

I have had clients who suffered terrible digestive pain that resulted from emotional upset. One man had extensive testing done at Mayo clinic to find that nothing was wrong with his digestive organs. It was stress. Another woman had liver pain that occurred with every meal attended by her mother-in-law. How can you avoid stress during meals? Try to eat at regular hours of the day. Avoid a big meal before bedtime. To avoid cramps during meals, avoid extreme temperatures from hot spices and iced drinks, and enjoy quiet pleasant surroundings and no heavy discussions. After eating, breathe into the lower abdomen. Take a walk or sit quietly. Free the passage from the small intestine to the large intestine by pushing with your palms from the navel downward toward the right groin. Anytime we free the natural flow of our energy and vitality, we begin the healing process. Digestion begins in the eyes. We see delicious foods and enjoy their colors. Their fragrance refreshes our senses. We taste them and feel their healing comfort in our digestive and emotional center reach every cell.

CHAPTER SEVEN

Female Issues

Men who have a pierced ear are better prepared for marriage.
They've experienced pain and bought jewelry.

—Rita Rudner (American comedian, 1953–)

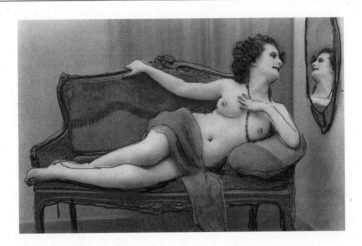

RITA RUDNER CAME TO NEW YORK AT AGE FIFTEEN, DANCED ON BROADWAY, became a stand-up comic at twenty-five, and at forty-nine adopted a daughter. Upon turning fifty she remarked, "Now I dwell on the fact restaurants are getting darker and how very uncomfortable underwear has become." Being female, having a sense of humor helps. This chapter covers the "Ughs!" of fertility, ripening, and withering into a state of grace: menstruation, childbirth, and menopause.

Women and Herbs

What can women do to prevent common female discomforts? Women owe a lot to herbs. There have always been wise women herbalists. Traditional Asian doctors had germ theories, and women's health herbal formulas and many anti-inflammatory antibiotic herbs have been in use for centuries, such as andrographis (*Andrographis paniculata*), now commonly used to treat flu. During my own menopause, I found taking an occasional capsule of andrographis to be comfortably cooling and calming. That herb's cooling, cleansing, and calming actions improve inflammatory PMS and cramps. That simple anti-inflammatory treatment did not complicate my already mixed-up hormones. Long-term use of anti-inflammatory herbs is not usually recommended, and andrographis can increase the chance of miscarriage during pregnancy. But its antibacterial, antiviral, antifungal, and antiparasitic detoxifying properties are quite useful for chronic inflammatory skin conditions, hepatitis, wounds, and as an immuno-stimulant to avoid colds and flu.

Andrographis, a shrub, is used in China, India, and throughout subtropical and Southeast Asia. In traditional Chinese herbalism, it is used to support healthy digestive, cardiovascular, and urinary systems. In Sweden, it is used for immune support. Research has shown andrographis to be a useful anti-inflammatory for diabetes, fevers, upper respiratory tract infections, cancer prevention and treatment, herpes, malaria, and rheumatoid arthritis. Andrographis extract calms behavior in animals and apparently perimenopausal women. It may be useful for nervous tics. The herb improves sleep and lowers body temperature. It is great for hot pounding menstrual cramps with clots, or hot flashes. I will cover many useful women's herbs in detail later in the chapter.

How to Choose Your Herbs

Instead of taking an aspirin, let's get to the root of your pain in order to prevent irregular periods, fertility problems, and fibroids. Before choosing the correct herbal treatment for female discomforts, you have to recognize your imbalance. Do not be confused by your symptoms. Just answer this: does your pain, hormonal/fertility problem, or menstrual period feel hot or cold?

Periods Hot and Cold

In the previous chapter, we learned to observe the tongue in order to check our internal temperature, level of metabolism, and vitality. Now you can observe your tongue and symptoms to get a sense of why you may have menstrual discomforts.

What Is a Healthy Period?

I have to answer the question because so many women suffer discomforts they consider normal. A healthy period comes on time, separated by about twenty-eight days in a regular cycle. There may be slight cramping or a light discharge during the middle of the cycle, but the period ought to last three to four days and stop without much pain or problems such as temper tantrums, complexion blemishes, insomnia, and overly swollen breasts. The lack of symptoms indicates good health, adequate blood production, and smooth, easy qi circulation. When fatigue, stress, and bad habits interfere, the period may arrive early or late, become too heavy or sparse, and generally be a pain.

Hot Periods

Is your tongue red and dry? Are the edges around the sides more bright or red and cracked or swollen? If so, your tongue shows respectively inflammation, blood and moisture deficiency, and liver irritation or congestion. Do you feel flushed and feverish or headachy during PMS? Your cramps will feel hot, pounding, relentless, and severe. Your period may come heavy and early. It may send you to bed for a few days each month. This example is extreme, but many women suffer from intense internal heat (inflammatory pain), especially if they smoke, overindulge in spicy hot foods and alcohol, become dehydrated from excess sweating, or have a chronic feverish condition that weakens their blood production and digestion, such as diabetes. If you have heavy, lumpy, smelly blood or a difficult period with clots, inflammation has lodged in the uterus and over time may end up giving you endometriosis or other complications.

The proper treatment is cooling, moistening foods and herbs to detoxify the blood and support vitality. I like treatments that are simple and inexpensive. Start by using detoxifying herbs for two weeks before you expect your period. For example, drink up to one-fourth cup per day of aloe vera juice. If you do not like the taste, add lime juice, or add aloe to apple juice. If you usually have clots in the period, add one to two capsules of myrrh daily for two weeks before the period. Stop taking the purifying herbs during the period. You will experience a heavier period from the cleansing herbs. That is normal and beneficial. If you still have a pounding headache, bad breath, testy PMS, and cramps during the period, then continue with the aloe between periods as long as it feels soothing and cooling. Do not be alarmed if during your next period you lose very large clots. That is part of the cleansing process, and it is better to have them outside than inside. The period will become regulated with a couple of months of this cooling, cleansing treatment, and you will have saved yourself the trouble of a medical procedure, or worse, a tumor.

If, after the period becomes more normal and regular, you still have a thick odorous vaginal discharge or pain, check with a health professional that you do not have a sexually transmitted illness or a yeast infection. Very painful periods and spotting, which is bleeding between normal periods, may also indicate a fibroid or other problem that requires diagnosis and treatment.

Cold Periods

Is your tongue pale, puffy, scalloped, or bloated? Do you feel weak and washed out during and after your period? Is the blood thin, watery, and pale? Does the flow begin late, last a while, stop, and then start again? Are the cramps sickening and draining? Do you have an upset stomach, dizziness, or exhaustion during and afterward? Have your periods stopped completely for several months or years with no warning (not menopause)? Have you lost your period because of surgery or illness? Have your periods become thinner after changing to a raw foods diet? Do you spend energy weeping around the time of your period? Have you lost interest in sex, in socializing, in being a woman? "Internal cold" is a term used by traditional Chinese doctors that does not refer to a cold temperament or so-called frigidity. It means your blood, urine, and bowel movements are watery, and that you have a tendency for chills and facial pallor, not fever. You may feel less sociable and more emotionally vulnerable because of physical weakness and blood loss.

There are times when an herbal tonic is needed to build blood and vitality in order to regulate your period and mood. Overwork is a big energy drain for women. So are childbirth and moving to a new city, job, or relationship. These events cost us blood and energy that must be replaced monthly. Remember in the previous chapter when I described how digestion is key to vitality and emotional balance? Diet and digestion are major factors in maintaining a healthy, comfortable period. Xiao Yao Wan, the digestive remedy, is also recommended by TCM doctors for supporting normal blood production and menstrual regularity. It contains ginger and several blood-enhancing herbs. Also see Young Yum pills on page 264.

A nourishing diet of soups, teas, and foods cooked with tonic herbs is very helpful for warming vitality and building blood. Tonic herbs may include Chinese ginseng (also known as red or panax ginseng) or a combination of ginsengs such as Ginseng Complex made by Vitamin Shoppe, ginger tea, and one-fourth teaspoon of steamed tienchi ginseng powder made into a tea. See page 160 for additional information on raw and steamed tienchi ginseng.

Three Blood-Enhancing Beverages for Health and Beauty

Many discomforts associated with menstrual pain, hormonal shifts, and fertility problems, including amenorrhea (loss of the period), can be avoided if you have adequate blood production. Are your gums very pale? That shows low blood quality and production. Do you feel listless, tired, short of breath, cranky, or anxious after losing blood during the period? Is the flesh under your fingernails white? Improving health means having the ability to make healthy blood and having good circulation. Having healthy blood requires energy, oxygen, and the sun's ultraviolet light that increases our vitamin D protects life.

Facial pallor is a sign of ill health from so called "internal cold." Signs of "internal heat" include a red complexion, acne, chronic thirst and hunger, dry skin, reduced body fluids, and a body odor from inflammation and dehydration. Blood is a fluid required by every tissue of the body and a cooling balm for mind and spirit. The following three foods work in different ways but are useful for either case of blood deficiency—hot or cold periods. They are black cherry concentrate, tang kuei root, and Tibetan goji berry. Upon observing your symptoms, you will be able to combine these foods with herbs and spices to either warm or cool them as required.

Black Cherry: An Iron-Rich Food

Black cherries are a favorite source of iron and, therefore, blood for anyone with weakness, joint pain, and fatigue. Black cherry is a specific anti-inflammatory treatment for gout, a severe joint pain that usually starts in the big toe.

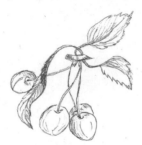

Black Cherry Beverage

Add one teaspoon of black cherry concentrate, available in health-food stores and online, to a glass of water or seltzer daily. This treatment supports complexion and hair beauty, while it regulates the period. For hot types, enjoy this often. For cold types, add a little fresh, sliced ginger or cinnamon powder to this beverage.

Tang Kuei

Tang kuei (also known as *Angelica sinensis*, dong quai) is estrogenic, a tasty semisweet, blood- and circulation-enhancing herbal root that makes a nice addition to chicken soup. The sliced root can be simmered to make a tea. It feels warming and energizing yet grounding. It is most useful for women with "cold periods" who are pale, chilled, weak, and overworked. Since it increases circulation in the uterus, it helps regulate sparse periods. Chinese herbalists have an expression—"cold uterus"—which refers to infertility with "internal cold" symptoms including blood and energy deficiency. They warn women to eat more cooked foods and avoid cold baths. In a glass, earthen, or ceramic-coated pot, simmer a tang kuei root in spring or purified water for an hour. Drink a glass of the beverage, and you can cook the root again until soft and eat that too. If it feels too warming, add aloe juice and lime. Tang kuei should be avoided by anyone with a fever, inflammatory symptoms, or someone with an active cancer or following a course of cancer chemotherapy.

Goji Berries

Many herbalists think Tibetan goji berries should be taken by everyone over age forty. Everyone needs enhanced vitality, immunity, and nutrient-rich blood provided by these power-packed little red berries. Goji berries have been used to protect the liver, improve circulation, and help prevent cancers. Steep a cup of tea using a handful of Tibetan goji berries in hot water and enjoy it during the afternoon or at bedtime for a relaxing sleep. If it is too cooling for you and results in diarrhea, add fresh ginger. You might also combine goji berries with warming tang kuei. If that is too cooling, relaxing, or draining, add up to ten drops of panax ginseng extract.

Adzuki Beans for Weak Qi (Low Energy), Water Retention, and Chronic Fatigue Pain

Do you feel waterlogged around the time of your period? Do your breasts, abdomen, and joints swell? Do you find it difficult to breathe, climb stairs, and have a normal sex life because you feel too tired? Those are signs of weak qi. Small red adzuki beans are prized in TCM for their ability to support qi and rid the body of excess water. They are considered to be warming or *yang*. Adzuki beans can be made into a soup with orange peel and dried lotus nuts. Hard beans like adzuki and lotus nuts absorb excess water in the body. Sometimes you can find delicious, soft little sweets, adzuki bean paste wrapped in rice dough, sold at the checkout counter of Chinese supermarkets. Here is a simple recipe for daily use.

Red Adzuki Bean Soup
Serves 6–8

Ingredients
1 cup adzuki beans
¼–½ cup dried lotus seeds
6–8 cups water
1 strip dried tangerine peel (chen pi) or fresh organic orange peel
stevia extract, an herbal sweetener, or brown sugar, as desired
a handful of dried alaria seaweed for flavor and minerals (optional)
cardamom powder to taste

1. Soak the adzuki beans in water overnight to soften. (The beans will expand considerably.) Drain.

2. About 2 hours before making the soup, place the dried lotus seeds in a bowl with enough water to cover.

3. In a medium saucepan, bring the 6 cups of water with the tangerine peel to a boil. (The soup can be thicker or thinner as desired. You can start with 6 cups of water, and then add more boiling water at the end with the sweetener if you want it thinner.)

4. Turn the heat down, add the adzuki beans and lotus seeds and simmer, partially covered, for 1–1½ hours, until the beans are softened to the point where they are just beginning to break apart. Add alaria seaweed, if using, after 1 hour.

5. Add the sweetener and stir until dissolved. Taste and add more sweetener if desired. Add cardamom powder to taste. Remove the dried tangerine peel before serving. Serve the red bean soup hot or cold.

Herbal Combinations for Menstrual Discomforts, Regularity, and Fertility

For prolonged menstrual discomforts and irregularity, it is best to consult a professional herbalist and follow up with regular checkups to see if the herbs are working well over a period of several months or longer. Hormonal issues are complex, involving physical and emotional elements that take time to regulate. If the herbs and dietary changes unleash painful emotions or excess bleeding, inform your health adviser so the dosage and formula may be adjusted.

Here are a few suggestions of Chinese herbal pills to illustrate how such female herbal formulas work and what you might expect. Please do not use them without guidance.

- **Blood deficiency herbs**: Eight Treasures (Health Concerns), Liu Wei Di Huang Wan and Sexoton (two Chinese patent remedies, the first cooling, the second warming)
- **Blood and qi deficiency, fertility herbs**: Fertile Garden (Health Concerns), Xiao Yao Wan (Chinese patent remedy also used for digestive bloating and chest pain)
- **Cooling (anti-inflammatory) herbs**: Coptis (also known as huang lian), Oldenlandia Diffusa tea sweetener, skullcap extract
- **Pain herbs that enhance circulation**: Channel Flow, Crampbark Plus (Health Concerns)
- **Anti-infection for vaginal irritation herbs**: Clearing (Health Concerns)

Health issues that may trouble menstruation include blood deficiency; chronic irritation/infection; circulation problems affecting the uterus, lower abdomen, and associated meridians; and hormonal insufficiency. Blood deficiency symptoms, as I have said before, may include chronic fatigue, dry itchy skin, reduced appetite, cold limbs, seeing spots in front of your eyes, shortness of breath, dizziness, delayed irregular menstruation, or loss of the period (amenorrhea).

Herbs that enhance blood and qi (vital energy in internal organs and meridians) will strengthen endurance and lift your spirits. For example, a combination of white atractylodes, rehmannia, white peony, tang kuei, and ligusticum will build blood by enhancing the function of the spleen/pancreas. Additional herbs such as ginger, red date, and baked licorice are added to enhance qi. Codonopsis, an inexpensive ginseng used to lift prolapse conditions such as excess menstrual bleeding or diarrhea, may be added. Health Concerns makes Eight Treasures pills that contain these and other ingredients. Chinese patent remedies Liu Wei Di Huang Wan (also known as Six Flavor tea), which is cooling, and Ba Wei Di Huang Wan (also known as Eight Flavor tea pills, Sexoton), which is warming in order to address backache and diarrhea, are also blood-enhancing. (Note: if you have active herpes zoster, avoid Chinese herbal formulas that contain rehmannia, which may aggravate an outbreak.)

Letha's Advice: Individual Dosage Works Best

Traveling third-class around south China during the mid-1980s, alone and eating a meager diet, I became rundown and consulted a traditional Chinese hospital herbalist. He observed my pale tongue, deep, thready pulse, and lethargy. In China, herbal doctors usually recommend concentrated herbs that work powerfully and quickly. He recommended that I take fifteen small black pills of the moistening blood tonic Liu Wei Di Huang Wan twice daily. It worked. I felt and looked better and stopped taking the herbal pills after several days. If I had continued consuming such moistening nourishing herbs, they would have given me diarrhea and chills. In other words, I took the herbs in a concentrated dose *while they worked*. Based on your energy level and health condition, your herbalist can help you to decide the best dose that feels comfortable and works well. Otherwise, you might start with four to five Chinese patent remedy pills twice daily, a smaller dose if you are very sensitive, and adjust the dose as needed.

Candida

Candida, a yeast infection, was introduced in the chapter covering digestion because diet is so important for preventing and curing it. However, the yeast is always with us. It can be increased from a hormone imbalance caused by stress, oral contraceptives and contraceptive devices, high estrogen levels, or having sex with someone infected. Candida infections cause painful vaginal sores internally making sex impossible. Three quarters of women experience vaginitis in their lifetime, and 30 percent of vaginitis is caused by *candida*. Vaginitis accounts for ten million office visits per year.

For vaginal yeast infections, with your clean finger put one-fourth teaspoon of plain yogurt into the vagina overnight as needed for a few days. Another method is to moisten with aloe and insert one capsule of acidophilus into the vagina (or as an anal suppository) at night and wear protection because the watery yeast discharge is unpleasant. Thrush, candida yeast in the mouth, results from medicines and long term weakening illness including HIV. Medicines for candida and thrush (candida in the mouth) take a long time to work and the outcome is not certain. If will help to simultaneous follow the dietary recommendations in the previous chapter covering digestion. All yeast-causing foods, including breads, pastries, fruits, most fermented foods like cheese, sweets, and alcohol must be avoided. Those foods are also pain triggers so you will do yourself a favor by avoiding them. Add one drop of Australian tea tree oil to a cup of warm water several times daily.

Fertility Herbs

Fertility is an important sign of health during our twenties and thirties. Unfortunately, women are often forced into unstable relationships, overwork and worry, bad habits, and medications that reduce menstruation. Diet and herbs aimed to support fertility replenish blood and the tissue and function of the liver, kidneys, and adrenal energy, and regulate the circulation of qi. The same herbs support comfortable, regular periods, and reduce breast distention, depression, and emotional liability. They include Fertile Garden pills made by Health Concerns. Fertile Garden contains blood-enhancing herbs ligustrum, tang kuei, peony root, and lycium (goji). Loranthus stem, cuscuta seed, and ashwagandha support adrenal vitality. Hormonal herbs include shatavari and false unicorn. Shatavari is wild East Indian asparagus, which contains useful rejuvenating female hormones. There are no contraindications for this formula and it can be used as a tonic between periods for women in their middle thirties and early forties. Even if fertility is not an issue, you will enjoy looking and feeling your best.

PMS Depression

Depression around period time seems worse than usual. Maybe it's because we are feeling it deeper in our female identity as hormonal changes release blood. Xiao Yao Wan, though primarily a digestive formula, can be used to reduce PMS bloating, cramping, chest pains, depression, anxiety, and temper. It regulates our emotional center. Taken over a period of months, it may be helpful to prevent breast distention and breast and uterine fibroids. Tang kuei, in this and many other women's formulas, is estrogenic, while it supports circulation and blood.

Do you feel especially weepy or short of breath around period time? It may be from the hormonal shift or low vitality. Homeopathic pulsatilla is useful for people who feel low, feel as though they lack oxygen, who often complain or ask for emotional support from friends, and who weep watching television commercials. It feels strengthening and drying for crying jags. It also helps reduce PMS bloating and water retention.

Cooling Herbs for Menstrual Pains, Fever, Blemishes, and More

Aside from drinking aloe daily until your tongue turns from dry, red hot to a normal moist pink, you may want to add some cooling, moistening herbs that feel comfortable and rejuvenating. A cooling herbal formula may contain coptis (also known as golden thread or huang lian), used to calm nervous headaches, stomach ulcers, complexion blemishes, hypertension, and fevers. It reduces cholesterol and improves atherosclerosis. Studies have found that berberine, an anti-inflammatory in coptis, can lower blood sugar in diabetes. Coptis, like many cooling herbs, is very bitter, but you can find pills containing this valuable herb in Chinese herb shops and online.

Oldenlandia Diffusa tea sweetener is an easy way to use anti-inflammatory herbs as a tea sweetener or cooking ingredient. Chinese groceries and herb shops sell this "instant beverage" made from oldenlandia and skullcap (*Scutellaria baicalensis*), two anticancer herbs native to south China. Chinese skullcap has been used in traditional Chinese medicine to treat allergies, infections, inflammation, cancer, and headaches. It may also have antifungal and antiviral effects. Animal studies suggest that this bitter herb may help reduce symptoms of diabetes and hypertension (high blood pressure). The extract is too bitter tasting to use alone.

Channel Flow is a pain formula made by Health Concerns. Its ingredients relieve joint, muscle, abdominal, and gynecological pain and cramps, as well as headache, arthritis, and fibromyalgia. It is a relaxing formula that includes corydalis, angelica root, and peony for nerve pain. Cinnamon and tang kuei enhance circulation. Salvia root protects the heart and circulation. Myrrh and frankincense help prevent and dissolve fibroids. This can be taken along with medicinal mushrooms or other tonics for cancer prevention.

Crampbark (*Viburnum opulis*) is a time-honored Native American women's remedy for menstrual pains. It is warming and relieves spasms by enhancing circulation. Chinese herbalists combine it with zedoaria root (e zhu) to reduce fibroids. Additional ingredients such as cyperus, tang kuei, and cinnamon may be added to increase circulation and reduce pain. Health Concerns' Crampbark Plus is a strong formula that can be used by women who need stimulating, warming herbs. If it is too warming, it can be modified by using it along with aloe, which is cooling, alkaline, and cleansing.

Chronic Bladder Infections, Vaginal and Urethral Irritation, Mouth Sores

They may seem unrelated—mouth sores and vaginal inflammation—however, herbs used to clear inflammation from heart, lungs, liver, stomach, and bladder work well for both problems. Chinese "heat-clearing" formulas may include astringent herbs that absorb excess moisture, such as lotus seed, along with cooling herbs such as American ginseng and ophiopogonis tuber (mai men dong). A formula called Clearing by Health Concerns contains cooling, diuretic plantago seed, poria, and smilax (also known as tu fu ling or sarsaparilla), a hormonal herb and detoxicant useful for urinary tract infections. For this problem, if a simple beverage made using health-food store nonsweetened cranberry concentrate does not reduce symptoms, medical examination may be necessary. Clearing, the Chinese herbal pill, may reduce symptoms, but medical follow-up with tests for sexually transmitted diseases and other issues is important.

Menopause Discomforts

The line between youth and age has blurred. Today, menopause is no cause for alarm as it once seemed. Only the challenge of uncertainty makes some women decline. An end to menarche makes travel and taking charge of relationships easier. That extra testosterone that surges around age forty-five comes in handy for mountain-climbing. The downside—hot flashes, night sweats, and inflammatory aches—are shared by younger, less fortunate smokers, pungent spice-eaters, caffeine addicts, and night owls. The answer to aging is to support rejuvenating fluids, reverse inflammatory discomforts, and get on with life and love.

Letha's Menopause Advice: Go for the Obvious

Begin simply with the easiest, least expensive, most practical solutions to health and beauty issues. Since menopause involves loss of fluid and blood that leads to heat symptoms, start by staying cooler. Turn your thermostat down to around sixty-eight to seventy degrees. Wear light cotton sleepwear and a cooling essential oil fragrance such as sandalwood or rose. Instead of heavy oily creams and cosmetics that clog pores and hamper breathing and circulation, stay cool with a cold green-tea skin spray or try the juice of two ounces each of raw cucumber and raw potato. Apply the topical juice to refine and cool complexion irritation. Curb your inflammatory caffeine and chocolate (hidden caffeine) habits. Drink black cherry concentrate in seltzer or water instead of wine or other alcohol. Enjoy cooling, rejuvenating Tibetan goji berry tea. Stay cooler by avoiding arguments, late nights, spicy hot foods, and saunas.

Menopause Herbs for Balanced Beauty

Liu Wei Di Huang Wan (Six Flavor Tea pills) which I mentioned earlier reverses what Chinese doctors call "afternoon fevers" and night sweats, diabetes, hypertension, and chronic hunger and thirst. Moistening herbs that support blood and liver are useful for dry skin. The only caution about using this remedy is that it contains rehmannia (shou di huang) which in large doses may encourage a herpes outbreak. Other anti-inflammatory herbs for internal use that I mentioned above, including coptis, skullcap, Oldenlandia Diffusa instant beverage, and andrographis capsules, are all cooling and detoxifying for a variety of discomforts.

Three Immortals pills by Health Concerns is especially formulated to treat inflammatory menopausal symptoms such as those already mentioned plus palpitations, vertigo, tinnitus, depression, insomnia, lower back ache, hot burning palms and soles of the feet, constipation, break-through bleeding between periods, bleeding gums, and lowered sex drive. It contains testosterone-precursor herbs epimedium and morinda, as well as blood tonics tang kuei, eclipta, ligustrum, and lycium. It also has herbs to reduce fever conditions (hot flashes), anemarrhena and phellodendron. To make the change easier, it supports vitality as well as counters heat.

For chronic weakness, fatigue, and lower backache, Ayurvedic doctors recommend using tonic herbs such as ashwagandha tea, often recommended for women during the final trimester of pregnancy in order to strengthen muscles and shorten delivery. As an energy and muscle tonic, add one-fourth teaspoon of ashwagandha powder with an equal amount of shatavari powder in warm water daily as a tea.

The Heart-Energy Connection

I illustrated a common case of low vitality-related poor circulation leading to chronic shoulder pain in the chapter covering headaches. Women may experience irregular heart rhythms or congestive heart problems without directly feeling heart or chest pain. This is important because the qi circulation of heart, chest, breast, and upper back and shoulders are all linked energetically. The deeper pathways of surface meridians lying on the neck, shoulders, and chest pass though the digestive and heart centers. Pay attention to such pains. Are the pains sharp or sudden or dull and long-lasting? Does pain travel down the left arm? Does chest or shoulder pain accompany fatigue, overexertion, or emotional stress? If upper body discomfort corresponds to low vitality or lack of sleep, an herbal tonic may bring improvement. If emotional upset makes you feel choked and vulnerable, the Tibetan Precious Pills for emotional balance described below can greatly help.

Make it a healing practice to get enough rest, observe a proper diet, use balancing herbs, get lymphatic drainage or other healing massage, and enjoy the

How to Use Tibetan Precious Pills

Below are my suggestions for Precious Pills that may help to ease female issues and improve general well-being. I have additional suggestions of Tibetan Precious Pills in chapters dealing with emotional trauma and complexion issues. It is best to consult with a Tibetan doctor for specific problems, but Precious Pills may be taken by healthy persons as a tonic.

Using Tibetan Precious Pills, many people find it comforting to follow the traditional practice: for three days during and following taking the pill, abstain from eating meat, fish, eggs, hot spices, caffeine, alcohol, and smoking. What is left to eat? Cooked whole grains, tofu, walnuts, vegetables, and green tea. Think of it as a cleansing fast. Avoid sex, cold showers, and arguments. This is a detoxifying treatment from everything that overexcites or causes emotions to rise. The normal dose is usually one or two per week, for a course of treatment such as one month or more. However a Precious Pill may be taken during the full moon or a special holiday.

On the day you take the pill, open the cloth container carefully without exposing the pill to sunlight or bright light. Place the pill whole (or broken in pieces with a hammer) into a porcelain cup. Add four ounces of hot boiled water. Cover the cup with the saucer from the teacup. Allow it to steep for several hours or overnight. I usually take my pill at bedtime and cover with blankets. I repeat a mantra: "Om Mani Padmi Hum!" and empty my thoughts, waiting for a calming vision, a glimpse of the wholeness I hope to achieve.

calming practices described in this book. Also make sure your heart is safe by having regular checkups. Pollution underlies many stress-related health problems today. Abnormal heart rhythm may be hormone- or thyroid-related or from other factors that may eventually lead to lymph congestion, fibroids, high cholesterol, or chest pains.

Weight Loss, Menopause, and Pain

Carrying extra weight stresses muscles and joints and increases chronic pain and fatigue. Menopause is not the only time to address excess weight, but we know it is harder to get rid of fat after age forty. Boost metabolism with cleansing, cooling, hormone-supporting herbs added to a slimming tea. The Well-Known Tea combines Chinese oolong tea with coptis to help prevent hot flashes, salvia and hawthorn to protect the heart, raphani to protect liver function, and alisma as a diuretic. Oolong and black tea can help you break a coffee habit. Both coffee and tea have advantages for weight loss, but their caffeine may be irritating for some. You can find valuable diet advice, herbs, and recipes in *Feed Your Tiger*, especially the baseline diet and the sections for Dragons (edema and low energy and compromised immunity) and Bears (sweet tooth and diabetes).

Menopause, Longevity, and Enlightenment

Do you try to transform challenging experiences including female discomforts into positive ones? If so, you are among the enlightened. One positive aspect of menopause is that with age, we are expected to gain experience and wisdom. If we are to fulfill our destinies as women, we will encourage within ourselves, refine, and relish our God-given gifts. Our bodily structures present a *karma* pregnant with possibilities: an openness to life, love, nurturing, generosity, and kindness. With that awareness, we may become a vessel of spirit open to high aspirations and good works. To fully appreciate our potential, we need to address body, mind, and spirit with a potentiating approach to wellness and personal development. Such an approach has been practiced by Tibetan medicine over the millennia. Asian herbs, precious metals and gems such as gold, silver, turquoise, and opal, used to make Tibetan Precious Pills, are gathered during times when nature's positive influences are intensified, during the full moon and on sacred dates in places known to have healing powers. Tibetan physician-monks chant many prayers over the herbal pills and send them into the world with their blessings. We are fortunate to have access to this treatment approach in the West. However, you do not have to be Tibetan or Buddhist to benefit from herbal treatments formulated to bring about physical, emotional, and spiritual balance. Some people take Tibetan precious pills to celebrate an event such as a birthday, the full moon, or a change in their life situation. The calming, centering influence of the herbs enhances personal harmony.

Normally, Tibetan doctors rarely visit from India. We may have to wait weeks for an appointment. However, a monastery, Tibetan medical clinic, and Tibetan botanical research center with resident Tibetan doctors and monks is located on Orcas Island, near Seattle. The Tanaduk Botanical Research Institute was established to support the preservation of the ancient art of Tibetan and traditional Himalayan Medicine. The intention is to conserve the botanicals used in Tibetan medicine by cultivating them and the societies they live in, both in their native habitat and on conservation sites in the West. In addition, research is conducted on all phases of the botanicals used, from planting to harvesting to their efficacy when used in medicinal formulas.

The Tanaduk Tibetan medical clinic has helped many to regain health and balance with diet advice and herbal treatments. Tibetan Precious Pills are available from Nepal and India and some are now made in American. They are sold from the clinic website, www.tibetandoctors.com, along with guidance for their use. Personal consultation is available. But if traveling to the area is impossible, a detailed questionnaire, patient photos, and interview available online help the doctors decide the proper treatments.

Amla 25

Named for the East Indian berry amla (*Emblica officinalis*) that has great rejuvenating properties because of its high tannin content, this rejuvenating pill enhances health while it beautifies complexion and hair. Amla berry is used to cool and cleanse the body, reduce hair loss, acidity, water retention, and complexion problems. Amla 25, the herbal combination in pill form, can be used to decrease high blood pressure and pain in liver and gallbladder, on the right side at the ribs. Amla 25 calms the mind and nourishes the body.

The biomedical applications for Amla 25 include chronic hepatitis, cirrhosis of the liver, intercostal neuralgia, hernia, Addison's disease, chronic gastritis, menstrual disorders, dysmenorrhea (painful periods), gastric upsets, diabetes, multichemical sensitivity, and chronic fatigue. Like other Tibetan Precious Pills, Amla 25 helps detoxify the body from foods, drugs, chemicals, and environmental poisons. Use two pills twice daily with hot water.

Emotions and Health

Some women wear feelings like perfume on the skin. They may withdraw to safety or into a soliloquy of illness. Actually, our emotions have deep origins in our blood, bone marrow, nerves, and vital energy that support life force. Are you sometimes too upset to work, think clearly, sleep soundly, and enjoy satisfying relationships? Tibetan medicines address the entire spectrum of human behavior in ways that bring about health and balance. Here are two Tibetan Precious Pills that I will also recommend in Part Three.

Agar 35

Agar 35 is the most common and widely endorsed traditional Tibetan compound for all types of anxiety, stress, and fatigue. By balancing all three humors (wind, bile, and phlegm), energy is increased and stress is relieved. This formula addresses many symptoms, including insomnia, overactive mental states, uneasiness, nervousness, jittery nerves, mental upset, lower back pain, feeling tense, dizziness, tinnitus (ringing in the ears), and pain in the upper back from excess of nervous irritation. It is effective for pain that wanders throughout the body and whose origin is difficult to determine. It improves shortness of breath and difficult breathing. The herbal pill brings support to the kidneys, liver, blood, and overall circulation.

Agar 35 is especially useful for general anxiety disorder (GAD), obsessive-compulsive disorder (OCD), and post-traumatic stress disorder (PTSD). The treatment principles for this multielement pattern are said to "course the liver and rectify the qi, fortify the spleen and supplement the qi, nourish the heart and quiet the spirit, transform phlegm, clear heat, and quicken the blood." That means it improves the liver's ability to detoxify the blood and fluids. It enhances qi to correct chronic weakness and poor metabolism. It improves absorption of nutrients by supporting spleen and pancreas function. It soothes anxiety and strengthens the heart structure and function. It helps reverse congestion and water retention that may impair digestion and circulation. It reduces chronic inflammatory pains and depression.

Non-habit-forming but surprisingly powerful, Agar 35 is a safe, effective means of dealing with life's aggravations and turmoil. This formula is especially supportive to meditation practitioners and people who are overworked and mentally exhausted. Use one to two pills once daily in morning or evening with hot water.

Happiness of Mind

Agar 35 is often used along with another Tibetan Precious Pill called Happiness of Mind, a traditional Tibetan compound widely recommended for a wide range of imbalances, such as depression, stress, and mood complaints. These range from mild, moderate, and even severe depression to seasonal affective disorder (SAD) and "the blues." Happiness of Mind produces results for most people in a few days, often in hours. Used to manage stress, anxiety, and depression on a daily basis, many people find their overall quality of life increases. It supports the kidneys, liver, blood, and overall circulation. This formula is especially supportive for meditation practitioners and for anyone dealing with major life-changing stress. One to two pills are recommended once a day, morning or evening.

Massage and Baths

Here are simple things you can do at home to make yourself feel more comfortable during PMS and menstruation. For intense menstrual pain in the lower abdomen, sit comfortably in bed with one leg bent at the knee. Lean hard with the palms of your hands on the inner thigh of the bent leg. For support, place the bent leg on the bed. Press and hold for the count of five and repeat, moving from the groin to the inner knee area. Then reverse to sedate nerve pain on the opposite leg. This moves inflammatory pain from the abdomen on its way downward to the feet. Finish this self-massage with a foot soak and massage. Soak the feet in warm water, adding fresh lemon juice. This reduces fever conditions and inflammatory pain. Massage both feet, top and bottom, and wear warm cotton socks.

Baths and Oils

Neem is a wonderful, refreshing, and highly detoxifying tree leaf known in India for reversing complexion problems and parasites. The leaf is too bitter to consume as a tea. The link below provides capsules. I also like to add one tablespoon of powdered neem leaf to tepid bath water. Soak up the green freshness for fifteen minutes, then rinse with cool water. Add two drops of pure neem oil to a cotton swab and swab the inside of your nose in order to cool, cleanse, and refresh vision and soothe nerves that lead to the brain. The neem oil treatment can help you breathe during very dry weather or radiator heat. The earthy aroma of neem oil feels grounding for erratic or overemotional energy. Do not consume neem oil by mouth. Applying it in your nose will make your eyes appear less red and irritated. If you prefer using another oil, olive and sunflower oils are cooling for anger. Light sesame oil is nourishing and helps ground anxiety. It smells nice and refreshes mature skin to help prevent wrinkles. It is always better to treat a discomfort with a pleasure.

How Well Do You Prevent Chronic Pain?

MARK WHICH OF THE FOLLOWING LIFESTYLE CHANGES YOU HAVE BEGUN, THEN find your score at the end.

I have started to reduce my pain by:

- ❏ interrupting work every hour in order to stretch or walk around
- ❏ drinking more water
- ❏ eating more fruits and vegetables
- ❏ getting to bed earlier and staying in bed up to seven hours, whether or not I sleep
- ❏ walking more often
- ❏ using stairs instead of an elevator
- ❏ swimming or doing other gentle exercise, once or several times a week
- ❏ adjusting my diet in order to lose weight if necessary
- ❏ using a support belt or other wrap or cream for painful areas
- ❏ using a massage machine on painful areas
- ❏ using a magnet strap or belt to increase circulation for painful areas
- ❏ getting treatments by a chiropractor or body work specialist
- ❏ giving myself an oil massage every day or a few days a week
- ❏ taking relaxing herbal or mineral baths
- ❏ using herbs or foods recommended for pain
- ❏ paying more attention to the weather and dressing to avoid spasm

If you marked off three checks, you passed. If you marked off five checks, good for you! You pass with a B+. Seven or more checks and you've earned an A.

Part Two

Heal Quickly
and Painlessly

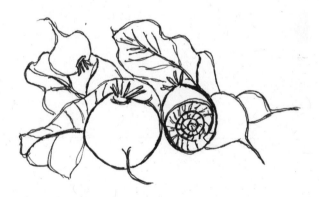

CHAPTER EIGHT

Home and Field Injuries

The two enemies of human happiness are pain and boredom.

—Arthur Schopenhauer (German philosopher, 1788–1860)

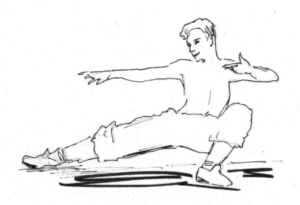

SCHOPENHAUER BELIEVED THE WORLD IS NOT A RATIONAL PLACE BUT AN EXPRESsion of blind, striving will. He lived a quiet contemplative life, according to his temperament, sacrificing pleasure in order to avoid pain. Those of us who work around the house cooking, building, and decorating or men and women in the battlefield would agree: life is not always rational, and boredom—call it inattention—does great harm. Whether kitchen burns, hammer blows, cuts, bug bites, or gunshot wounds, mental fuzziness allows injury to happen. This chapter will help you survive with life and limb from home and field injuries. Chinese martial arts Dit Da Jow ointments and plasters are of particular use to anyone who suffers muscle pains, bruises, sprains, puncture wounds, and broken bones.

Burns

According to the American Burn Association, approximately five hundred thousand people are treated yearly for burns. Among them, 70 percent are males aged eighteen to thirty-five years with wounds occurring in a residential setting. The highest numbers of scalding victims are kids aged one to five years and adults over sixty-five. Burns can result from exposure to chemicals, bare electrical wires, radiation, light, heat, and friction. First-degree burns affect the upper layer of skin, making the skin red and causing pain. Second-degree burns affect deeper tissue, cause blisters, and take longer to heal. Infection is a possible result of burns. Watch for pus formation and inform your doctor, who may prescribe antibiotics. Most authorities recommend dousing a first-degree burn with cold water, but there are better remedies in your kitchen. Never apply butter or anything oily to a burn, because it can deepen and aggravate the burn and the pain.

Tea

One of the best simple remedies for superficial burns is tea. Cold, strongly brewed, strained black tea makes a good wash for kitchen and ironing burns. It is astringent, which means it prevents oozing wounds. It is antibacterial and begins the healing process, making new cells for skin-damage accidents. Pour it on without rubbing and repeat this every five or ten minutes until the skin feels soothed. I always keep my tea in a porcelain (not metal) teapot overnight. The following morning, the cold, strained tea makes a refreshing facial astringent. Use it for tired skin as well as for burns.

Aloe

Aloe vera gel kept in the refrigerator also feels good on burns and cuts. Aloe vera is one of the only plants in nature that repairs itself. Cut a piece of aloe leaf and within a day it will have grown over the wound to repair the cut. Aloe is alkaline and full of amino acids; hormones; sterols to reduce inflammation; vitamins A, B, C, and E; choline; folic acid; and minerals including calcium, chromium, copper, iron, magnesium, manganese, potassium, phosphorous, sodium, and zinc. Vitamins A, C, and E provide aloe vera's antioxidant activity to neutralize free radicals.

The B vitamins and choline are involved in amino acid metabolism. Vitamin B12 and folic acid are required for producing blood cells. Folate, the form of folic acid naturally found in plants, is safer than any nutritional supplement because it works with the total plant to produce results. Nutritional supplements have been known to contain contamination or cheap substitutions. For example, most of the folic acid supplements available in American health-food stores originate in China. It is better to have your own plant or a reliable source of organic aloe vera gel, for internal and external use.

Spread the aloe gel on a burn and, unless it is deep, do not cover the burn with gauze because it may stick to the wound. A good combination for an allergic or other itchy skin rash is aloe gel mixed with a dash of antibiotic turmeric powder. It turns skin and clothes yellow, but takes away the sting and itch.

Cuts, Scrapes, and Superficial Wounds

Let's define a cut as a narrow tear in the skin, for example made by a kitchen knife, a razor blade, or a piece of broken glass. If it is deep, there may be damage to underlying muscle, tendons, and nerves. A scrape may result from rubbing the skin against a rough surface such as pavement. The outer surface of the skin may not be broken, but since small blood vessels are ruptured, the skin may ooze blood. A puncture wound is deeper, caused by a nail, pin, or other sharp object. Deep cuts and puncture wounds require medical attention because they can result in infection. If the wound develops pus or you have a fever, signs of infection, see a doctor as soon as possible. Small cuts and punctures usually heal by themselves in a week to ten days.

Wash the injury with cold water. Remove loose debris such as slivers and glass with tweezers cleaned by washing in soap and water and then dipping in alcohol or by placing the tweezers' tips in a flame. Allow a puncture wound to bleed for a few minutes in order to clean the site. Otherwise, stop the bleeding. Apply pressure with a clean cloth or paper towel. Stopping the bleeding may take as long as ten minutes. Do not remove the bloody cloth but apply a new one on top. If the blood spurts like a fountain, a blood vessel is damaged and the wound requires immediate medical attention.

Spit

The cavemen had it right. One home remedy recommended in a study published by the *Lancet* is saliva. Researchers found that nitrites in saliva react with the skin to make nitric oxide, which kills bacteria and speeds healing. Other popular cleansers, including alcohol, iodine, Mercurochrome, and hydrogen peroxide, are irritating and should be avoided. For small cuts and scrapes, antibiotic ointments are usually unnecessary, but keep them clean with Betadine (povidone-iodine) ointment.

You can apply a gauze bandage or Band-Aid that doesn't stick to your skin, changing it at least once daily if the cut is in an area exposed to dirt. An ointment that keeps a bandage from sticking to the wound is petroleum jelly. New soft skin will form under the petroleum jelly covered with a bandage. Applying drying antiseptic liquids to cuts and wounds toughens the scar.

Check with a health-care specialist if bleeding comes in spurts; if the wound is deep or irregular so that you need stitches; if your face is cut and requires plastic surgery; if you injure yourself with a garden tool or dirty object; if you have been exposed to someone with a staph infection and may have shared food, sports equipment, or clothing with that person; if you have not had a tetanus booster within the past five years; or if signs of infection develop. They are redness, swelling, discharge, fever, or red streaks spreading from the wound site. (The same applies to bug bites.)

Do not pick at scabs, but allow them to do their work by covering the wound. After bleeding and pain have stopped, the scab has fallen off, and a scar has begun to form, you can apply an antiscar cream. Available in most pharmacies, they may contain irritants such as extract of onion, silicone, or other ingredients that keep the skin pliant while minimizing scaring.

Bug Bites

Mosquitoes

With bugs, the best defense is avoidance. Mosquitoes love the smell of sweet fruits and bananas coming through your pores. They will follow you to bite your acidic blood. They dislike the smell of B vitamins, so take a large dose before going outside during the season. You might also mix mint, lavender, and citronella essential oils as a fragrance. Add five to ten drops of each to a teaspoon of kitchen oil, such as olive, canola, or sunflower, and apply it to exposed areas. Wear clothing as protection. An old Vermont method is to rub the skin with sheets of fabric softener, but I prefer essential oils to such chemicals. You might stick some sheets of fabric softener into your clothing instead of wearing it on skin. For itchy mosquito bites, the simple home remedy is to apply a drop of plain liquid ammonia. Avoid the eyes and other sensitive areas. Bugs bites can also infect, so be watching for the signs.

Spiders, Wasps, Bees, and Others

I once sat next to a young Army medic on an airplane, who told me our troops in Iraq were more concerned about an especially ugly, deadly spider whose bite caused great swelling and pain. The resulting infection might be fatal if not medically treated. For such bites, including bee and wasp stings, I also recommend the following Chinese herbal capsule as a first line of defense. It is Yunnan Paiyao (also known as Yunnan Baiyao or Yunnan white powder), made in

Yunnan, China, and available in Chinese herb shops and online. The Chinese People's Liberation Army uses it for deep puncture wounds, infections, surgery, and gunshot wounds. It stops hemorrhage from deep wounds and internal bleeding. It also reduces swelling and pain from bug bites by helping to normalize circulation while it repairs injury. The contents of Yunnan Paiyao capsules can be poured into deep wounds in order to bring out the infection from deeper layers of skin. The capsule is also taken orally to stop hemorrhage and internal bleeding.

Yunnan Paiyao aerosol spray is very good to keep on hand. Do not spray it on open wounds because it may burn. The spray activates blood circulation, relieving pain and eliminating swelling and blood stasis. It is used for the treatment of bruises, contusions, parenchymal contusions, muscular aches, and pain due to rheumatic arthritis. Yunnan Paiyao analgesic tincture offers temporary relief of minor aches and pains of muscles and joints due to simple backache, arthritis, strains, bruises, and sprains. Yunnan Baiyao Woundplast bandages are used for the treatment of small open and surgical cuts. They are hemostatic, analgesic, and antiphlogistic, aiding in stopping bleeding, reducing pain, and speeding clotting time.

You can find Yunnan Paiyao in all Chinese herb shops and supermarkets. There are many websites that sell the capsules and powder, but my favorite online source of Yunnan Paiyao and other herbal products for injury is Modern Herb Shop, run by Suigetsu Dojo, a traditional Japanese martial arts school located on Long Island in New York. The Japanese kanji for Suigetsu (Sui = Water, Getsu = Moon) represent clarity of mind, integrity of spirit, and devotion to purpose. They apply those principles to the Modern Herb Shop. They do not have a storefront, but you can order herbal products and martial arts gear online from them. The website for products is www.modernherbshop.com, and the website for the dojo is www.suigetsu.com.

Here is a chart showing some popular martial arts treatments for various sorts of injuries. They work fast and are safe to use except on open wounds.

Common Chinese Pain Liniments and Balms for External Use		
Name	Actions/Uses	Main Ingredients
Po Sum On Chinese massage oil	For sore, tight inflexible muscle, stiff knees, sore joints, and tight backs. Can also be used for chronic coughs (massage throat front and back of chest), giddiness, common cold, muscle sprains, minor bleeding, sea sickness, mosquito bites, itching, and burns. Rub oil on affected parts as frequently as possible to produce good results.	Menthol 13%, Vaseline, beeswax, white paraffin wax, stearic acid, peppermint, cinnamon, tea oil, licorice, and scutellariae root (skullcap).
Die Da Wan Hua oil	An excellent liniment for injuries where a hardened mass has formed. Also applied to traumatic swelling, infected burns, and open wounds.	Active: Turpentine oil 6% Inactive: Camellia (Chinese name for Tsubaki oil), (Chinese name for *Cleistocalyx operculatus*) flower, dock root (yang ti huang), dragon's blood resin (xue jie), drynaria (gu sui bu) rhizome, kudzu flower (ge hua), lacca secretion (zi cao rong), lineate supplejack (Chinese name for *Berchemia lineata*) root, ragwort (Chinese name for *Senecio palmatus*), safflower (hong hua) flower, safflower (hong hua) oil, and winter sweet (Chinese name for *Calycanthus praecox*).

Name	Actions/Uses	Main Ingredients
Zheng Gu Shui	"Rectify Bone Liquid" penetrates to the bone level to promote healing and stop pain. It is well known for its effectiveness at healing deep bone bruises and fractures.	Notoginseng Sheg Tian Qi 25%,Tiglium Wu Ma Xun Cheng 18%, Croton Ji Gu Xiang, Angelica Bai Zhi, Fleminingia Qian Jin Ba, Inula Da Li Wang, Mentha Bo He Nao, and Camphora Zhang Nao.
White Flower analgesic oil (also called Pak Fah Yeow)	Can be applied to joints and lower backache for arthritis, neuralgia, rheumatism, and lumbar pain. It dispels blood stasis, bruises, and swelling injury	Active ingredients: Wintergreen 40%, menthol 15%, and camphor 6%. Inactive ingredients: eucalyptus 18%, peppermint 15%, and lavender 6%.

Carpal Tunnel, Sprains, and Bruises

Chinese traditional hospitals and martial arts clubs often make their own herbal Dit Da Jow medicines for relieving pain and injuries. Dit Da Jow (also known as Die Da Jiu; Dit Da Jao) literally means "hit-fall wine." Most martial arts shops sell liquids, of various strengths, called Dit Da Jow. The liniment, a customized blend of herbs considered the number one remedy for bruises of all kinds, is rubbed into the skin to heal bruises, sprains and strains, carpal tunnel inflammation, shin splints, and other injuries. Pain disappears quickly because stuck qi and blood (making bruises) are moved by the medicinal ingredients. There is an old saying in Chinese: "*Tong Ze Bu Tong, Ze Tong Bu Tong,*" which means, "Where there is pain there is no flow; where there is flow there is no pain." For useful tips on using and storing Dit Da Jow plasters see: www.eastmeetswest.com /dit-da-jow/, a website devoted to martial arts information. Here is an example of one user's experience with Dit Da Jow:

> The best way to use Dit Da Jow if you are training in the martial arts is to apply some to the areas of the body that are going to make contact, let's say if you're punching a bag or makawari, apply some to your hands prior to training, like twenty to thirty minutes, then apply some more right after training; just enough to fill your palm should be sufficient. If you are kicking a bag then of course your shins would need more. For the everyday person who bruises easily, apply twice a day morning and night on the areas you need. I have found it is best to apply and let air-dry instead of wiping it with a

cloth; this will allow for more of the Dit Da Jow to penetrate the skin and help the healing process.

The Modern Herb Shop Dit Da Jow Bruise Liniment contains cooling herbs to reduce swelling and inflammation as effectively as ice and warming herbs that kill pain, promote circulation, and break up accumulations of stagnant blood and fluids. The combination provides an overall synergistically balanced formula to speed healing. It has been aged a minimum of six months, unlike many commercial formulas that are aged only a few weeks. Their Extra-Strength Jow has been aged more than one year.

Apply externally, avoiding broken skin, as soon as possible after the injury and two or three times per day or more for the next twenty-four to thirty-six hours. For bruises, put a small amount in your palm and pat gently into the injured area. Then use your thumb or three fingers to massage sore spots and break up lumps of accumulation. Start lightly and gradually work the liniment in more deeply as the pain subsides. For pulled muscles and sprains, massage the liniment into knots in the muscle. Try to break up knots by following the direction of the muscle fibers (longitudinally). Also massage into the muscle attachments.

Broken Bones

Bone-knitting powder has been used for centuries by martial arts physicians and the warrior monks of Shaolin to treat injuries from combat and training. The herbs in this powder specifically strengthen bones, tendons, and ligaments. For this reason, "bone-knitting" powder can be used to treat recurring sprains due to overstretched ligaments. When ligaments become overstretched, the joints they hold in place become less stable, which in turn can lead to joint damage.

This amazing powder, made by Modern Herb Shop, is recommended for bone fractures, dislocations, torn or damaged ligaments (such as neck, ACL, or medial collateral ligaments), torn cartilage (such as the meniscus), as well as torn tissue and overstretched joints that become unstable. This formula is also great for recurring sprains and fractures that are slow healing. This combination of nine herbs helps the body to clear any residual blood stagnation, promotes circulation, prevents atrophy, repairs damaged tissue, "tonifies the kidneys" (in traditional Chinese medicine, this refers to increasing adrenal energy), which in turn, strengthens and heals broken bones and encourages the body to heal itself. The regular formula contains bones or animal ingredients, but there is also a vegetarian version, which is slightly less effective.

The powder is taken internally from the third week of injury for up to four weeks. Mix one-fourth to one-half teaspoon powdered herb with enough water, juice, or strong liquor to mix it up to swallow; or mix with honey to make a small ball and swallow. Take twice daily for up to four weeks. The package contains approximately 50 grams powdered herbs per jar—enough for eight weeks. **Cautions: do not take this formula if there is infection present**. It is also not recommended for broken ribs (use Rib Fracture Formula instead). Do not take if pregnant or nursing.

Medicated Oil for Fractures

Zheng Gu Shui, or Rectify Bone Liquid, penetrates to the bone level to promote healing and stop pain. See the chart on the preceding pages. It is effective for healing deep bone bruises and fractures. In case of fractures, set the bones first. Soak the fracture immediately and continuously with this liquid for pain, bruising, swelling, and healing. Soak cotton balls or gauze with Zheng Gu Shui and apply, wrapping the cotton loosely with gauze. Leave on one hour for upper body, an hour and a half for lower limbs. Shorten the time for children. Do this two times a day until the bone is healed. It is useful before or after exercise for soreness and to strengthen tendons. It can be added to bath water. **Caution: do not apply to broken skin or open wounds.**

Letha's Advice: A Chinese Fix-Everything Oil

The Chinese love to formulate herbal potions to simultaneously accomplish a wide variety of curative effects. Here is a good one: Kwan Loong Pain-Relieving Aromatic Oil. It is used for fast, effective relief of dizziness, headaches, motion sickness, a stuffed-up nose, stomachaches, sprains, and rheumatic pains, and it speeds healing of insect bites. You can sniff it for nasal congestion headaches or spread it on skin lightly with a sterile cotton ball.

The active ingredients are methyl salicylate and menthol, with eucalyptus oil, light mineral oil, and spike lavender oil as inactive ingredients. Adults and children twelve years of age and older can apply a few drops to the affected area and rub gently three to four times daily. For children under twelve, consult a physician. Avoid the eyes.

Non-Chinese Pain Remedies for Injury

Xtra Mint Muscle Rub: Sprains, Aching Muscles, and Joints

My friend Judy sprained muscles in her neck after hitting her head when she fell in the shower. She was dizzy and in great pain, but a CT scan showed no permanent injury. I gave her an innocent-looking salve called Xtra Mint Muscle Rub, made with wild-crafted herbs and essential oils by The Twelve Tribes, a born-again Christian community I know from Vermont, who have communities scattered throughout the world. The rub worked wonderfully well to ease Judy's muscle pain and feeling of injury. (Note: relieving stiff neck and shoulder pain with such a relaxing, balancing remedy may also improve sleep.) The ingredients are castor oil, beeswax, sweet almond oil, lanolin, eucalyptus, wintergreen, menthol, peppermint, clove bud, and nutmeg (essential oils). "The Tribe," as we call them, makes quality, wholesome cosmetic creams, lotions, and bath and body products without additives and chemicals. The delightfully polite and industrious community has restaurants and clothing stores in New England. Their products are sold online at www.commonsensefarm.com.

Homeopathic Arnica: Bruises and Pain

Most pharmacies carry arnica cream or ointment for pain and bruising. Actually, the ingredient is *homeopathic* arnica because arnica, a wild desert flower, is an irritant. Mexican herbalists brew a tea of arnica flowers for asthma, but the most common use in North America is a skin treatment for bruises. Plastic surgeons who know something about natural remedies recommend its use after surgery. It does not stain or sting. It can be used for chronic aching muscles that feel better with massage.

Papaya and pineapple enzyme pills are useful, if you don't mind eating a handful several times a day. Papain and bromelain are anti-inflammatory for injuries and digestive, which helps overcome dietary abuse. Clearing the body of toxins with digestive enzymes often improves circulation and speeds healing. One powerful combination is Super Enzyme Caps made by Twinlab, a maximum-strength dietary supplement that contains pancreatin, betaine hydrochloride, pepsin, bromelain, and papain.

CHAPTER NINE

Sports Injuries

Have you noticed that whatever sport you're trying to learn, some earnest person is always telling you to keep your knees bent?

—Dave Barry (American journalist, 1947–)

SPORTS AND RECREATIONAL ACTIVITIES ACCOUNT FOR 21 PERCENT OF ALL TRAU-matic brain injuries among American children, but authorities don't agree on the most injury-prone sport. Some say it is basketball, others football. One thing everyone agrees on is that knee injuries are the most frequent, painful, and hard to treat. Ask any skier. For that reason, this chapter is mostly about knees, with shorter sections for hip pain and tennis elbow. That should help protect runners, golfers, skiers, dancers, game players, and walkers of all ages.

If God intended us to have trouble-free knees, we would look like wood storks. Unfortunately, our knees, the largest, most poorly constructed joints in the body, hardly bear our weight. The knee joint, like the elbow, depends on muscles for stability and alignment. The hamstrings and quadriceps serve both the hips and knees. Large demands are placed on these muscles, and they are prone to dysfunction. The knee is ill-equipped to handle stress placed on short, tight leg muscles. Injuries to the knee cause changes in our gait and leg alignment which affect posture. You may be surprised to learn how posture affects the knees.

Your Back and Knees

Working with a computer, reading, or watching television, while sitting for hours in a chair, damages the knees, because keeping the spine vertical or slumping in a chair weakens the muscles in our back. Those muscles become stiff and short, which causes a stress overload for the joints they serve, especially the hips and knees. We feel that stress when rising from a chair. Our knees are supposed to provide stability and flexibility for the body, allowing our legs to bend, swivel, and straighten. However, if they lack proper nourishment and blood circulation, knees become stiff, swollen, and easily injured. The knee is made up of bones, cartilage, muscles, ligaments, and tendons, all working together. So a knee injury could stress or damage any of these parts. Doctors and sports enthusiasts warn against knee injuries, recommending that we wear correct exercise shoes for support, warm up before exercise, and cool down afterward with stretches, yoga, and Pilates exercises. That is good advice, but let's get more specific.

Sliding Scale for Knees

This sliding scale advice section goes from really easy health tips to more complex treatment, including exercise. Foods to avoid are hot and spicy, drying salty foods, dairy foods (a pain trigger for many people), and alcohol. Drinking lots of water is supposed to hydrate muscles, tendons, bones, and joints. However, for many people, that just means more visits to the toilet. We need special targeted herbs that keep joints moistened and supportive tissue strong and flexible. That's how Asian medicine excels by offering specific treatments for specific areas of the body.

Injury Prevention: Juicy Joints

Be sure to read the previous chapter covering useful pain liniments. They can help to eliminate knee pain and stiffness and avoid injury. For example, apply a pain liniment or Dit Da Jow bruise liquid to your knees as part of your stretches and warm up before walking or other exercise.

Guan Jie Yan Wan

Some people have special knee problems. The Chinese patent remedy Guan Jie Yan Wan, translated as "close down joint inflammation pills," can be used by people with either cold or hot symptoms, which include respectively a pale tongue, chills, and weakness or a red tongue with inflammatory pain. The pain may be medically diagnosed as arthritis or rheumatism. If your knees hurt during bad weather, this is your remedy. One major ingredient, erythrinae bark, treats lower back and knee pain. Other ingredients, including barley, ginger, and cinnamon, reduce leg swelling. Stephania and achyranthes, often used for leg pain, lead the other herbs to where they are needed in the body—to the knees. The usual dosage is eight pills, three times daily between meals. You can take more as needed. (Remember: at mealtimes, use digestive remedies. Treat other problems between meals.)

Letha's Advice: Yucca—It's Estrogenic

Some forty to fifty varieties of yucca grow wild in desert areas. Its tall, elegant stalk blooms every several years. Cassava (also known as yuca or manioc), often confused with yucca, belongs to the *Euphorbiaceae* (spurge) family native to South America, and is cultivated as a crop for its edible starchy root. Cassava is the third-largest source of carbohydrates for meals in the world. You can buy cassava roots in some supermarkets and Latin American street food shops. You have to peel off the tough brown bark and boil it like a potato, but the root does not offer adequate lubrication for joints. Yucca capsules are a concentrated herbal medicine that reduces joint pain and swelling.

Nature's Way describes their capsules this way: "Yucca stalk (*Yucca schidigera*) supports joints and blood sugar problems. Beneficial saponins are found in the yucca plant's stalk and root." Saponins, as the name implies, are slippery like soap. They make the joints juicy. The standard dose is two capsules yielding 980 milligrams of yucca stalk, which is 1 gram of carbohydrates. However, you know the best dosage depends on your pain. Yucca is estrogenic, soothing, moistening, and cooling for painful knees. It shrinks swelling and makes knee joints feel juicy when used in large doses of ten to fifteen capsules per day. If the dose is too high, resulting in cramps and diarrhea, then reduce the dose to whatever is comfortable for you. If you have slow digestion, frequent nausea, or diarrhea, you will need to start with the standard dose along with a digestive remedy such as one-fourth to one-half teaspoon of ginger powder in warm water. Avoid all estrogenic foods, even coffee, if you have an active estrogen-sensitive cancer.

Knee Stretches for Three Minutes

We love anything that works fast and well! Dr. Joseph Weisberg, PT, PhD, and Heidi Shink wrote *3 Minutes to a Pain-Free Life: The Groundbreaking Program for Total Body Pain Prevention and Rapid Relief*. I was impressed by reader comments online from people whose pain improved after using their exercises. Wonderful! You don't have to be a jock to do them. I have modified the moves to make them even easier to do.

Natural Squat: If you can squat with your feet flat on the floor, you are in good shape. My arthritis prevents it. So I passed up this movement. If you can hold a squat for thirty seconds without outside support by holding on to something, it strengthens the lower back and pelvis, hips, leg muscles, knees, and ankles. The modified form is easy. Hold a door knob with both hands. Gently, slowly lower yourself about three inches by bending the knees. Hold for the count of ten. Lower yourself another three inches for another count of ten. Feel the pull on thigh muscles becoming toned. Slowly raise yourself. Repeat a few times.

The Split: There are two ways to do this. One way, if you are stronger, is to stand, spreading your legs as far as you can while keeping your feet parallel. Hold this position for fifteen seconds. Then bend at the waist and lean forward as far as you can, keeping your knees straight. Hold this position for fifteen seconds.

The second way to do the split works well for seniors or others who need additional support for the movements. The exercise targets the lower back, hips, hamstring and inner thigh muscles, groin, and knees. The muscles near the hip need to be strong enough to support the hip joint as well as to protect the knees. Sit comfortably on a chair and spread your legs as far apart as you can. Place your heels on the floor and point your toes upward. Keep your knees slightly bent. Hold this position for fifteen seconds. Then bend at your waist so that you grasp your shins and look at the floor. Hold this position for fifteen seconds. Modified: bend over and grasp your knees.

The Sitter: This is for knee pain, inflammation, spasms, limited mobility, sprains, strains, arthritis, bursitis, synovitis, and tendinitis. Sit on a chair and lift both feet about two inches off the floor. Cross your right ankle over your left and press it against the left ankle as hard as you can. Resist the downward push for five seconds. Relax and switch feet. Do the entire procedure six times for a total of thirty seconds per leg. Repeat this daily until your symptoms are relieved. Modified: sit as described and do the cross-ankle exercise without lifting your feet off the floor.

Two Homeopathic Remedies

Homeopathic remedies can offer quick relief without complications. In cases where inflammation must be reduced quickly or ice must be used, homeopathic iron ferrum phosphate 30C is useful. After initial inflammatory pain and swelling are reduced with homeopathic ferrum phosphate 30C, homeopathic arnica 30C can be used to reduce bruising and increase circulation. Follow directions for use on the label, and do not mix homeopathic remedies with foods or beverages. They can be used until the symptom improves; then the treatment will continue to work on its own. A potency of 30C is for acute injury, and 6X is used for chronic injury. The letters X and C are used to describe the dilution of the remedy. A remedy that has been diluted ten times is X and one hundred times is C, which means that it enters the bloodstream quicker. Although you may feel much better using natural therapies, give yourself adequate time to heal before returning to activities.

Medical Diagnosis and Treatment of Specific Types of Knee Injuries

Below is a brief summary of typical approaches taken by many medical doctors. X-rays, MRIs, and CT scans may be necessary as well as examination by a doctor. Do not limit your treatment options. Exercise or physical therapy is now recommended more often than rest in many cases of acute pain. Platelet-rich plasma (PRP) and stem-cell injections are now preferred in many cases over surgery.

Muscle Tendon Injuries

These strains are usually treated with ice, elevation, and rest. Sometimes compression with an Ace wrap or knee sleeve is recommended. Crutches may be used for a short time to assist with walking. Doctors recommend an over-the-counter anti-inflammatory for pain, but I prefer applying a cooling rub, either Chinese White Flowers or White Tiger Balm, to ease muscle stiffness, as it reduces inflammation.

The mechanism of injury is either hyperextension, in which the hamstring muscles can be stretched or torn, or hyperflexion, in which the quadriceps muscle is injured. The patellar or quadriceps tendon can be damaged or ruptured. Surgery may be recommended if you cannot extend the knee. Usually tears of the hamstring muscle are treated conservatively without an operation, allowing time, exercise, and perhaps physical therapy to return the muscle to normal function.

Medial Collateral Ligament (MCL) and Lateral Collateral Ligament (LCL) Injuries

These ligaments can be stretched or torn when the foot is planted and a sideways force is directed to the knee. This can cause significant pain and difficulty walking as the body tries to protect the knee, but there is usually little swelling within the knee. The standard treatment for this injury may include a knee immobilizer, a removable Velcro splint that keeps the knee straight and keeps the knee stable. RICE (rest, ice, compression, and elevation) are the mainstays of treatment. However, Dr. Matthew Gammons, MD, a sports medicine doctor working at a thriving New England ski area, advised me that these injuries are generally best treated in a brace that helps stability and allows motion as opposed to an immobilizer. For MCL injuries, he uses PRP (platelet rich plasma) injections, which use the patient's own blood platelets to speed healing. PRP is covered in chapter 18.

Anterior Cruciate Ligament (ACL) Injuries

If the foot is planted and force is applied from the front or back to the knee, then the cruciate ligaments can be damaged. Swelling in the knee occurs within minutes, and attempts at walking are difficult. The definitive diagnosis is difficult because swelling and pain make it hard to test if the ligament is loose. Long-term treatment may require surgery and significant physical therapy to return good function of the knee joint. Recovery from these injuries is measured in months, not weeks. I heard from Dr. Gammons that this is the most frequent knee injury resulting from skiing accidents. According to him, "ACL tears are akin to cutting a rope that is stretched across a room. The two cut ends will not lie near enough to each other to reconnect."

Meniscus Tears

The cartilage of the knee can be acutely injured or gradually tear. When acute, the injury is a twist; the cartilage that is attached to and lies flat on the tibia is pinched between the femoral condyle and the tibial plateau. Pain and swelling occur gradually over many hours as opposed to an ACL tear, which swells quickly. Sometimes the injury seems trivial, but chronic pain develops when walking uphill or climbing steps. The knee may give way, resulting in falls. An MRI may be used to confirm the diagnosis. Knee surgery is famously difficult, slow healing, and may lead to scarring that continues pain. Therapies that may speed healing include LED light therapy, PRP injections, and Dit Da Jow pain ointments.

Fractures

Fractures are relatively common. The patella, or kneecap, may fracture from a fall directly onto it. If the bone is pulled apart, surgery will be required for repair, but if the bone is in good position, a knee immobilizer may be all that is required. The head of the fibula on the lateral side of the knee joint can be fractured either by a direct blow or as part of an injury to the shin or ankle. This bone usually heals with little intervention, but fractures of this bone can have a major complication. The peroneal nerve wraps around the bone and can be damaged by the fracture. This will cause a foot drop, so do not be surprised if the physician examines your foot when you complain of knee problems.

With jumping injuries, the surface of the tibia can be damaged, resulting in a fracture to the tibial plateau. Since this is where the femoral condyle sits to move the knee joint, it is important that it heals in the best position possible. For that reason, after plain X-rays reveal this fracture, a CT scan is done to make certain that there is no displacement of the bones. Occasionally, this type of fracture requires surgery for repair. Fractures of the femur require significant force, except for people with osteoporosis (thinning bones). In people with knee replacements who fall, there is a potential weakness at the site of the knee replacement above the femoral condyle, and this can be a site of fracture. The decision to operate or treat by immobilization with a cast is usually made by an orthopedist.

Patellar Injuries

The patella can dislocate laterally (toward the outside of the knee). This occurs more commonly in women because of anatomic differences in the angle aligning the femur and tibia. Fortunately, the dislocation is easily returned to the normal position by straightening out the knee, usually resulting in the kneecap popping into place. Physical therapy for muscle strengthening may be needed to prevent recurrent dislocations.

Patellofemoral syndrome occurs when the underside of the patella becomes inflamed if irritation develops as it rides its path with each flexion and extension of the knee, and it does not track smoothly. This inflammation can cause localized pain, especially with walking down stairs and with running. Treatment includes ice, anti-inflammatory medication, and exercises to balance the quadriceps muscle. Severe cases may require surgery to remove some of the inflamed cartilage and realign parts of the quadriceps muscle.

Acupuncture for Knee Pain

Acupuncture, now considered a medical specialty used by the World Health Organization (WHO), was considered witch-doctor treatment (except in Asia and Latin America) when I studied it some thirty years ago. The knee conditions generally responsive to medical acupuncture include knee osteoarthritis, bursitis, tendinitis, strains, and local contusions, as well as improvement in motion with conditions such as hamstring and quadriceps strains.

In a study conducted by the University of Maryland School of Medicine that included 570 patients receiving either acupuncture or sham acupuncture treatments for knee osteoarthritis, the acupuncture patients received improvement in function and pain relief in comparison to the sham treatments (Berman et al. 2004).

To simplify, it appears that putting a needle through the skin or using a cold laser serves to improve local blood flow to an area that may have relative ischemia (a lack of blood flow), that then benefits greatly from a local improvement in circulation. This is particularly true for conditions that involve strain and swelling. With the addition of electrical stimulation, which is frequently used in conjunction with acupuncture, there is proof of local production of beta-endorphins, the body's natural painkilling and pain-modulating substance.

Home Acupuncture Treatments

If ice or anti-inflammatory medicines are recommended, acupuncture may be useful. The points are easy to find. Use a cold laser that does not puncture the skin—not needles—in order to avoid pain, bruising, and possible infection. You can order an inexpensive laser adequate for acupuncture treatments online. See the Recommended Natural Product Sources section at the back of the book. Links for recommended companies are also provided at www.asianhealth secrets.com.

Locate the painful points. Do not move the kneecap, but touch lightly all around the edges of the kneecap. Often the acupuncture points treated to reduce pain and swelling under the kneecap are located in the impressions in front and below the kneecap and surrounding the kneecap. Touching will indicate how sensitive the points feel. Place the laser against these points, pointing the light toward the center and underneath the kneecap. Hold the laser light there to the count of twenty or up to three minutes; then move on to the next point. Repeat this once or twice daily as needed. Important: never point a laser light toward the eyes or heart. Use it for local pain and swelling at the front and back of the knee. If pain continues or gets worse after treatment, get a medical diagnosis to be sure you are treating the right problem. If using a laser is out of the question for you, apply a cooling Dit Da Jow bruise liniment or White Flowers, described in the previous chapter.

Letha's Lazy Exercise Advice for Pain Prevention

The *Calgary Herald* reports, "An astonishing 50 percent of runners in Canada will grapple with a running-related injury every year. Of those injuries, 60 percent will involve the knee." How can runners protect their knees? According to Matt Fitzgerald, senior editor at Competitor Group, who has written *Brain Training for Runners* and *Racing Weight*, "Core training is essential for runners." What is "core training"? Think of an apple core. It holds the seeds. Here is how I firm my core.

I am really lazy, a nonexerciser, except for an occasional leisurely dip in a swimming pool. I perfected my technique by watching sea turtles slowly glide through the water. I was happy to learn from my chiropractor that the core, including abdominal muscles that support the front and back, can be strengthened by sitting on a big rubber ball. "Balloon sitting" became a favorite pastime while I wrote health articles for my website.

Core Exercises for Athletes

Matt Fitzgerald, an exercise expert, offers advice to improve muscle tone. Do not try his suggestions if you are out of shape. According to Matt, "A strong core enhances running performance and may reduce injury risk. The best core exercises for runners are those that mimic the specific ways the core muscles are required to work during running." They include the supine march, standing trunk rotation, and suitcase dead lift. It is best to get personal attention from a trainer in order to avoid injury. Here is a summary.

Supine March

The supine march tones the transverse abdominis, a deep abdominal muscle that needs to hold the right amount of tension to prevent excessive movement of the pelvis and lumbar spine during running. Lie face up on the floor with both knees sharply bent and your feet flat on the floor. Press your low back into the floor. While concentrating on keeping your low back pressed into the floor, lift your left leg straight up until your left foot comes even with your right knee. Then slowly lower the foot back to the floor. Repeat with the right leg. Continue until you begin to feel an abdominal tension, up to twenty repetitions per leg.

Standing Trunk Rotation with Cable

Among the biggest energy wasters in running is excessive rotation of the hips, pelvis, and/or spine. The standing rotation with cable isolates and intensifies this particular challenge. This is a gym exercise. I would not attempt it without guidance. Matt says, "Stand with your left side facing a cable pulley station with a handle attached at shoulder height. Grasp the handle with both hands and both arms fully extended. Begin with your torso rotated toward the handle and tension in the cable (i.e., the weight stack is slightly elevated from the resting position). Rotate your torso to the right while keeping your arms fully extended and the handle in line with the center of your chest. Keep your eyes focused on the handle as you rotate and your hips locked forward. Return to the start position without allowing the weight stack to come to rest. Complete twelve repetitions, then reverse your position and repeat the exercise."

Suitcase Dead Lift

The suitcase dead lift trains the oblique muscles on the sides of the torso to keep the torso vertically in line. The low back muscles are also challenged in a running-specific way in this exercise. Stand with your arms hanging at your sides and a dumbbell in one hand. Push your hips back, bend the knees, and reach the dumbbell down as close to the floor as you can without rounding your lower back. Now stand up again. Don't allow your torso to tilt to either side while performing this movement. Complete ten repetitions, rest for thirty seconds, then repeat the exercise while holding the dumbbell in the opposite hand. (I was hoping this exercise involved a suitcase and travel, which unfortunately it does not. I suggest this exercise can be done in a modified way sitting in a chair—especially useful for those of us who lift a cup of coffee more often than gym weights.)

Hips: The Chair Dilemma

Compared to the knees, hip joints are naturally sturdy and stable and located deep enough in the body to avoid injury. Despite their structural advantages, hip-replacement surgery is the number two most common joint replacement surgery each year, after knees. Most of the damage to hips is done little by little, by day-to-day wear and tear—neither from trauma accidents nor from trauma but from neglect.

Dr. Joseph Weisberg, PT, PhD, believes the hip joint's biological needs are severely underserved. "The hip is rarely taken through its full range of motion, and the muscles that serve it are rarely maintained at their optimal length." The demands placed on the hip are enormous. It is subjected to the pull of the most powerful muscles in the body and is under nearly constant pressure. But that is not the only reason we have painful hips.

It makes sense that our hip pain also results from sitting. After all, we do it much of the time. Sitting eliminates exercise and tenses lower back muscles, which impact the groin and buttocks. Here is a simple exercise that mobilizes the hip, causing the joint to be lubricated with synovial fluid. That increases movement and flexibility. In the long run, it makes the hip and lower back less vulnerable to injury. You may notice the difference in your golf swing. Another nice thing about this exercise is that you can do it sitting in your chair.

Chair Hip Roll

Sit with your butt on the edge of a chair that is firmly planted and support yourself with your arms. With legs extended and knees straight, place your heels on the floor two feet apart. Slowly roll out your legs so that the outsides of your feet touch the floor. Your toes are pointing away from each other. Then reverse and slowly roll them inward so that the insides of your feet touch the floor. Your toes are pointing toward each other. Roll back and forth with your feet fifteen to twenty times for about thirty seconds daily.

Tennis Elbow

Epicondylitis, an inflammation of the muscles and tendons of the forearm better known as tennis elbow, results from repeated twisting of the forearm and can cause considerable pain even with simple movements such as lifting a cup. Dr. Matthew Gammons informed me that epicondylitis is better termed epicondylosis, because there is not inflammation but ongoing degeneration. This is why laser or PRP therapy may help heal tennis elbow, because they both try to stimulate healthy tendon formation.

Rest, warmth, stretches, and anti-inflammatory injections from a doctor may help temporarily, but the only treatment found to permanently relieve pain is acupuncture. But there is a simple home treatment you can use as well, to help reduce pain from tennis elbow.

Letha's Advice: Simple Home Treatment for Tennis Elbow

You can locate the painful points at the elbow very easily for yourself. Place your arm on a table and bend the elbow to place your palm flat. Douse three cotton balls with Chinese White Flower analgesic liquid and place them on the points at the elbow, hand, and pointer finger shown in the illustration. Apply medium pressure for the count of ten and release. Repeat this for up to fifteen minutes. The treatment is not as deep or effective as acupuncture, but it will bring needed blood circulation to the area to improve pain and mobility.

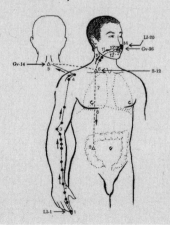

Laser Treatment of Tennis Elbow

A cold laser treatment makes injury, acupuncture pain, and infection impossible. If you have an at-home laser kit, use the acupuncture points described for tennis elbow, holding the laser light on each point for the count of twenty. Never look directly into the laser or point it toward the eyes or heart. Then move the arm slightly and repeat the treatment once or twice more. You can do this daily or on alternate days as needed until the spasm pain is resolved and mobility has recovered. Do not treat the area for longer than five minutes a day. You can apply White Flower analgesic liquid to the area if a cooling treatment feels better, or Po Sum On oil if warmth feels better.

A photon diode light stimulator can also be used. Beauty spas use light therapy to even skin color and reduce blemishes, but more recently other diodes have been used for pain. You can easily find them to buy online. Hold the light close to your painful area for the recommended time and feel a release of muscle tension. Pain management using infrared diode light therapy temporarily increases local blood circulation where applied and temporarily relieves minor muscle and joint aches and pains. The machine uses a balanced array of both visible (660 nanometer) and infrared (940 nanometer) diodes for maximum therapeutic and healing properties. I will detail the use of laser and light therapies later.

Bunions

A chapter on leg and foot pain is not complete without a word about bunions. They are very common among women, especially those of us who wear high heels or stuff our tootsies into dainty stylish shoes. Bunions are similar to bursitis in that the protective sac that holds the big toe joint in place becomes irritated from supporting body weight that has been shifted to the toes. Medical treatment of bunions is painful, to say the least. Most alternate health treatment is not much more comfortable. A massage person or chiropractor may give your big toe a yank. A foot doctor may put the big toe into a splint to keep it immobile because the tip is reaching for the second toe and the joint is sticking out away from the foot. That is the beginning of a bunion, extra bone growth at the joint. A foot surgeon may cut off the bunion and put a metal implant in place. All these treatments are very painful and hard to walk on while healing.

Our answer is simple and much more pleasing: Wear comfortable low-heeled shoes most of the time. If you do wear high heels, after you remove them, stretch out the leg muscles by standing for ten to fifteen minutes with your toes two inches higher than your heel. Massage your feet and toes daily with an oil that enhances circulation to lubricate the toe joints, such as Die Da Wan Hua oil, recommended for sprains. If it feels comforting, you might soak two cotton balls with the oil, tape them over the bunion, and wear them and cotton socks to bed.

If you already use a laser for painless acupuncture treatments, stimulating the entire bunion can help to break down the extra calcium and sometimes help relieve the pain. If you prefer a cooling homeopathic remedy to reduce joint redness and swelling, I recommend homeopathic Apis mel 6X to 30C strengths, used as directed. Avoid eating sugar, unripe citrus, and hot spices if you have inflammatory joint pains and bunions.

Stay Cool

Exercise and sports are dehydrating to the entire body, including the joints, bones, and muscles. I see people carrying water bottles at the gym. Why not drink something better for stamina than water or sugary drinks? Add black cherry concentrate to your water bottle in order to increase iron, a nourishing, anti-inflammatory food. To benefit from the natural boost to metabolism gained from a workout, eat a small meal within thirty minutes of ending exercise. Include foods that reduce pain. They are anti-inflammatory foods, muscle relaxants, and analgesics.

- Anti-inflammatory foods are high in unsaturated fats and produce anti-inflammatory prostaglandins: flaxseed, pumpkin seeds, salmon, sardines, tuna, and walnuts are a few.
- Muscle relaxants include dark leafy greens, especially broccoli and spinach, as well as artichokes, nuts, sunflower and sesame seeds, soy milk, and sweet potato—all sources of magnesium, which helps prevent cramps and headaches.
- Natural analgesics include very irritating foods. Try two drops of cayenne pepper extract on your tongue. It gets the brain to produce endorphins, natural painkillers. Cayenne (*Capsicum annuum*) is traditionally used in herbal medicine as a circulatory tonic. The active ingredient in cayenne is a pungent substance known as capsaicin. Capsaicin appears to alter the action of the bodily compound (called "substance P") that transfers pain messages to the brain, reducing pain and inflammation by short-circuiting the pain message. Avoid peppers if you have chronic digestive irritation or ulcers. Or apply a cream that contains capsaicin to aching joints.

Note: I think capsicum (capsaicin, Capzasin) is too irritating for people with thin, fragile, or mature skin. Never apply it to broken skin. If you can easily see your veins, I would avoid using capsicum products externally. I tried a "deep penetrating and odor free" roll-on (with 0.15 percent capsaicin), recommended for arthritis pain relief, simple backache, muscle strains, muscle sprains, bruises, and cramps. I felt nothing for about an hour. Then it burned deeply and ferociously for hours, even after I washed it off. The acid had deeply penetrated beyond my natural defenses. It turned my Hungarian "blue blood" red hot.

CHAPTER TEN

Computer-Related Injuries

There is no coming to consciousness without pain.

—Carl Jung (psychologist, 1875–1961)

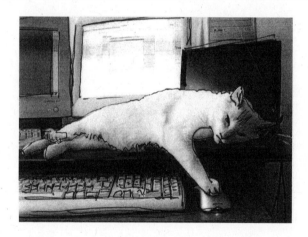

DO YOU TURN TO YOUR COMPUTER FOR COMFORT AND COMPANIONSHIP? Computer speak, LOL emails, computer games, and social networking are a way of life. A study done in cooperation with several Chinese universities and the University of Florida, published in January 2012 by the medical journal *PLoS ONE* and by *Forbes* online, reports that a new health challenge called IAD, Internet Addiction Disorder, changes the brain structure and chemistry of people addicted to computer use. The gray matter is reduced in certain areas, and other areas of the brain usually stimulated by drugs such as heroine are stimulated by computer use. Long hours at the screen can cause pain and stiffness in the entire body because of sitting under tension. However, the most crippling pain for many people is in the wrists.

Carpal tunnel syndrome is a painful, disabling disorder caused by the impingement of the median nerve that supplies function and feeling to the thumb, index, middle, and one-half of the ring finger. According to an April 2000 article titled "The Incidence of Recurrence after Endoscopic Carpal Tunnel Release," carpal tunnel syndrome is the most common nerve compression disorder of the upper extremity. Surgical treatment for carpal tunnel syndrome is the most frequent surgery of the hand and wrist, with 463,637 carpal tunnel releases annually in the United States, accounting for $1 billion in direct costs. The United States Department of Labor, Occupational Safety and Health Administration (OSHA), reports that repetitive strain injuries are the nation's most common and costly occupational health problem, costing more than $20 billion a year in workers' compensation.

In many cases, it is caused by an imbalance of muscle groups surrounding the median nerve. When left untreated, the condition leads to pain, numbness, tingling, pins and needles, stiffness, tenderness, swelling, lack of coordination, loss of grip strength, and muscle atrophy. In more severe cases, pain travels from the median nerve up the arm, creating referred pain and dysfunction throughout the forearm, shoulder, upper back, and neck.

Despite decades of research, the cause and physiology of carpal tunnel syndrome are not well understood by many physicians and therapists. Research shows that factors may include heredity, environment (workplace stressors), and illness (diabetes, renal failure). It is controversial. Who can say whether a "hereditary problem" is due to genes or an inherited diet and lifestyle? Although some of these problems are unavoidable, there are still some easy, effective ways to prevent carpal tunnel syndrome.

Prevention of Carpal Tunnel and Repetitive Stress Injuries

Therapeutic chairs, keyboards, computer mice, wrist rests, and wrist braces and splints are common options, although relief is often short-term. For long-term relief, stretches and exercises help eliminate pain and promote muscle balance with and around the carpal tunnel. This in turn relieves pressure on the median nerve and alleviates the disabling carpal tunnel symptoms. Here are a few general suggestions to improve circulation.

- Try to reduce unnecessary strain to the hands and wrists.
- Stay physically fit to keep repetitive strain injuries at bay.
- Doctors recommend exercising the muscles in the hand, wrist, forearm, and shoulder to promote optimal muscle balance to prevent

carpal tunnel syndrome from occurring. I prefer a soothing massage using a stimulating massage oil or five drops of essential oil of rosemary added to one teaspoon of olive oil.

The Heart/Arm/Wrist Connection

The heart and healthy blood vessels, free of excess cholesterol, are important for maintaining upper body comfort and health. They impact the chest, shoulders, arms, and even the hands. One thing a heart specialist checks is whether or not your hands are often numb. The following herbs help maintain circulation health and may also improve pain, tingling, and numbness.

A diet and herbal regime that protects circulation and the heart benefits general health, reduces pain, and protects against repetitive stress injuries. That means whole grains, fruits and vegetables, seaweeds, nuts, flaxseed oil, and pumpkin seeds.

We will cover herbs that regulate heart circulation vitality in chapter fifteen. They include hawthorn berry and dan shen root (*Salvia miltiorrhiza*), which we have covered and will revisit when discussing heart health and emotional balance. Those herbs reduce harmful cholesterol and normalize the heartbeat to improve upper body comfort. For health maintenance, especially if you are overweight or suffering from chronic heart failure, you might take two capsules of hawthorn once or twice daily and add one-fourth teaspoon dan shen powder to a cup of water.

I add one-fourth teaspoon of dan shen powder to a cup of tea or water daily to keep my heart and circulation healthy. I find it also improves my right-hand numbness. Researching the Chinese herb dan shen in connection with heart health, chest circulation, and prevention of upper-body repetitive stress injuries, I found an interesting abstract at www.pubmed.com by Korean researchers. Dan shen, besides its action that tones the heart muscle, regulates abnormal heartbeat, reduces harmful cholesterol, and supports thyroid activity, also impacts proliferation of cancer cells. In plain English, it helps stop breast cancer from spreading. Do you keep your emotions in your chest and shoulders? Dan shen between meals will help free your breathing and ease tensions.

Ginger Powder for Inflammation and Circulation

Another herb that increases qi circulation, the energy flow in meridians, as well as increases digestive energy, is ginger powder. It has been recommended as an anti-inflammatory for chronic pain, but I suspect that like myrrh and its cousin guggul, ginger also helps reduce cholesterol and tones blood vessel elasticity. I add one-fourth teaspoon ginger powder to warm tea twice daily, especially when I am at the computer for a long period of time, and find it reduces arthritis pain and stiffness throughout the body. Avoid ginger if you have stomach ulcers or excess acidity.

Prevent Computer-Related Injury: Ergonomic Advice

- Try an ergonomic ("ergonomic" means specially designed for comfort) keyboard that has a curved design, and use a trackball instead of a mouse.
- To prevent injuries from computer use, make sure your computer equipment and furniture fit you properly and that you use correct typing and sitting positions.
- Make sure the top of your computer screen is aligned with your forehead.
- Sit up straight with your back touching the back of your seat. Chairs that provide extra support, especially lumbar (lower back) support, are helpful. Avoid slouching over your keyboard or tensing your shoulders, which can place unnecessary stress on your neck, back, and spine. An exception may be if you have sciatica, a crippling pain that reaches from your lower back to your ankle. In that case, it may feel better to sit with your buttocks at the edge of your chair. Experiment to see which position feels better for your lower back.
- Let your legs rest comfortably with your feet flat on the floor or on a footrest.
- Use a light touch when typing. Place the keyboard close to you so that you don't have to reach for it.
- Fingers and wrists should remain level while typing. Try a wrist rest for extra support. Your wrists and forearms should be at a ninety-degree angle to the upper part of your arms. Elbows should be placed close to the side of the body to prevent bending the wrists side to side.
- Be sure to take breaks to stretch or walk around about every thirty minutes, even if you don't feel tired or in pain. I prefer lying flat and using a massager machine on my lower back and legs.

Carpal Tunnel Pain Relief with Modified Acupuncture Treatments

Acupuncture is now high-tech, simplified for home treatments presented in this book and affordable. I sympathize with people who for one reason or another are afraid of acupuncture needles. An inexpensive, small cold laser and a muscle stimulating machine (a.k.a. TENS stimulator) are easily available online and can do the work of acupuncture to ease chronic pain. The same meridian points are used as for regular needle acupuncture, but instead of needles a cold laser, diode light therapy, or electric stimulation are used. You can easily find these points because they hurt. Electronic muscle stimulators (EMS) stimulate, reeducate, massage, and build muscle. Electrode pads are placed directly on the body areas that need to be stimulated. By dialing the voltage, you can choose the appropriate pressure on the muscles to create medical and cosmetic effects. The low voltage is used on smaller, involuntary muscle groups that cannot be stimulated in other means. For pain treatments, the low voltage setting of the EMS also stimulates the brain, like a TENS unit, that sends impulses through involuntary muscles stimulating them as well. EMS are used for conditioning and toning muscles. Some medical conditions treated include muscle spasms; long-term disuse after fracture or prolonged bed rest; strengthening for joint or muscle injury; immobilized limbs and atrophy prevention; Bell's palsy; improving muscle tone; muscle spasticity following a stroke; and fitness training. Many athletes incorporate EMS into a training program for muscle strength, fast recovery, and rehabilitation. Does it work for cellulite? We need to try it and find out.

Contraindications: Do not use any electrotherapy device (EMS or TENS) for the following: for patients with cardiac pacemakers of any type; over the carotid sinus area, near or around the eyes, near or around the heart, transcerebrally (around your head), or transthoracically (around the chest); to remove pain syndromes until etiology (the cause) has been established; on pregnant women; over or near a known or suspected malignancy; on patients who have skin diseases; on patients who have implants of any electrical nature; and on patients with cardiac disease.

An acupuncture treatment for chronic pain and injury that may be applied to computer generated pain has been proven effective by Dr. Margaret Naeser, PhD, Lic.Ac. (licensed acupuncturist), Research Professor of Neurology, Boston University School of Medicine and Department of Veteran Affairs (VA) investigator. The treatment is useful for carpal tunnel syndrome, post-stroke spasticity, and Raynaud's syndrome, a condition that includes numb fingers and discoloration (white or blue fingertips). In this chapter, I have modified the treatment for easy home use, and have had splendid results for clients with carpal tunnel syndrome and arthritis wrist pain.

You will need two medical devices: a small TENS or muscle stimulator (costing about $100) and a small handheld cold laser (costing less than $200). For serious long-term cases of carpal tunnel syndrome, you may need as many as three treatments per week for up to three months for full results. However, the expense and trouble are small compared to surgery. See the Recommended Natural Product Sources section at the back of the book or www.asianhealth secrets.com. Often you can achieve good results after one treatment, but the treatments detailed here should be continued on a regular basis once or twice a week for several months to insure proper healing.

Note: Before you buy any machine and do any acupuncture treatment, consult with your acupuncturist, who can determine if this treatment is suitable for you, advise you on the location of points, and follow up to make sure the treatment is working effectively. During the period of treatments, you will very likely experience energy shifts in circulation. That may result in temporary pain, numbness in the fingers, or a slight nerve tingle. That is normal and passes quickly. However, people who have a weak heart, are heart surgery patients, or have other major health issues should proceed only under the direction of a qualified acupuncturist.

Survey the Damage

First find out what hurts or feels numb. Can you make a fist? Some people, after suffering a stroke or an injury or repeated computer use, cannot open or close their fist. Check your hand mobility. Do your fingers feel numb? Numbness may result from pinched nerves in the neck. But if you are a computer addict, the numbness is more likely the result of inflammation of nerves running through the carpal tunnel between the tendons on the inside of your wrist and forearm. If finger/arm numbness continues in the long term or is related to chronic fatigue or chronic heart failure, it may also be improved by taking one to three hawthorn capsules or one-half teaspoon of dan shen powder in water daily. Those herbs encourage a stronger, steady heart rhythm.

Decide on a convenient time and place for the treatments. You might enjoy doing them while watching television. To avoid indigestion, do not treat pain in the extremities, such as carpal tunnel pain, within two hours of a meal. Wash your hands with soap and water before and after the treatment. Washing before allows the stimulator pads to stick to the acupuncture points. Washing afterward reduces possible skin irritation. To ensure better adherence to the skin, it may be necessary to moisten the TENS or muscle stimulator pads with a few drops of water.

Place the stimulator pads on each side of the wrist on top and inside, near the palm. On top of the wrist choose either triple heater 4 or 5. Acupuncture point triple heater 4 (yangchi) is at the wrist crease, and triple heater 5 (waiguan) is about one inch above the crease of the wrist on the top side of the hand. Waiguan (English translation: "outer pass") is located on the forearm, two centimeters (about an inch) above the transverse crease of the wrist between the ulna and radius. It is an important point for connecting the outer and inner meridians running along the side of the head, chest, and legs. It is used to treat fevers, headache, eye pain and swelling, tinnitus, and deafness. It can be used to treat pain in the ribs and spasms of the upper extremities.

The other stimulator pad is placed on the palm side of the wrist crease between the two tendons at pericardium 7 (daling; English translation: "big mound" or "big tomb"). It is located in the depression in the middle of the transverse crease of the wrist, between the tendons of m. palmaris longus and m. flexor carpi radialis. The carpal tunnel lies in between these two tendons on the inside of the wrist.

Traditional Chinese acupuncture doctors describe the function of daling as to "clear the heart and calm the spirit." It reduces "fire from heart, and calms the mind." That means it may be used to ease palpitations and anxiety. It is a main point to treat insomnia, while it "expands the chest, dispels fullness from the chest." And depending upon the other points used with it, daling is indicated for cardiac pain, vomiting, heart discomfort (palpitations), and psychosis. It is also used for gastric pain, epilepsy, pain in the chest and sides, panic/fear, insomnia, tonsillitis, swollen armpits, skin disorders, bad breath, and arm pain.

Daling can be combined with other points to treat diseases and pain of the wrist joint, pain at the root of the tongue, lack of energy, constipation, cholera, numbness of fingers, headache, fever without sweating and with headache, inflammation of eyes, yellow sclera, dry mouth, dark reddish urine, and hot palms of hands. As you can see by the list of uses, daling is an important point to bring inflammation from the upper body and chest down to the hands and out of the body.

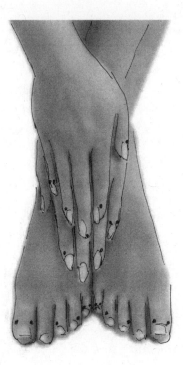

Ting Points

After you have placed the stimulator pads on both sides of the wrist, gradually turn on the power high enough to feel the vibration. Allow that to stimulate both sides of the wrist for less than a minute. Then turn down the stimulation until you cannot feel it. With a TENS unit, that setting should be around only 300 or 500 mA, or less. Allow that barely perceptible stimulation to continue for twenty minutes.

During that time, use your cold laser to stimulate the acupuncture points located at the tips of each finger that is numb. These end points of major acupuncture meridians are called ting points. Each fingertip has a ting point. Stimulate each point for three minutes. See the illustration. The points are located on the right hand at the lower left corner of the fingernail for the thumb and pointer finger; the lower border of the middle finger; and the lower right border of the fingernail for the fourth and fifth fingers. The ting points are located at the corresponding points on the left hand: at the lower right corner of the thumbnail and pointer fingernail; the lower border of the middle fingernail; and the lower left corners at the fingernail of the fourth and fifth fingers.

The total time of treatment should be fifteen to twenty minutes. According to Dr. Margaret Naeser, "If positive response is observed with three minutes of laser stimulation per point, during later treatments, only one or two minutes could be tried, in an attempt to reduce the total treatment time." She also reports, "Poor results are often observed if the patient's wrist joint has previously been injected with Botox; or if the patient takes certain medications, e.g., Tegretol, phenobarbital, or steroids (prednisone)."

Margaret A. Naeser, PhD, Lic.Ac., graduated from the New England School of Acupuncture in 1983 and is a licensed acupuncturist in Massachusetts (Dipl. Ac., NCCAOM). In 1985, she was invited by the Shanghai Medical University to exchange research information in stroke and acupuncture. While in China, she studied the use of acupuncture and laser acupuncture in the treatment of paralysis in stroke patients. In 1997, the National Institutes for Health (NIH) sponsored a Consensus Development Conference on Acupuncture. Her topic was "Neurological Rehabilitation: Acupuncture and Laser Acupuncture to Treat Paralysis in Stroke and Other Paralytic Conditions and Pain in Carpal Tunnel Syndrome." From 1993 to 2001, she conducted laser acupuncture research to treat carpal tunnel syndrome at the V.A. Boston Healthcare System. Anyone who says that the use of acupuncture for pain treatments has not been adequately studied should have his head examined.

If you prefer using massage instead of acupuncture to treat carpal tunnel syndrome, apply White Tiger Balm or White Flower Analgesic oil to the painful points described on the previous page at the inside of the wrist, between the tendons at the carpal tunnel, and along the fingers on the palm side. Massage from the wrist to the tips of each finger. The direction of an anti-inflammatory treatment for pain is always away from the source of pain (the wrist) toward the extremities. This massage approach will take much longer and will not be as effective as acupuncture, but may improve pain and numbness to some degree.

Use a Foot Rest

Sitting at a computer freezes us in an unnatural position of pain, reflected throughout the nervous system. Use a foot rest, not for your feet, but to position the lower back in order to avoid stress injury pain. See the chapter on back pain. When muscles in the lower back lack adequate blood circulation, when they collapse into your chair, the discs may become dry, and stress injury to the spinal column becomes possible. A foot rest positions your legs to more closely resemble squatting, which is a more natural position that helps remove stress from the colon, pelvis, and lower back.

Choose the right height. You do not need to create a deep squat. Often, lifting your feet three inches off the floor by placing them on a box is enough to create the desired angle. You can feel a comfortable squat if your knees are slightly higher than your groin. A pencil placed on your thigh should roll toward the groin, not fall toward the floor. Some experts believe that cultures in which people squat have fewer back problems and pain. Find a happy medium for comfort: try a higher or lower foot rest to see if you feel less fatigued. Position the foot rest under your desk so that you can sit comfortably. Remember to get up and walk around if possible every hour to avoid getting stuck into a painful freeze. Do the chair hip rolls described on page 130.

Aching Shoulders and Neck

Staying hydrated or walking around the room in order to keep your knees from locking does not help your neck. Here is a nice simple tea that brings needed blood circulation to tired shoulders.

Have this tea between meals. Add one-fourth teaspoon each of turmeric powder and cinnamon powder to a cup of warm water and drink it slowly.

Rubs for Pain Relief

Many people get pain relief by applying a cooling or warming ointment. To enhance circulation, several Asian pain preparations feel both cool and warm. Chinese White Flower is one. Apply some White Flower analgesic liquid to a cotton ball and apply it to your stiff joints. It is useful for headache and stiff neck. It does not stain clothing. Apply it to the hairline at the neck, on top of the shoulder, at the center of the shoulder blade, at the elbow crease, and at the wrist. Its ingredients, including lavender, smell fresh and invigorating. If you want a stronger warming pain rub, try Red Tiger Balm at the temples, back of the neck, top of the shoulder, and wrists.

Letha's Advice: A Big Percussion Massager

I don't go anywhere without my HoMedics massager, which I bought at Walmart. I stick it into a suitcase whenever I travel. It has two rotating heads and adjustable speeds and strength. Run it along the top of your shoulders, down the arms, at each underarm to encourage lymphatic drainage, across the collarbone, and pause a moment where the thymus is located. It is beneath the Adam's apple under the collarbone. The thymus stops working around age thirty, but in childhood it protects immunity. Use the massager to loosen aching back muscles, buttocks, thighs, and legs. Bring new life and qi movement to shrinking limbs trapped under a desk.

CHAPTER ELEVEN

Surgery and Recovery

All pain is either severe or slight; if slight, it is easily endured; if severe, it will without doubt be brief.

—Marcus Tullius Cicero (Roman statesman, 106 BC–43 BC)

CICERO WAS OBVIOUSLY A PHILOSOPHER, NOT A CHRONIC PAIN SUFFERER. BUT his life serves as a useful example. His writings refute both the Epicurean philosophy (the gods are indifferent to human suffering) and the Stoic philosophy (the gods reward the good and punish the bad). During the chaotic latter half of the first century BC, troubled by civil wars, Cicero championed traditional republican values. After making speeches against Mark Antony, Cicero was murdered in December 43 BC. His life and death mark the decline and fall of the Roman Republic. Today, we take the responsibility of preventing pain and illness upon ourselves, but we need also to negotiate with the powers that be, the medical establishment.

There are a growing number of surgeons in the United States who use nonsurgical techniques. Be sure to ask about different options available to you when considering surgery. They may include the use of radio frequencies, high-energy sound waves to treat varicose veins, back pains, or heart irregularities, and cryotherapy, the use of extreme cold to freeze

Surgery Shorthand

A week or two prior to surgery, simply avoid taking vitamin C, aspirin, and garlic (blood thinners), and take 60–80 milligrams of vitamin K per day to prevent excess bleeding and 60 milligrams daily of zinc to help avoid stress. If possible, enhance circulation with gentle massage and light exercise. Practice relaxation techniques. Discuss your herbal treatments with your surgeon. After you return home following surgery, check your blood pressure daily, watch for signs of infection, and stay in touch with your doctor until you feel stronger.

diseased tissue such as benign lesions. However, if you and your medical adviser decide surgery is the best solution, do not delay. Surgery can be life saving.

This chapter aims to make the pain of surgery and recovery as brief, easy, and rewarding as possible. Your presurgery planning requires discussion with your doctors, because most do not know the effects of foods on surgery and they tend to mistrust herbs. The Preparation for Surgery protocol laid out in this chapter can help. It is, among other things, a lesson in natural blood thinners. Blood-thinning drugs, foods, and herbs increase bleeding during and bruising following surgery.

It is also important for us to note the drug interaction effects of our favorite health foods. Eliminating all blood-thinning foods and supplements limits your diet to cheeseburgers—murder for cardiovascular health. Some dietary compromises are necessary. In addition, this chapter details quick recovery treatments, including a section on Yunnan Paiyao, a marvelous Chinese herbal remedy that may be taken prior to and following surgery, that prevents hemorrhage and reduces bruising, swelling, and pain.

Preparation for Surgery

Stop Smoking Now!

No need to explain this. Smoking chokes circulation and ruins vitality, endangers survival, and lengthens recovery. So quit any way you can. Acupuncture works for some people. Chew gum, cinnamon sticks, tang kuei root (it builds blood and increases T-cells), osha root (it clears lung congestion), or any other suitable pacifier. The addiction is physical, mental, and social. Occupy your hands with something new. Take a good general nutritional supplement, American ginseng tea for dry mouth, and a tonic such as reishi medicinal mushrooms capsules to regain vitality and help prevent some of the thirteen or so cancers (mouth, throat, breast, etc.) linked to smoking.

Blood Thinners

The American Society of Anesthesiologists suggests that patients stop taking *all* dietary supplements and herbs two to three weeks before surgery. I caution readers who are energy- and immunity-challenged, heart patients, or elderly to continue taking herbs that support vitality and immunity, with the guidance of their health professional. For example, hawthorn protects our heart rhythm and in that way helps to maintain healthy circulation to enhance healing and reduce pain. Herbs and common foods to be avoided are blood thinners such as garlic because they can increase bleeding during and following surgery. Below is a detailed list of blood-thinning foods, herbs, and cooking ingredients.

Salicylates

Salicylates block vitamin K. Vitamin K increases blood coagulation. The best-known salicylate is aspirin, but many foods contain natural blood thinners such as vitamin C. They include most fruits (especially dried fruits), nuts, and some flavorings and preservatives. If you bruise easily, reduce your intake of the following foods and medicinal herbs. Also see Garlic, on the following pages. Herbs and spices high in salicylates include:

- Curry powder
- Cayenne pepper
- Ginger
- Paprika
- Thyme
- Cinnamon
- Dill
- Oregano
- Turmeric
- Licorice
- Peppermint

Traditional Asian medicine considers many spices to be "warming" because they increase blood circulation and speed metabolism. However, herbs and spices impact energy in specific areas of the body. For example, cayenne, cinnamon, and paprika stimulate blood circulation; ginger, licorice, peppermint, turmeric, and curry enhance digestion; and oregano and thyme, both antibiotic herbs, help clear lung congestion.

Fruits high in salicylates include:

- Raisins
- Prunes
- Cherries
- Cranberries
- Blueberries
- Grapes
- Strawberries

- Tangerines
- Oranges

Raisins, prunes, cherries, and blueberries, sources of iron, increase blood production. Strawberries and oranges are sources of vitamin C.

Other substance high in salicylates:

- Chewing gum
- Honey
- Peppermints
- Vinegar
- Wine
- Cider

In general, most meat, dairy, grain, and vegetable foods are not high in salicylates. Many types of fish do, however, have blood-thinning properties because of their omega-3 fatty acid content. Fish with high amounts of omega-3s include:

- Anchovies
- Salmon
- Albacore tuna
- Mackerel
- Lake trout
- Herring

Common Medicinal Herb and Drug Interactions

Most patients do not tell their doctor about the herbs and spices they use. The risk is that, because surgery involves anesthesia and an incision, natural supplements may affect the surgery and its outcome. Interactions of herbs and supplements with medications used during surgery—including anesthetics, epinephrine, muscle relaxants, and antiarrhythmics—have become commonplace. Deaths may result from anesthesia given to patients who are too elderly, weak, or sick to tolerate that medication. For that reason, it may be wise to continue with your energy tonics and heart health herbs other than garlic while preparing for surgery. Inform your doctor about the herbs you are taking.

"Despite the technological improvements, anesthesia is not completely benign, and mistakes are made," writes Dr. Karen B. Domino, professor of anesthesiology at the University of Washington School of Medicine in a 2004 *New York Times* article entitled "Anesthesia, Without a Knockout Punch." Dr. Domino believes the most common problems during surgery are from "drug errors, mistakes in the administration of fluids, and the misinterpretation of information delivered by the monitoring equipment." *Not herbal/drug interactions.* By the time you receive anesthesia, it is too late to discuss herbs. Herbs complicate surgery, but many improve healing. You have to take responsibility for using them. Here is a short list of complications associated with some of our more common medicinal herbs.

Garlic: A Blood Thinner
Possible complications: bleeding during and immediately following surgery.

In large doses, garlic may lower blood pressure and interfere with blood clotting. This increases the risk for serious bleeding during surgery. Garlic can increase the effect of warfarin (also known as Coumadin), a drug used to prevent blood clotting. In combination with chlorpropamide, garlic may cause low blood sugar.

Ginkgo: Dilates Blood Vessels
Possible complications: bleeding during and immediately following surgery.

Ginkgo interferes with blood clotting and dilates blood vessels. This may lead to increased bleeding during surgery and just after surgery. Ginkgo may also lead to abnormal bleeding when used in conjunction with the prescription drug warfarin or with aspirin.

Cloud Ear Mushroom: A Blood Thinner
Possible complications: bleeding during and immediately following surgery.

Cloud ear (also known as *Auricularia polytricha*, wood ear, tree ear, dry black fungus, silver ear, and mok yee), an edible fungus used in Chinese hot and sour soup, is among the best blood thinners. According to Dr. Andrew Weil, MD, it has an action "comparable to Coumadin without the drug's known side effects." I normally soak this black fungus, which resembles crinkled paper, in water. It puffs up much larger. I keep it in the refrigerator until it's time to cook it. Then I slice some into boiling water to cook along with pasta or oatmeal. Avoid it prior to surgery.

Ginseng: Stimulating and Drug Interference
Possible complications: bleeding during and immediately following surgery.

Ginseng (also known as panax ginseng, Chinese ginseng, red ginseng, or ren shen) can interfere with normal blood clotting. In addition, it has significant stimulatory effects on the central nervous system. It is considered a warming tonic: for some overheated people, it can cause headaches, nervousness, and sleep abnormalities or insomnia. Ginseng can cause hypoglycemia. Ginseng interferes with some prescription drugs. It enhances the effect of warfarin and may result in unwanted and dangerous bleeding. When taken with phenelzine, it can cause insomnia and psychological effects from hyperstimulation.

Kava: A Sedative

Possible complications: may increase the sedative effect of anesthesia.

In the South Pacific islands, kava is used socially for relaxation. It can increase the effect of alcohol, sedatives, or anesthesia. Kava has also been associated with liver damage, with some fatalities. The exact mechanism of action is still being studied. Because kava interferes with cytochromes, it has the potential to interact with a fairly large number of drugs.

St. John's Wort: Drug Interference

Possible complications: may cause acute rejection of a transplanted organ by interfering with antirejection medications; rejection may begin within twenty-four hours of taking St. John's wort.

St. John's wort, usually recommended for depression, interacts with many drugs. It rapidly decreases the plasma levels of cyclosporine, a medication commonly used to prevent rejection of a transplanted organ. It can decrease the plasma levels of the asthma medication theophylline, HIV medications (indinavir), heart medications (digoxin), and antidepressants (amitriptyline). It decreases the anticoagulant properties of warfarin, acenocoumarol, and phenprocoumon. When used with selective serotonin reuptake inhibitors, such as sertraline, paroxetine, or nefazodone, it can cause serotonin syndrome. Serotonin syndrome is a potentially life-threatening drug reaction that causes the body to have too much serotonin, a chemical produced by nerve cells. It most often occurs when two drugs that affect the body's level of serotonin are taken together.

Valerian: A Sedative

Possible complications: may increase the sedative effect of anesthesia.

Valerian is typically used to induce sleep. This property may dangerously enhance the effects of anesthesia. When taken with opiate medications, it may increase the risk of excessive central nervous system (CNS) depression. Valerian may also cause excessive CNS depression when taken with benzodiazepines such as Valium and Xanax, some of the most commonly used medications in psychiatry. Heart failure patients should especially avoid using sedatives.

Vitamin E: A Blood Thinner

Possible complications: bleeding during and immediately following surgery.

Taking vitamin E in excess of the recommended dosage interferes with the blood's ability to coagulate. Large doses of vitamin E decrease platelet adhesiveness, a property necessary for plugging holes in capillaries and triggering the clotting process. Foods high in vitamin E may not *necessarily* thin the blood. For example, spinach and broccoli also contain significant amounts of vitamin K, which tends to clot the blood.

Alcohol: Possible Blood Thinner

Possible complications: bleeding during and immediately following surgery.

Most of us have heard that drinking red wine reduces cholesterol. Flavonoids in dark grape peel are cleansing. To a certain extent, blood thinning may also result from alcohol consumption. A study that appeared in the October 2005 issue of the journal *Alcoholism: Clinical & Experimental Research* stated, "Alcohol consumption is inversely associated with both platelet activation and aggregation." Another article, published in 1986 in the same journal, found signs of vitamin K deficiency in a study of twenty male alcoholics.

Topical Blood Thinners

Possible complications: bleeding during and immediately following surgery.

Not only foods, but also what you rub onto your skin, may thin your blood. The *New York Times* reported in 2007 the death of a high-school track star from an overdose of an over-the-counter sports rub containing methyl salicylate. Methyl salicylate at high enough doses rubbed into the skin can act as an anticlotting agent, which in turn may result in internal bleeding and related health issues.

Letha's Advice: Prepare Yourself Emotionally for Recovery

I once met a woman who said she "dissolved a tumor by meditating on the painful relationship that gave her the tumor." Daily, over many months, she visualized the lump becoming smaller until it was gone. I know a famous healer in Israel, Suzanna Marcus, who cured herself of cancer, avoiding surgery, by following a raw foods cleansing diet and most importantly, she said, by "cleansing and healing her relationships." These are extraordinary people. You will find comfort in reading Suzanna's book *6 Months to Live 10 Years Later,* described as "a riveting memoir for those who face life challenges in health, relationships, work, or faith, but also for those who are well and want to remain so." You may wish to read poetry, find comfort in prayer, take a walk in nature, or have a swim. In whatever you choose to prepare yourself emotionally for surgery, whether prayer or medication, a massage or a run in the park, grant yourself the strength, confidence, and permission to recover. It is amazing what spirit and will can do.

Prepare Your Body and Home for Surgery and Recovery

Joint replacement and surgery to repair torn knee ligaments from skiing, running, dancing, and active sports are among the most common surgeries. I met with Maureen Gibeault, PT, Director of the Vermont Sports Medicine Center, in Killington, Vermont. She is a pleasant, strong, and reassuring physical therapist who immediately creates an atmosphere of comfort and confidence. I asked her how someone planning to have joint surgery should prepare. She advised:

> The most important thing anyone can do before surgery is to improve overall health. If they smoke: stop. If they are overweight they should get on a structured healthy diet and weight loss initiative. This diminishes stress on the joints. Specifically, a swimming program is effective for many health aspects, prior to joint surgery. Swimming enhances cardiovascular fitness, flexibility, and muscle tone, all without adding stress to an already impaired joint. Begin exercises that you would be doing postoperatively within the constraints of your joint disease and pain level. In doing so, you begin the motor learning process and awareness preoperatively, and also can gain strength preoperatively. Doing upper-body exercise and gentle weight training helps prepare the arms for use of crutches, walkers, and canes. It is also generally good for your heart. All exercise programs should be approved by the doctor.

Review your home environment for hazards after you come home from the hospital. Remove area rugs that may cause tripping. Make sure you have a railing into your home or going to your second floor. Get bathtub or shower chairs and a raised toilet seat with arm rests to make your bathroom more accessible and safer.

Get a Massage

There is no substitute for healing touch. A comforting yet stimulating massage improves circulation and mood. If possible, schedule one or several massage treatments in the weeks prior to help prepare for surgery. The exception is an active cancer, for which it is important to avoid spreading the problem. The type of massage you choose depends upon your pleasure and needs. A gentle massage such as Swedish massage or a Reiki treatment, which barely touches the skin, is comforting for some. If you have aching pain that feels better with a heavy touch, shiatsu or Chinese tui na may work better. A firm, deep massage sedates nerve and muscle pain. Moving stuck circulation, even if it results in temporary discomfort as your energy shifts, will greatly benefit healing. If you feel exhausted and chilled after a massage treatment, drink a warming cup of ginger tea.

An experienced massage therapist may be able to help you avoid complications such as bruising. See Dit Da Jow Chinese martial arts liniments to reduce bruising pain on page 117. Avoid a therapist who gives the same treatment and speech to everyone. Yours is a sensitive problem that requires gentle, experienced care and follow-up.

Hospital Preparation

This is more important than you know! Hospital-acquired infections (HAIs) are known to kill more Americans each year than AIDS, breast cancer, and auto accidents combined! HAIs such as ventilator-acquired pneumonia, bloodstream infections, urinary tract infections, and surgical site infections are not systematically studied or counted; however, the Centers for Disease Control and Prevention in Atlanta estimated in 2002 that there were about 1.7 million cases per year, including 99,000 deaths in the United States. The CDC estimated the cost of treating HAIs at $28 billion to $35 billion in 2007. After 2008, Medicare stopped reimbursing hospitals for HAI costs, placing the enormous burden onto financially challenged hospitals.

Throughout the world, hospitals are in financial trouble. That often leads to reduction in cleaning staff. To make matters worse, the overuse of antibiotics has created hospital supergerms that are immune to medication. An article in *Plastics Engineering* states, "Plastic surfaces on medical devices and equipment in hospitals and clinics make great breeding grounds for bacteria, including some of the nastiest germs around. The typical solution to infections in hospitals is antibiotics for patients and biocidal cleaners for the hospital room. The unintended consequence, however, is that bacteria may develop resistance, particularly to antibiotics, making them far more dangerous, like MRSA (methicillin-resistant *Staphylococcus aureus*), the so called 'flesh-eating' germ, or multi-drug-resistant 'gram-negative' bacteria." MRSA is a particularly strong threat to surgery patients because of open wounds, but everyday cuts and bug bites also make us vulnerable.

Up to now MRSA has been passed by touching something or eating food that has been touched by an infected person or from skin-to-skin contact with an infected person. Medical sources report that approximately half the staff members of most hospitals have been exposed to and may carry MRSA, compared to 30 percent of the general population. MRSA is now also airborne, passed from person to person by coughing and sneezing. A separate strain of antibiotic-resistant staphylococcus MRSA has developed outside the hospital and is stronger and more resistant to antibiotics than the original strain. Most at risk of developing MRSA are people who are weak, the elderly, babies, and people with a compromised immune system such as HIV patients. However, the newer strains of MRSA attack healthy persons and are unchecked (out of control) in certain areas of the world. A respected New York dermatologist told me, "We see tons of MRSA in New York because people easily become infected when they share equipment in gyms and yoga centers."

Herbs for MRSA

While working on the final edit of this book and vacationing in Florida, I was diagnosed with MRSA after a bug bite became infected. I was not near a hospital but next to a swimming pool at a posh hotel. The current medical treatment that I underwent was ten days of a sulpha drug. A doctor explained that since MRSA staph germs were already immune to most *modern* antibiotics, the older sulpha drug might work against it. After the medical treatment was partially successful and I continued to develop the rash, I added the San She Dan (Trisnake pills) described in the chapter covering skin remedies because that cure for itchy skin rash was even older than the sulpha drug. To make the herbal formula stronger I added neem capsules, another herbal antibiotic. The final answer for prevention and treatment of superbugs is individual depending upon a person's immunity, age, and lifestyle. Improved hygiene has become more important than ever. Some of the better supermarkets now provide hand sanitizers for people using shopping carts. Use them. It is also a good idea to keep some alcohol-based hand sanitizer wipes in your pocket or purse, and when possible, use gloves when using public transportation.

The MRSA problem has become important enough to attract research money, and new treatments in the UK are attempting to knock it out with nanotechnology. See chapter 18 for the future of pain medicine. Other ways to prevent infections such as MRSA are on the horizon.

A conference held in May 2011 in Boston covered the latest developments to the medical plastics industry. The hot topic was silver, used for many years as an antibacterial. Meanwhile, China is using natural antimicrobials like chitosan, a derivative from crab shells, and bamboo fiber. More far-out are hospital surfaces and public restroom counters that have microembossed patterns similar to sharkskin. Bacteria, for some reason, seem to shun surfaces that resemble sharkskin. The countertops are made by Sharklet Technologies Inc. in Aurora, Colorado (www.sharklet.com). While scientists debate whether or not colloidal silver harms the environment and make countertops that resemble sharks, you must take active steps to protect yourself and family from hospital-acquired infections. You will most likely choose your hospital and doctor because of location and convenience. But you can also prepare yourself, your room, and your surgical team to ensure a safer outcome for surgery.

- Wash your entire body with an alcohol-based antibiotic soap and water for several days prior to surgery.
- Cover cuts or bug bites immediately with a silver gel antibiotic ointment and a sterile bandage to avoid exposure to supergerms.
- If your immunity is challenged and you are weak or elderly, it is wise to take the current medical treatment for MRSA for one week prior to surgery. Adding an antibiotic, anti-inflammatory herbal combination such as those described in chapter 12 can speed healing and reduce pain.
- Make sure the hospital staff washes their hands before and after examining you. Keep a hand-sterilizer liquid in your room.
- Have sterile face masks available for visitors who may have a cold.
- Spray furniture and bathroom surfaces with antibacterial colloidal silver spray.
- Essential oil of lavender is calming and antiseptic. Put a drop on your arm if you find it relaxing. You may prefer to have familiar scents from your garden, such as rose oil, which is cooling, or rosemary oil, which is stimulating.
- Consider using colloidal silver internally during the time you are hospitalized.
- Build resistance and endurance: For patients who are too weak or ill to eat, a homeopathic combination of cell salts called bioplasma is very supportive of health and well-being. It is a combination of twelve minerals essential for cellular health. The tiny pills dissolve on the tongue or in water. Do not mix homeopathic remedies with medications, colloidal silver, or food, but wait at least two hours after eating, brushing your teeth, and using medicines.
- Put yourself squarely on your doctor and medical team's radar by discussing the operation and follow-up.

The Surgical Safety Checklist

Let's say you prepped yourself to avoid hysteria and your hospital room to avoid germs. The problem of human error, such as wrong-side surgery and drug-dose mistakes, should not be ignored. The World Health Organization (WHO) has created a surgical safety checklist for medical hospital staff that reduced the rate of death after surgery from 1.5 percent to 0.8 percent and the number of complications from 11 percent to 7 percent. However, a representative from the WHO informed me that this official version of "Who is this patient and what are we doing with him today?" is used by very few, if any, hospitals in the United States.

Since most surgery teams meet each other and the patient shortly before an operation, and because they are overworked and may have other things on their minds, it pays for you to take an active part in the preparation. This is strongly recommended by Dr. Kenneth Kizer, former CEO of the safety advocacy group National Quality Forum. Below is Dr. Kizer's checklist for patients to use with their doctor and nursing staff before surgery. Kizer suggests:

1. Ask **"What are you going to do to ensure that you don't operate on the wrong site?"** While this sounds a bit like asking the doctor, "Do you know your business or are you just visiting?" it is still a good idea to discuss your surgery and follow-up in a friendly manner well in advance of surgery.

2. **Request a "time-out" just before anesthesia.** The Joint Commission's Universal Protocol recommends that the operative team communicate to ensure they are all in agreement. However, this may not be possible, especially with emergency surgery.

3. **Say: "My name is John Smith, and my birthday is January 21, 1976."** I suggest that you simply introduce yourself to nurses during intake questions and make some comment about your surgery. They are the ones who keep track of who and where you are in the presurgery and recovery process.

4. **Don't rush through the informed consent form.** Dr. Kizer says rushing through the informed consent form is a missed opportunity to find potential errors.

5. **Make sure your doctor initials your surgery site.** The American Academy of Orthopaedic Surgeons urges its members to sign their initials directly on the site before surgery.

6. **Trust your gut.** If you have bad feelings about the surgery, Kizer advises that you tell your doctor. You do yourself, your family, and the hospital a great service by taking an active role in the operation.

Patients about to go under the knife are not in a mood to question their doctor. They need to feel confident. They may be doped by drugs and worried about their condition. Waiting until the last minute to ask questions is a mistake. I hope that you and your relatives already have a positive, open relationship with your surgeon, and that you chose him or her because of experience, training, and other reasons for your respect.

On the lighter side, I enjoy joking with my favorite surgeons before and during a procedure. I already mentioned my longtime friend and expert plastic surgeon in New York, Dr. Gerald Ginsberg, MD, FACS, Director of Plastic Surgery at New York Downtown Hospital. Another friend you will read about in chapter 18, "The Future of Pain Medicine," is orthopedic surgeon and author Dr. Alan Lazar, MD, FACS, in Plantation, Florida. Both men are brilliant, experimental when creating new surgical procedures, good guys, and funny. Their vast experience and great bedside manner made us instant friends. We always discuss exactly what will happen during surgery. It is part of our special way of feeling in tune. I can stay awake during surgery and report what I am feeling, because I use the Chinese patent remedy Yunnan Paiyao to avoid bleeding complications.

Prevent Excess Bleeding, Bruising, and Pain During and Following Surgery

Yunnan Paiyao

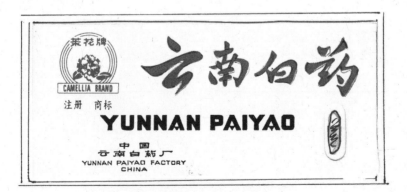

Throughout Asia and the Americas, Yunnan Paiyao is a famous Chinese over-the-counter vegetarian herbal "wonder drug" used for wounds and bruises. It reduces the bleeding, pain, and swelling of injuries, deep wounds, and surgery. The Chinese People's Liberation Army uses Yunnan Paiyao capsules internally for injuries resulting from explosions and gunshot wounds. It stops hemorrhage and normalizes blood flow fast! You can use it for any sort of internal bleeding such as stomach ulcers or menstrual flooding. Taken internally, it reduces swelling and redness from bug bites.

Yunnan Paiyao means "Yunnan white powder" and is made in Yunnan province, China. The formula combines two forms of tienchi ginseng (also known as sanqi), a cardio-tonic used to normalize blood flow, repair damaged blood vessels, and reduce cholesterol. Yunnan Paiyao repairs blood vessels and stops hemorrhage because it combines tienchi along with astringent, detoxifying herbs such as myrrh and *Daemomorops draco* from Sumatra and China, an herb called "dragon's blood" in Latin America. Yunnan Paiyao reduces the size, seriousness, and lightens the color of surgery bruises fast. Your surgeon will be amazed.

On the battlefield, you can pour the Yunnan Paiyao powder from capsules or the powder sold in a small jar directly onto open wounds to help resolve pus and stop excess bleeding. At home: have you cut yourself shaving? Why use a chemical on shaving cuts? Dab Yunnan Paiyao powder on the cut with a cotton swab. Has a hornet sting caused swelling? Swallow a couple of capsules of Yunnan Paiyao two to three times daily, and the swelling will resolve in a day or so.

Yunnan Paiyao for Surgery

Just before surgery, swallow the tiny red pill that is provided with the Yunnan Paiyao capsules or powder. Yunnan Paiyao will not interfere with surgery drugs or painkillers. However, if you will be given a blood-thinning drug following surgery in order to avoid a blood clot, discuss with your doctor whether or not you should use Yunnan Paiyao. It is not a blood thinner but does enhance circulation. Yunnan Paiyao is not habit-forming. You can read more about it in the chapter "Yunnan Paiyao: A Chinese Miracle Cure" in *Asian Health Secrets: The Complete Guide to Asian Herbal Medicine*. I have recommended Yunnan Paiyao for many clients and friends who have avoided disfiguring scars and deep wounds because it speeds healing. Barring an active cancer, you can even take it on a regular basis with a sip of wine to treat chronic gastritis and improve general circulation. At my website I posted an article "Yunnan Paiyao = Strong Medicine" and hundreds of people commented, giving positive examples of how they regularly use and love Yunnan Paiyao for themselves.

Yunnan Paiyao is so strong that it contributed to saving my brother Eric's life when he cracked up his motorcycle one day while he was attending chiropractic college. At the hospital, the staff watched him nearly bleed to death as he lost many units of blood. They planned to remove his spleen, which was split in pieces. Although he was an athletic body builder, his abdomen was largely swollen with blood. I FedExed Yunnan Paiyao to him overnight. He swallowed the red pill and took capsules and soon the hemorrhage stopped, his swollen abdomen shrank to normal, he and his spleen survived, and he went on to become a busy, successful doctor of chiropractic medicine.

Another man in his forties injured his pelvis in a skiing accident that required eight hours of surgery. He took Yunnan Paiyao capsules for several months following the surgery and said he loved the pain relief the Chinese herbs gave him. He returned to sports, which brings up an important point. Warning: Although you may be pain-free after surgery from using natural remedies, give your body a chance to heal completely; return to normal activities and follow your doctor's advice before jumping back into sports and other physical activities.

Note: it is best to avoid eating salads and fish when taking Yunnan Paiyao. It may be okay to separate them by a couple of hours. However, cold foods require strong digestion. If Yunnan Paiyao upsets your stomach or makes you feel dizzy, take it with warm cooked food.

Other Postsurgery Treatments

Homeopathic Arnica montana 30C

A few surgeons know about natural treatments for bruising, including homeopathic arnica. It does not quell infections like Yunnan Paiyao does, but the remedy does increase circulation and, therefore, helps resolve bruises and pain. Take homeopathic remedies as directed by your homeopathic specialist. Never use a remedy with food, beverages, or toothpaste, but separate their use by at least two hours.

Resinall E and Resinall K

Health Concerns in Oakland, California, makes these two formulas, the first being pills and the second a liquid taken internally and applied externally. Resinall E Tabs are based on digestive enzyme therapy and contain bromelain, rutin, papain, trypsin, chymotrypsin, and herbs, including dragon's blood (Chinese xue jie), tienchi, catechu herb, corydalis, carthamus, myrrh, frankincense, and borneol resin. It treats pain and swelling due to traumatic injuries, sprains, strains, fracture, broken bones, bleeding, and bruising. It is taken by athletes before and after events such as running, football, and boxing in order to reduce swelling. It can be used by people with arthritis to help resolve pain. The enzymes and herbs promote tissue regeneration, stop excess bleeding, and activate circulation.

Resinall K liquid also stops pain and swelling of traumatic injuries as well as working topically for fungal infections (athlete's foot), bacterial infections, eczema, and dermal ulcers, and chronic pain. It contains herbs, including tienchi ginseng and myrrh, that enhance circulation and corydalis to treat pain. Place one-half to one dropper under the tongue between meals for pain. You can also apply it topically with cotton three times daily as needed. It does stain clothing.

Note: avoid Resinall E and Resinall K during pregnancy. If you use either one for more than two weeks, add an energy tonic to avoid fatigue.

Build Blood and Energy to Speed Recovery from Surgery

Some people die a few days following surgery because they are not strong enough to survive the shock. The heart tonic herbs in chapter 15 would be very helpful for anyone who experiences chest pains, weakness, or blood pressure changes following surgery. Be sure to inform your doctor of the problem and the herbs and medicines you are using. For a speedy recovery and to enhance general wellness, Asian traditional medicine is particularly good at providing life-saving tonic herbs known as adaptogens. They help body, mind, and spirit to heal and work more efficiently. Adaptogens such as the ginsengs support many functions such as breathing, digestion, and heart and sexual health, and as such they have been frequently used by athletes to recover energy after competition. Adaptogens can also be used to tone vitality and prevent fatigue and illness. In this section, I describe the actions of famous tonics, including several ginsengs and a healing fungus. Another useful enzyme helps dissolve scars while it enhances circulation and detoxifies the body after surgery. Also see chapter 17 for suggested additional uses of general herbal tonics.

Raw and Steamed Tienchi Ginseng

If you are using Yunnan Paiyao to recover from surgery, you do not need to take additional tienchi ginseng because it is already part of the formula. Tienchi (also known as sanqi, *Panax notoginseng*, *Panax pseudoginseng*) is a special ginseng that works as a cardio-tonic that reduces cholesterol, helps regulate heart rhythm, and heals blood vessels to protect against hardening of the arteries. Like other ginsengs it contains ginsenosides that tone energy and endurance. It also contains flavonoids, glycans (panaxans), maltol, peptides, polysaccharide fraction DPG-3-2, saponins, vitamin A, vitamin B6, other B vitamins, and zinc.

Most Western medical sources describe its actions as antihemorrhagic and antiarrhythmic for the heart. However, traditional Chinese medicine sources are more specific. There are two forms of tienchi—raw and steamed—and their actions are different. Both support the heart and reduce cholesterol.

Dosage: an easy way to use tienchi is to add one-fourth teaspoon of the appropriate powder—either raw tienchi or steamed tienchi—to warm water as tea or juice, once or twice daily as needed long-term.

Raw Tienchi Ginseng Powder

Raw tienchi powder is "cooling," which means it reduces bruises, inflammation, and fever, and may be laxative to some people. It makes us feel cooler and can be added to water or soup daily to reduce cholesterol and regulate hypertension. It is useful for diabetes because it reduces chronic hunger and thirst and, like other adaptogens, can help regulate blood sugar.

Use raw tienchi powder if you have a red, dry tongue, quick pulse, fever conditions, night sweats, hypertension, diabetes, hot palms or soles of your feet, thinning hair, or flushed appearance, or you feel uncomfortable in hot climates.

As a cooling tonic, raw tienchi powder is known to improve the following.

Blood Conditions

- Hematemesis (vomiting of blood)
- Hematoma (tumorlike mass produced by coagulation of extravasated blood in a tissue or cavity)
- Hematuria (blood in the urine)
- Hemoptysis (coughing and spitting of blood, result of bleeding from the respiratory tract)
- Hemorrhage and pain caused by trauma
- Metrorrhagia (uterine bleeding at irregular intervals)
- Blood circulation through the body
- Bleeding
- Traumatic injury with bruising

Cardiovascular Conditions

- Angina pectoris
- Arrhythmia
- Myocardial ischemia
- Circulation

Immune Conditions

- Defense system balance

Other Conditions

- Chest and abdominal pain
- High blood cholesterol
- Alzheimer's disease
- Physical functioning depending on what the individual needs (e.g., it will lower high blood pressure but raise low blood pressure)
- Recovery from illness or surgery, especially for the elderly
- Swelling
- Weight loss

Steamed Tienchi Ginseng Powder

Steamed tienchi is considered "warming" and "blood-enhancing," which means it is best used by someone who tends to have chills, weakness, pallor, or fatigue after blood loss. Steamed tienchi, as a cardio and circulation tonic, has many of the same uses as raw tienchi (on page 164), but should be avoided by people with fevers, hot palms and soles, night sweats, chronic thirst, dry skin, or dry cough. Use steamed tienchi ginseng powder if you have a pale tongue; slow, deep pulse; listlessness; chronic chills; a thin, watery, irregular period; or you feel exhausted and/or depressed after blood loss.

General Precautions for Use of Either Raw or Steamed Tienchi Ginseng

Tienchi ginseng is a stimulant, and taken at high doses it may increase nervousness and insomnia. Other, rarer side effects may include anxiety, diarrhea, euphoria, high blood pressure (for steamed tienchi), vomiting, and vaginal bleeding (for steamed tienchi.) It should be taken with food to avoid hypoglycemia (low blood sugar), even in nondiabetics. Caution: raw and steamed tienchi should be discontinued at least seven days prior to surgery, because they may act as a blood thinner. Tienchi should not be used during pregnancy or when breast-feeding. Ginsengs may exaggerate the effects of morphine and monoamine oxidase inhibitors (MAOIs) (antidepressant medication), especially phenelzine. Interaction with ginseng may cause symptoms such as headaches, manic-like episodes, and tremulousness.

Do not use ginsengs without first talking to your health-care provider if you are taking any of the following medications:

- Blood-thinning medications
- Aspirin (ginseng may inhibit platelet activity)
- Warfarin (ginseng may decrease effectiveness)
- Caffeine or other substances that stimulate the central nervous system
- Haloperidol (antipsychotic medication)

Ginseng Complex Capsules

If you cannot decide whether or not you need a warming or cooling ginseng to work as an adaptogen, try a combination of both, such as Ginseng Complex, made and sold by Vitamin Shoppe. Start slowly by taking one capsule once daily with a meal, then increase to two or three daily as needed. It combines several useful adaptogens:

- American ginseng—cooling, moistening, useful for diabetes
- Korean ginseng—warming, stimulating for energy
- Red Chinese ginseng—warming, stimulating
- Eleuthero (Siberian) ginseng—for extreme climate changes, stress, nerve pain
- Royal jelly—source of predigested B vitamins for enhanced endurance

Cordyceps Medicinal Fungus Capsules

This medicinal fungus has been in use in China for centuries, but has recently become more popular. The Chinese love to use their silkworms, caterpillars, and bugs as medicines. They use everything that walks, runs, or flies because these too can benefit qi. If you found raw cordyceps in a Chinese herb shop, you might never buy it because it looks like dried worms. It is not. After a caterpillar leaves behind its cocoon home, a fungus grows on it, and that becomes dong chong xia cao—*Cordyceps sinensis* (also known as caterpillar fungus, Cs-4, dong chong zia cao, hsia ts'ao tung ch'ung, vegetable caterpillar).

Cordyceps, available in health-food stores and online, is considered a sweet and slightly warming tonic that supports the qi (vitality) of the lungs, liver, and adrenal glands. The purified fungus sold in capsules can be used for impotence and a sore or weak back. According to Chinese medical sources, cordyceps is used for strengthening the immune system, for reducing the effects of aging, promoting longevity, treating lethargy, and improving liver function in people with hepatitis B. It is also used to treat coughs, chronic bronchitis, respiratory disorders, kidney disorders, frequent nocturia (nighttime urination), male sexual dysfunction, anemia, heart arrhythmias, high cholesterol, liver disorders, dizziness, weakness, tinnitus, wasting, and drug addiction. It is mainly used as a stimulant, a tonic, and an adaptogen to increase energy and enhance stamina.

Dosage: start with one capsule, or about 500 milligrams daily. Avoid cordyceps or any medicinal fungus or mushroom if you are allergic to dietary mushrooms. Use Cordyceps as you would any other energy tonic before or after surgery. It can be taken along with daily vitamin supplements or foods.

General Postsurgery Tonic Dosage Advice

With stimulating adaptogens such as cordyceps and "warming" ginsengs such as steamed tienchi powder, red, Korean or Chinese ginseng, start with a low dose. Following surgery or childbirth, we need to slowly come back to health and vitality. A higher dose of a stimulant can further stress the body and cause insomnia, so start with a low dose. For example, start with one-fourth teaspoon of tienchi powder or one capsule of the above adaptogens. Using more or combining several is not necessarily beneficial. It is better to carefully observe your reactions, take time to heal, and use the treatment most suited to your needs. If using a tonic makes you feel dizzy, take it with food. If raw tienchi powder gives you diarrhea, it is too cooling and moistening for you at this time. You can reduce the dose and adjust your diet, omitting excess raw foods.

Postoperative Inflammation and Scars

Serrapeptase (serratiopeptidase) is a proteolytic enzyme that digests protein. It is produced by bacteria in the gut of silkworms and is used to digest their cocoons. When this enzyme is isolated and enteric-coated in a tablet, it has been shown to act as an anti-inflammatory and a pain blocker, much like aspirin, ibuprofen, and other nonsteroidal anti-inflammatory drugs (NSAIDs). Preliminary research indicates that serrapeptase may help inhibit plaque buildup in arteries, thereby preventing atherosclerosis (hardening of the arteries) and a resulting heart attack or stroke. Therefore, much like aspirin, this naturally derived enzyme may work to prevent inflammation, pain, heart attack, and stroke. Unlike aspirin and other over-the-counter NSAIDs, serrapeptase has not been shown to cause ulcers and stomach bleeding. This is good news for people who need daily protection against plaque buildup.

However, there are several cautions: serrapeptase should be avoided by pregnant women, people with gastrointestinal ulcers, and those who use anticoagulant drugs such as Coumadin (warfarin).

Serrapeptase works in three ways:

- It reduces inflammation by thinning the fluids formed from injury and facilitating the fluids' drainage. This in turn also speeds tissue repair.
- It helps alleviate pain by inhibiting the release of pain-inducing amines called bradykinins.
- It enhances cardiovascular health by breaking down the protein by-products of blood coagulation called fibrin. Serrapeptase is able to dissolve the fibrin and other dead or damaged tissue without harming living tissue. This could enable the dissolution of atherosclerotic plaques without causing any harm to the inside of the arteries.

Serrapeptase has been used in Europe and Asia for over twenty-five years. Because the enzyme digests or dissolves all nonliving tissue, including blood clots, cysts, and arterial plaque, it is used to treat a variety of conditions, including sprains and torn ligaments; postoperative swelling; venous thrombosis (clots in the legs); ear, nose, and throat infections; and atherosclerosis. Abroad, serrapeptase is marketed under a variety of name including Danzen, Aniflazym, and SerraZyme. In the United States, it has been used and marketed as Serrapeptase since 1997.

Health Concerns makes Serramend, a pill which is 10 milligrams of enteric-coated serratiopeptidase per capsule (not less than 2,000 units per milligram) derived from L serratia E-15. The dosage is one to two capsules two or three times daily between meals. Serramend is recommended as an anti-inflammatory that dissolves blood clots and plaque. It thins lung secretions to reduce chronic coughing. It reduces fibroids. In a study cited by Health Concerns, in a group of seventy women with cystic breast disease, 85.7 percent of the patients taking the enzyme had moderate to marked improvement. It can treat chronic lung (bronchitis), ear, nose, and throat disorders. After injury and surgery, it digests scar tissue and speeds healing.

The Long Term: Detoxify, Repair, and Rest

After surgery, your body will begin the healing process all by itself. You can help by resting, relaxing, and taking a few herbs.

Letha's Advice: An Easy Liver Flush

When you feel ready, you will definitely want to get rid of surgery and narcotic drugs after you return home from the hospital. With your doctor's approval, a simple liver flush can accomplish that. In addition, using olive oil reduces inflammatory pain. Here is a simple recipe for daily use. This is not the time to challenge vitality with a strong liver flush. This beverage tastes better cold, but to avoid headaches, do not drink any cold or raw liquids first thing in the morning.

Ingredients:
½ glass unfiltered apple cider
½ glass water
1 tablespoon extra-virgin olive oil

Stir it together and chug it down. You might do this before a meal. It will be laxative for some people. Continue this for a few days until you feel cleansed. Since it is a liver flush, you may notice the loss of gallstone sludge during bowel movements. If drinking this flush causes liver pain (at the right ribs), you may have stones or other liver complications. Therefore, stop using the flush if you feel too uncomfortable. Consult your natural health specialist and/or get tested for stones and other complications.

Another good digestive and balancing remedy for mind and body is the Chinese patent remedy Xiao Yao Wan pills, which contain herbs that both stimulate and cleanse the liver. They are ginger, mint, bupleurum, tang kuei, atractylodes, peony, poria, and licorice. Note: avoid tang kuei and licorice if you have an estrogen-dependent cancer. Those herbs are estrogenic.

Gotu Kola

Gotu kola (also known as marsh penny, Indian pennywort, and British pennywort) speeds healing for scars and wounds with infections that have not reached the bone. The herb can be used both internally and externally. Components of gotu kola have been shown to increase levels of antioxidants and help repair connective tissues.

Sunlight and Vitamin D3

Light and vitamin D made from exposing skin to sunshine heals wounds, reduces yeast infections, and helps prevent many serious illnesses, including cancers. Try to get twenty minutes of sunshine daily. Someday we may have

LED lights built into our homes, which result in less pain and fewer wrinkles. But there is something special about being outdoors in sunshine. We hear birds singing and feel a breeze. It deepens our breath, eases anxiety, and connects us with healing powers beyond the light socket.

CHAPTER TWELVE

Skin Issues

Beauty is a manifestation of secret natural laws otherwise hidden from us forever.

—Johann Wolfgang von Goethe (German playwright, 1749–1832)

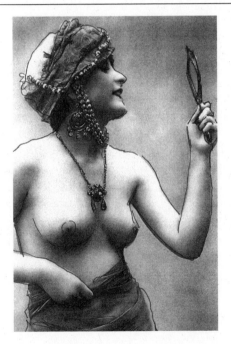

GOETHE, BEST KNOWN FOR WRITING *THE SORROWS OF YOUNG WERTHER* (1774) and his poetic drama in two parts, *Faust* (1806–1832), delved into alchemy, made important discoveries about plant and animal life, and evolved a non-Newtonian theory of light and color that influenced abstract painters Kandinsky and Mondrian. In *Zur Farbenlehre* (1810), Goethe wrote, "Every color produces a distinct impression on the mind, and thus addresses at once the eye and feelings." Goethe was moved by beauty. At the age of seventy-four, he fell in love with the nineteen-year-old Baroness Ulrike von Levetzow and proposed marriage. After she refused he wrote *The Marienbad Elegy*, his most personal poem. Unlike Werther, who committed suicide for love, Goethe died in Weimar at the ripe age of eighty-three. The Baroness never married. Who can say what our beauty may inspire?

Although skin problems may not cause pain like muscle strains or arthritis, they indicate injury and weakened immunity. Radiant-looking skin is proof that deeper energies such as nutrition, circulation, and elimination function well. A natural approach to complexion, beauty, and health impacts both inner vitality and outer complexion beauty with a cleansing diet, herbs, and treatments that affect well-being. Actor Redd Foxx said, "Beauty may be skin-deep but ugly goes clear to the bone." A Chinese herbalist would agree, adding that skin blemishes originate in the colon, stomach, liver, and lungs. Impurities, acids, and bacteria from poorly digested foods harm the blood and therefore the skin and our immune system. That is because skin, our outer shield against illness, is our largest organ of respiration. Beauty rises from the ground up, from healthy bacteria in the colon to the lungs and skin. Allowing one meal to be absorbed before eating another one improves digestion, breathing, and troubled skin, because poisons may be eliminated properly. Rich snacks harm digestive qi. However, digestive enzymes, taken with and *without* meals, increase absorption and reduce indigestion, joint aches, cellulite, and fibroids. Those are problems that take shape when "ugly reaches the bone."

The good news is that the same cleansing diet that reduces chronic pain, excess acidity and cholesterol, overweight, heart trouble, and cancer risk also clears the complexion. It is light, low in fats, with adequate fiber from complex carbohydrates, dark green leafy vegetables, moderate protein intake, and lots of green tea. Omega oils from fish, avoiding meat and cheese, work best. To clear your troubled complexion, avoid sweet acidic fruits (orange), excess nuts, oily or fried foods, hot spices, and all soda beverages. The baseline diet from *Feed Your Tiger* can be used to clear acne, allergies, and itchy rashes. For eczema and itchy dry skin rashes, avoid fried foods, honey, sugar, and oranges, because they are sweet, congesting, and acidic. Health Concerns makes Skin Balance herbal pills that are quite helpful in most cases.

Candida Yeast Skin Rash, Diabetic Sores, and PAD

Symptoms of candida (a very common yeast infection), fungus infections affecting nails, and diabetes often include chronic skin problems. A candida rash looks and may feel red-hot, like acne or diaper rash, and can cover the face, sexual area or entire body. Leg sores associated with diabetes are often painless from nerve damage. Slow-healing, painful, discolored sores on legs and feet, painful legs or buttocks from walking that improve with rest, and muscle loss in the calf are associated with late stages of peripheral arterial disease (PAD), resulting from plaque-clogged narrowed arteries in the arms or legs. PAD points to increased risk of heart attack and stroke. It is a problem often ignored in women and may affect many people after age fifty, especially smokers or people whose personal or family history includes diabetes, hypertension, or vascular problems.

Many people may develop a systemic candida yeast infection without knowing it. To clear a yeast rash, see the sections covering candida in chapters 6 and 7. In brief, omit foods that increase yeast, such as all fruits, mushrooms, sweets, candy, baked goods, breads, wine, and beer. Add one drop of antifungal, antibacterial Australian tea tree oil in a teacup of warm water daily. Wash affected areas of skin with tea tree oil diluted with a mild antibacterial soap and water. That advice alone can clear most yeast problems within a week. At the end of this chapter, I have included a section on effective food combining and a recipe to increase beneficial intestinal bacteria that will help prevent many complexion and other health issues. However, I have learned from clinical experience that health and beauty problems resulting from an unwise lifestyle are among the hardest to cure. In diagnosis, it is always easier to grasp an extreme case. For that reason, here is an interesting example given to prove a point: chronic skin problems start from deep within our energy and emotional imbalances.

Cynthia sent her friend Alice to me so that I might improve what she called "Alice's skin problem." She told me that Alice was in her seventies, lived alone in an expensive apartment, and wrote confessional poetry. Seeing Alice, I stepped back, shocked as a bag lady walked into the room wearing stuff she had picked up off the street, filthy shoes, and torn clothing. Her face was covered with oils and cosmetic creams and, not surprisingly, she had acne. She had smeared honey around her eyes that she said was to prevent blindness. She licked it with her finger. A shred of Kleenex was stuck on to her leg covering a wound. The overall appearance of her complexion looked reddish purple. I learned later it was from high cholesterol and energy and circulation problems.

Alice was bloated in the abdomen, but she insisted in a shrill voice that she was perfectly healthy. Traditional Chinese doctors observe qi in twelve meridians along the radial artery at the wrist. Her radial pulses were fast, wiry, and thin, indicating weakness and inflammation that had penetrated to affect internal organs. She had a slight odor of burnt garbage, indicating inflammation and liver congestion. She also smelled of rotten fish from rancid hemp oil she applied to wounds. But I confirmed inflammation by taking her radial pulses and observing her dark red, purple cracked tongue. She had a nail fungus for which she had tried various topical treatments without success. Because she had so many problems related to digestion, I suspected she had a systemic candida yeast overgrowth aggravated by her diet of fats, sweets, and rich health-food store snacks.

Not my usual client, she was unfortunately a sight not uncommon to big cities. Alone and depressed, Alice tortured her skin. Her face and tongue were fiery red from inflammation and congested digestion. She wanted to add more stuff, any skin cream I might suggest for her complexion, without improving her diet. A cleansing diet could lift her dark mood while improving her skin. I wondered, "Why do we torture the skin? It is an envelope of self-worth. Do women lacking love turn to illness for sensuality?" I shook off the feeling. I suggested a cooling, cleansing diet and herbal pills for Alice that could improve her complexion and many aspects of health and well-being. She refused. Alice's concern for complexion beauty was not misguided, but her approach missed the mark. That is because topical creams cannot reduce toxins in the blood that may harm body, mind, and spirit.

Another unusual example illustrates how the skin is part of a larger energy system. Alice came to see me again. This time her face was covered with large, angry red welts that resembled mosquito bites. When I asked what she had been putting on her skin, she replied that to treat her hemorrhoids she sat for hours on cotton balls soaked in vinegar. It was a treatment she had found on the Internet. I explained to her that the skin is part of an energy loop that includes the colon, lungs, and skin, and what she puts on her skin eventually goes inside. The vinegar made her entire body more acidic. I did not mention that excess acidity also increased her risk of cancer. I suggested that she stop sitting in vinegar and take Chinese herbal acne pills called Skin Balance, mentioned in this chapter. She took my advice about avoiding the vinegar treatment, and her facial skin rash went away.

Hemorrhoids are not really a skin problem but an internal inflammation problem that affects veins. Dr. Vasant Lad, author and Ayurvedic physician, recommends drinking aloe vera juice to reduce inflammation affecting the colon. That accomplishes many good things. It reduces acne, bad breath, constipation, and hemorrhoids. Alice did not try it.

Stubborn Skin Conditions and Messy Surroundings

Alice consulted another health professional experienced with difficult cases,

Christopher Phillips, CCH, RSHom (NA), a classical homeopath in New York City. He normally takes around two hours to interview a client in order to grasp the deeper aspects of the problem, discover its underlying cause, and choose the right homeopathic remedy. He always prescribes for the *person*, not the problem. I once heard Christopher describe the person for whom he might prescribe homeopathic sulphur. "The classic picture of a sulphur patient," he said, "is someone surrounded by mess and chaos, lost in intellectual musings and unable to realistically reconcile with her environment." Homeopathic sulphur may be used for stubborn, hard-to-treat skin problems. Sulphur, the nutrient in foods, makes new skin cells. Foods containing sulphur are listed in this chapter.

The connection between a qi energy imbalance and a person's physical symptoms, temperament, and lifestyle is fascinating. Homeopathy and herbal medicine are energy sciences that encompass many aspects of our lives while addressing our highly individual problems. They employ the art of looking, listening, and *sensing* another person to comprehend their discomfort. Alice may or may not be a sulphur patient. Many homeopathic remedies may affect her problems, but using a classical approach, one remedy at a time, can specifically impact underlying causes to treat problems deeper than skin. It often takes time for imbalances to surface and resolve. Working with someone as skilled and sensitive as Christopher, Alice made progress. Your skin problems are most likely not as serious as Alice's, and you can easily make progress clearing complexion blemishes with a light cleansing diet, select herbal treatments, and improved hygiene.

A Cleansing and Rebuilding Approach to New Skin

My background in Chinese herbal medicine naturally leads me first to cleansing foods and herbs for skin problems. I think of blemishes, rashes, and bumps as impurities trapped in the body. Chinese herbal medicine pays close attention to the energy of herbs, how the herb makes qi move in the body. Some foods and herbs move qi downward and inward through the meridians to impact internal organs, blood, and fluids. They may be antibiotic herbs, or those for reducing inflammation, or laxative or diuretic herbs. Other herbs move qi upward and outward in the meridian system toward the muscles and skin. For example, they may be herbs that increase sweating. That is an important difference when dealing with complexion. Think about this: do you want blemishes to shrink inward to become wastes or move outward like sweat on the skin?

Look at any typical Asian herbal formula for skin health and beauty: It contains bitter liver- and blood-cleansing herbs used to reduce inflammation, bacteria, fungal infections, and digestive acidity, as well as laxative herbs. That is where we want impurities to go—out of the body through elimination, not through sweating. However, foods and herbs such as hot spices and ginger increase a rash. Even certain cooling herbs—for example, chrysanthemum flower tea recommended for heat stroke, fever, or headache—increase sweating and bring out a rash. Herbs and foods that increase sweating are fine for eliminating chills, not skin rashes.

Letha's Advice for Troubled Skin: Aloe Vera Juice

Aloe is my first line of defense, useful for many aspects of well-being. The pulp and juice are alkaline, soothing, cooling, laxative and healing for internal and external skin irritations. Drinking up to one-fourth cup daily in water, unsweetened apple juice, or warm green tea can clear blemishes resulting from a too hot, spicy or fat diet; PMS; bad breath; and cramps that are accompanied by headache, fevers, flushed complexion and other signs of inflammation.

Here, beginning with the simplest suggestion and proceeding to more complex or odd, are popular herbal treatments to clear troubled skin, regulate metabolism, and protect immunity.

Simple to Complex Remedies for Acne, Rashes, Constipation, and Nerve Pains
Skin Balance by Health Concerns

Health Concerns in Oakland, California, purifies, tests, and combines Chinese raw herbs, used in traditional herbal formulas, with additional nutriceuticals to make health-food-quality Chinese herbal pills. For example, Skin Balance pills combine herbs that "clear liver heat" (dizziness, irritability, eye redness). The combination also "cleans blood," which means it reduces acidic impurities and eliminates what TCM doctors call dampness (when applied to skin, dampness means swelling, oozing, and slow-healing wounds.) The pills are recommended for itchy skin inflammation, psoriasis, eczema, rosacea, and hives, while they moisten and nourish skin dryness. The detoxifying ingredients are skullcap, oldenlandia, gentiana, raw rehmannia, viola (antibiotic), lonicera (antibiotic), lysimachia, coptis (reduces fever), tang kuei (enhances circulation and blood production), bupleurum, carthamus (safflower, enhances circulation), senna, and rhubarb (laxative). The recommended dose is three pills three times daily, but reduce the dose if diarrhea occurs. Avoid laxatives during pregnancy.

Lien Chiao Pai Tu Pien

These pills are a Chinese patent remedy that contains blood-cleansing herbs and dried rhubarb (not recommended during pregnancy). It is a popular Chinese medicine that "clears heat, resolves toxin, dispels pathogenic wind, dispels damp heat, disperses swelling, and cools blood." That means the herbs are anti-inflammatory (clear heat) and they quiet nerve irritations, spasms, pain, or itching (dispel wind). The formula also reduces oozing and infection (clears damp heat). "Cools the blood" means it reduces acidic impurities that lead to blemishes, boils, and rash. All in all, the pill is cooling, detoxifying, and useful for irritated, hot, slow-healing blemishes. Lien Chiao Pai Tu Pien herbal pills can be used for hives, boils, rash, poison ivy and oak, carbuncles, and acne. They may also be used for symptoms of measles, mumps, and chicken pox. The ingredients are forsythia bark (reduces fever), lonicera (a broad-spectrum antibiotic useful for fever, sore throat, and staph infections), rhubarb (laxative), paeonia (used in nervous disorders), skullcap (liver cleansing), gardenia, cicada (cools inflammation and reduces infections). The dosage is usually four pills taken with water twice or three times daily. Reduce the dose if diarrhea occurs.

Trisnake Pills

Snakes have been used in Chinese medicine for thousands of years, and there are restaurants and herb shops in South China that specialize in serving snake as a dish and snake wines. I had a rather chewy snake lunch at a posh Shanghai restaurant years ago, one of over six thousand restaurants that serve "dragon meat." Chinese herb shops may sell powdered black snake, used for chronic arthritic pain and inflammatory skin rashes. A dose of the powder is added to a little water to swallow. One of the earliest recorded uses of snakes in Chinese medicine was the application of sloughed-off snake skin, described in the *Shen Nong Ben Cao Jing* (ca. 100 AD). It was originally applied in the treatment of superficial diseases, including skin eruptions, eye infections or opacities, sore throat, and hemorrhoids.

Trisnake pills (Trisnakes Resolve Itching Pills, San She Dan) are a Chinese patent remedy that is very useful for itchy skin rashes, acne, slow-healing wet sores, inflammatory arthritis, and low immunity and poor circulation in the elderly. The pill combines the dried bodies of three types of snakes—pit viper (fan pi), krait (bai hua she), and black striped snake (wu shao she)—along with tonic herbs peony, dong quai, cnidium fruit, and ginseng. The nerve-sedative and circulation-enhancing aspects of snake are useful for arthritis, rheumatism, paralysis, and nerve pain (called wind or feng by TCM doctors). That same treatment is useful for slow-healing, itchy skin conditions, psoriasis, candida rash, and aging skin.

The overall effects of Trisnake pills are detoxifying and calming. The normal dose is five pills taken after or between meals twice daily. Avoid eating hot, spicy, or very bitter foods while using this pill. I refuse to give up my daily unsweetened tea, so the treatment may take longer than the usual month or two recommended. When I tried it the first time, the action was fast. I felt my qi circulation shift toward my ribs and legs. I felt sciatica more intensely for only a moment, and then a calm, happy, pain-free feeling swept over me that improved my sleep. While the pill moved my qi and reduced facial inflammation, a warm feeling came to areas of my face for a moment where inflammation had been. A Chinese herbalist friend told me she takes prepared snake gallbladder, sold with a little liquor in small bottles, during spring when winds are higher (when there are more allergies and irritants that may cause pain, rashes, and irritability).

Python Soup

I once described, only half seriously, a python pie recipe for a blog post I wrote. But here is a real recipe from one of my south Asian friends for python soup, which I hope becomes popular in south Florida, where Burmese pythons are devouring the Everglades.

Ingredients:

2½ pounds python steak

1 teaspoon lemon peel

10 stems lemongrass, peeled, tender parts finely chopped and pounded, stems reserved

5 shallots, peeled and sliced, peels reserved

7 cloves garlic, peeled and pounded, peels reserved

3-inch-long piece ginger, peeled and thinly sliced, peels reserved

2 tablespoons peanut oil

1 tablespoon turmeric powder

¼ teaspoon cumin powder

1 tablespoon sweet Hungarian paprika

⅛ teaspoon asafoetida powder (optional)

1 teaspoon curry leaves, chopped (optional)

¼ cup brandy

2 teaspoons salt

2 limes, cut in wedges

Chilies or black pepper seeds, pounded, to taste

First, boil/poach the steak with lemon peel, rough lemon-grass stems, and peels of shallots, garlic, and ginger in a couple of pints of spring water. When the flesh is soft, take the steak out and let it cool. Separate the bones from the flesh, and dice flesh. Next, sauté the shallots in oil on low heat until slightly brown, and add the ginger, garlic, and all other spices. (Asafoetida is an Ayurvedic medicinal herb that tastes pungent like garlic. It is used to treat spasms in the bowel, coughing, bronchitis, intestinal parasites, bloating, fungal and yeast infections, and chronic fatigue.) Continue stirring for a couple of minutes until an aroma rises from the pot. Add cooked diced python flesh. Add 1 quart water, and flavor with brandy and salt. Reduce heat and simmer for 10 minutes. Serve this hot with wedges of lime and chilies or pepper seeds and strong tea or a chilled glass of dry champagne.

Shingles (Herpes Zoster)

My favorite antibacterial, antiviral tea for detoxifying the body and reducing feverish conditions, irritability, and skin rashes is *Prunella vulgaris* (xia ku cao in Chinese). Some herbal experts say it reduces a herpes outbreak and reduces shingles pain. It grows wild in your lawn, like a spiral of little purple flowers and round green leaves. But I buy it dried in Chinatown. The tea is tasteless, and easy to brew, and feels cooling and relaxing. I especially enjoy its calming effects as a bedtime tea in spring. Over time, it helps reduce cholesterol and improves circulation. Steep about two tablespoons in a teapot and drink it warm or cool. Do not sweeten it, unless you add a pinch of stevia. You may combine prunella with dandelion herb to increase the cleansing effects.

Two Teas for Building New Skin

Dandelion herb and Japanese honeysuckle flower makes a slightly bitter tea that works fast to reduce skin redness and itching caused by eczema. Honeysuckle flower is an antibiotic herb used for fevers, sore throat, rash, and pneumonia and staph infections. Dandelion is a blood and liver cleanser useful as a diuretic and laxative herb that helps to dissolve gallstones, kidney stones, fibroids, and cholesterol. Steep a teaspoon each of honeysuckle flower and dandelion herb per pot of tea. If its taste upsets your stomach, add a slice of raw ginger. Both herbs are bitter. But do not add honey or the blemishes and acids will be brought out to the skin.

Oldenlandia Diffusa Instant Beverage (Tea Sweetener)

Sometimes Chinese herbalists use cane sugar to improve the taste of very bitter herbs. One popular instant beverage called Oldenlandia Diffusa, sold in the tea section of Chinese groceries, is recommended to clear complexion blemishes. It is so sweet that I use part of this packet of herbal granules as a beverage sweetener. The two anti-inflammatory herbs in Oldenlandia Diffusa (oldenlandia and skullcap) are used for skin problems and to help reduce cancer risk. It is a nice sweet addition to any tea or recipe that reduces acne at any age or PMS breakouts.

Purpura: Bleeding Under the Skin

Do you bruise easily? Some people who have poor circulation or who use blood-thinning medicines bleed under the skin. Purpura occurs when small blood vessels under the skin leak. Purpura spots can be very small blood spots, petechiae, or large ecchymoses. A person with purpura may have normal platelet counts (nonthrombocytopenic purpuras) or decreased platelet counts (thrombocytopenic purpuras). Purpura may be due to drugs that affect platelet function, rubella, fragile blood vessels seen in older people, and vasculitis (inflammation of blood vessels) such as Henoch-Schönlein purpura.

Henoch-Schönlein purpura in children often occurs after an upper respiratory infection. It causes skin rashes that bleed into the skin (small red petechiae and purpura of larger areas). Bleeding may also occur from the gastrointestinal tract and kidneys. Henoch-Schönlein purpura in adults has red to purple bumps on the legs, often accompanied by aching in the joints and fever. This condition follows an infection and may resolve without treatment. Skin lesions most commonly occur below the knee but may also be seen on the thighs, buttocks, and rarely on the arms.

Immune thrombocytopenic purpura (ITP) occurs when certain immune system cells produce antibodies against platelets. Platelets help your blood clot by clumping together to plug small holes in damaged blood vessels. In children, the disease sometimes follows a viral infection and usually goes away without treatment. In adults, it is more often a chronic disease and can occur after a viral infection, use of certain drugs, pregnancy, or an immune disorder. Adults are usually started on an anti-inflammatory medicine such as prednisone. In some cases, surgery to remove the spleen is recommended. If the disease does not get better with prednisone, other treatments may include injections of high-dose gamma globulin, drugs that suppress the immune system, or filtering antibodies out of the blood stream. Note: people with ITP should not take aspirin, ibuprofen, and warfarin (Coumadin) because these drugs interfere with platelet function and blood clotting, and bleeding may occur.

Purpura, Bruising, and Broken Capillaries: Persimmon Leaf Tea

Often in older people who have the characteristic puffy skin associated with "weak spleen," you see water retention in the legs, broken capillaries, and a ruddy complexion. In *Chinese Medicated Diet*, a textbook in a series published by the Shanghai College of Traditional Chinese Medicine, persimmon leaf tea is recommended for thrombopenic purpura, defined as dermorrhagia (fa ban), hematohidrosis (ji niu), and visceral hemorrhage (xue zheng), bleeding under the skin. Symptoms are excessive accumulation of "toxic heat" (inflammatory bacterial or acidic impurities) with purple ecchymosis (bruises resulting from trauma), nose bleeds, bleeding gums, blood in the urine, irritability, red tongue with yellow coating, and a wiry rapid pulse. In more extreme cases, there may also be excessive menstruation, afternoon fever, hot palms and soles, dizziness, or palpitations.

Persimmon leaf tea may work because it strengthens blood capillaries. In the 1980s, the Chinese Academy of Sciences found that persimmon leaf tea contains a large quantity of Vitamin C, tannins, flavonoids, rutin, choline, carotenoids, and amino acids. In addition, the tea contains magnesium, manganese, titanium, calcium, and phosphorous. Scientific research has shown that drinking persimmon leaf tea promotes a healthy metabolism. Rutin helps prevent arteriosclerosis (fragile capillaries). Flavonoids lower blood pressure and increase blood flow. According to Japan's *Longevity* magazine, drinking persimmon leaf tea can prevent melanoma. The tea's health benefits generate anticancer and anti-influenza virus interferons.

Persimmon Leaf Skin Treatment for Bruises and Aging Skin

If you have fragile, aging skin and broken capillaries, brew a pot of strong persimmon leaf tea by adding one teaspoon of the dried leaves for each two cups of boiling water. Allow it to stand overnight. Drink a cup or more of the tea daily. Fill a spray bottle with cold persimmon leaf tea and use it as a cooling skin spray. Add persimmon leaf tea to aloe vera gel and apply it with sterile cotton to clean skin. Avoid applying any skin preparation or cosmetic that contains alcohol or fragrance, often made using alcohol as a preservative. Alcohol weakens blood vessels.

Penny Frazier grows persimmon plants for the tea leaf and fruit. Her company Goods from the Woods is located in Licking, Missouri. She used to have a terrible pollen allergy that prevented her from going out in the fields for harvest. Drinking persimmon leaf tea cured her allergies. Other people have reported improvement of digestive complaints. The tea is slightly bitter and can be laxative in large doses. Penny has a blog at her website, www.wildcrops.com, that features news about piñon pine nuts, a fine source of protein and a tasty treat. Her company grows wild plants, specialty teas, fruits, mushrooms, and piñon nuts in season.

New Skin Foods: Minerals/Sulphur Foods

Foods high in minerals are helpful building blocks to better health, complexion, and beauty. A mixed mineral supplement that includes trace minerals is a good idea to use after digestion and elimination have improved and after the cleansing effects of bitter herbs have worked to clear your complexion. Otherwise, adding supplements may only add problems.

Sulphur forms an integral part of all human tissues, especially those high in protein, such as red blood cells, muscles, skin, and hair. Trace amounts come from foods, but most of the sulphur in our body is in the form of nonessential amino acids, such as taurine, methionine, and cystine. Sulphur is also a component of insulin, vitamin B1, and biotin. Sulphur protects our cells from the damaging effects of radiation and air pollution, thereby slowing down the aging process. It aids in the conversion of fats, carbohydrates, and proteins into energy, and as a component of collagen, helps to keep skin cells supple and elastic. Sulphur is required for the digestion of fats, activates enzymes, and helps regulate blood clotting. There is no recommended daily intake for sulphur, but deficiencies are rare. It is abundant in the diet. Toxic effects are nonexistent because excess sulphur is excreted in the urine. Foods particularly high in sulphur include meat and poultry, fish, eggs, beans and peas, brussels sprouts, onions, cabbage, garlic, wheat germ, and dairy products.

Food Combinations to Avoid

In general, it is best to avoid combining fruits with proteins and starches because of varying times required for their digestion. Fruits digest quickly and turn into sugar. Have them between meals with tea. Fruit combined with protein delays digestion and leads to bloating and indigestion. There is a science to food combining that goes beyond ethnic cuisines and traditions. Some fats, meats, and dairy foods, especially when they are unwisely combined, increase phlegmy congestion that underlies slow-healing blemishes, swelling, and oozing wounds. The aftereffects of poor food combining reach far beyond complexion problems.

I have studied with Dr. Yeshi Dhonden, the famous Tibetan monk and former physician to the Dalai Lama. Concerning cancer prevention, he said that certain food combinations are "fatal." They are too difficult to digest together so that they aggravate food allergies and increase congestion and metabolism problems that underlie tumors. The "deadly combinations" include fish and eggs as well as fish and milk, both combinations that increase digestive toxins. Dr. Dhonden said specifically, "Avoid eating meals and snacks that are too closely scheduled together. Allow the body to fully digest one meal before eating another." That simplifies food combining.

Pickled Vegetables for Complexion and Immunity

Digestion is only part of the picture. We absorb nutrients, including calcium, in a healthy gut that has adequate beneficial bacteria. Having healthy bacteria in the colon makes absorption of essential nutrients possible. That is why it is important to eat yogurt or take acidophilus capsules after using an antibiotic that kills both harmful and good digestive bacteria. Here is another way to insure proper digestion daily. The following recipe for pickled vegetables increases healthy digestive bacteria and has been used to eliminate warts and complexion problems for many people. It is recommended to eat one-fourth cup of pickled vegetables with each protein meal. It will be laxative for some people, and that also reduces skin problems and inflammation. Why bother to make your own pickled vegetables? It's fun, it's healthy, and gives you great-looking skin, a slimmer waistline, and improved zest for life.

By pickles I don't mean the kind you find sold in the supermarket that contain salt, vinegar, and preservatives. I mean naturally fermented vegetables that keep all their enzymes. Homemade pickles require fresh, clean organic vegetables. Cooking the vegetables beforehand will not work. Just rinse them in hot water or soak them for five minutes in water and apple cider vinegar and rinse well with clean water.

Get yourself a large, thick, glass canning jar that seals airtight with a red rubber tubing around the top. Thick glass will not crack when you clean it with boiling water to sterilize it. If you can't find jars with rubber tubing to make them airtight, use my method to make pickles and consume the vegetables within a couple of days.

Keep your hands and the jar clean when making the pickles. Store the pickled vegetables out of the refrigerator when they are fermenting, and keep them in the refrigerator after they have fermented and reached the flavor you want in a few days to weeks. Daily turn the jar upside down or shake it to get the juices to mix with the vegetables. Keep your hands out of the pickle jar. Use a clean fork to serve yourself. If you see mold or it smells bad, throw it out.

Wash your jar and vegetables. I pour boiling water and swish it around in the jar and pour boiling water on the sliced vegetables. The following recipe contains chopped cabbage because it ferments fast and naturally contains the enzymes necessary for fermenting. You don't need to buy a starter culture.

After thoroughly washing, pack the sliced vegetables tightly into the jar, leaving an inch free at the top of the jar to allow for the natural fermentation gases of vegetables to expand. I bring the spices to a boil in water and turn it off. Then pour the liquid and spices over the sliced vegetables to cover them. Seal the jar and let the vegetables do their thing. If you want to make rejuvelac (fermented barley water) and use some of the liquid to ferment your vegetables, your pickles will be ready faster. See the directions for fermented barley water in *Feed Your Tiger*. It's easy to make: soak organic barley in water for a couple of days to make the fermented liquid. Add sliced ginger and lemongrass for taste if you prefer. Drinking rejuvelac regularly improves digestion and speeds cleansing.

A golden rule for making pickles: thou shalt use neither salt, sugar, nor vinegar.

Let the vegetables ferment a day, and then smell and taste them. Adjust the spices. Leave them out to ferment longer if you want a stronger taste. The taste depends on the spices. Dill pickles take at least one week and lots of spices. Make up your own recipes, including some cabbage, garlic, and spices like coriander, cumin, juniper berries, turmeric, lemon juice, and a salt substitute such as dulse or kelp seaweed or a potassium salt substitute.

Basic Natural Dills

These look and taste like Grandma's but are made without preservatives.

Ingredients:

1–2 heads of green cabbage, chopped or thinly sliced
Raw garlic to taste
Coriander, cumin, turmeric, asafoetida, juniper berries, mustard seed (seeds or powdered)
Fresh dill herb if possible, or dried dill seeds
1 pound of small cucumbers or several large ones
1 handful of dried dulse seaweed per quart jar or a potassium salt substitute to taste
Juice of one lemon
Celery or onion, sliced (optional)

Thinly slice the cabbage and pack it into the bottoms of two 1 quart jars. Add the garlic and spices. Add sliced or small whole cucumbers so that they are tightly packed. Add the seaweed anywhere with the spices or on top. Add the lemon juice last.

Press down the vegetables so that they touch.

Place some sliced celery or onion on top if you like. The longer you ferment it and the more lemon juice, mustard seed, and dill you use, the more it will taste like dill pickles. It may look cloudy. That's okay if otherwise it looks and smells okay. Happy pickling!

Nail Fungus

Nail fungus is an unsightly problem that is more common among older people who have diminished blood circulation or poor immunity and may wear sweaty covered shoes or nylon socks. Moisture, darkness, and warmth breed germs. Anyone can get a fungal infection or a plantar wart, a viral infection that looks like a flat crusty patch, while walking barefoot in an area where germs live. Swimming pools, locker rooms, and public showers may all have the problem. Washing with soap and water, making sure shoes are clean, and adding an anti-fungal powder inside shoes are adequate prevention in many cases. However, a nasty inconvenience becomes a real problem if a nail fungus, mold, or yeast infection is accompanied by diabetes, a compromised immune system, leukemia, or AIDS, or for people who've had an organ transplant. Nail fungus is hard to treat and can reoccur. Dirt that collects under the nail and fungus can spread to other toes and fingers. Most of us touch foods and spread those germs to other people without thinking. In serious cases a fungus, mold, or yeast can become systemic. It harms digestion, skin, and energy.

If you have diabetes, your blood circulation and the nerve supply to your feet may become impaired. You're also at greater risk for cellulitis, a potentially serious bacterial skin infection. Therefore, any relatively minor injury to your feet, including a nail fungal infection, can lead to a more serious complication, requiring timely medical care.

Nail Fungus Risk Factors

According to the Mayo Clinic, factors that increase risk of developing nail fungus include:

- Perspiring heavily
- Working in a humid or moist environment
- Having the skin condition psoriasis
- Wearing socks and shoes that hinder ventilation and don't absorb perspiration
- Walking barefoot in damp public places, such as swimming pools, gyms, and shower rooms
- Having athlete's foot (tinea pedis)

- Having a minor skin or nail injury, a damaged nail, or another infection
- Having diabetes, circulation problems, or a weakened immune system

A nail fungal infection may begin as a white or yellow spot under the tip of your fingernail or toenail. As the nail fungus spreads deeper into your nail, it may cause your nail to discolor, thicken, and develop crumbling edges—an unsightly and potentially painful problem. You may even lose the nail.

Western Medical Treatment and Side Effects

If you have athlete's foot as well as nail fungus, you should treat the athlete's foot with topical medication and keep your feet clean and dry. To treat nail fungus, your doctor may prescribe an oral antifungal medication such as terbinafine (Lamisil) and itraconazole (Sporanox). These medications help a new nail grow free of infection, slowly replacing the infected portion of your nail. These medications are taken for six to twelve weeks, but you won't see the end result until the nail grows back completely. It may take four months or longer to eliminate an infection. Recurrent infections are always possible, especially if you continue to expose your nails to warm, moist conditions.

Antifungal drugs have side effects ranging from skin rashes to liver damage. Doctors may not recommend them for people with liver disease or congestive heart failure or for those taking certain medications. Another possibility is an antifungal nail polish called ciclopirox (Penlac). You paint it onto your infected nails and surrounding skin once a day. Or your doctor may recommend surgery to remove the nail.

Letha's Advice: Home Treatment for Nail Fungus

The Mayo Clinic suggests soaking your feet in vinegar and applying Vicks VapoRub, without knowing why Vicks might work. But unfortunately, absorbing vinegar through the porous skin of hands and feet can eventually give you a serious red blemish outbreak that resembles bug bites. Vicks may work somewhat because camphor in it is cooling. It is a slow, painful treatment at best. However, no dermatologist will mention anything about an antiyeast/antifungal diet. They are allowed to treat skin, not diet. But a fungus is a fungus inside and out: repeat it like a mantra. If you are weak or tired, or have had surgery, your immune system is challenged. Therefore, avoid foods that make yeast, mold, and fungus grow. They are sweets, sugar, fruits, fermented foods, breads and baked goods, tofu, wine, and beer. See the antiyeast diet suggestions on page

171. Remember to try Australian tea tree oil internally as mouthwash or added to water as tea. A cocktail made with gin, vodka, or scotch and no sugar may give you less trouble than a beer. Alcoholic beverages that are higher than forty proof breed no germs.

Antibacterial/Antifungal External Application and Tea

Wash with soap and water, dry your nails, and apply Australian tea tree oil to nail fungus daily. Add one drop of essential tea tree oil to a porcelain cup, not foam or plastic. Drink it in your coffee or brush your teeth with tea tree oil. Take acidophilus daily to repopulate your digestive tract with beneficial bacterial.

A Foot Patch

Assume a nail fungus may stay around awhile and may even go deeper to cause harm. You need to take active steps to enhance immunity. One way involves deep cleansing. Online and in Chinese or Japanese health shops, you can find convenient-to-use patches that you apply to the bottoms of your feet in order to detoxify the body while you sleep. Our bodies produce toxic wastes as a by-product of metabolic processes. Fatty wastes, uric acid crystals, and metallic residues normally accumulate in the joints and soles, preventing normal blood circulation and thus causing various problems such as arthritis, inflammation of the joints, swollen legs, skin allergies/diseases, and high blood pressure, among others, that seriously affect health. With regular application of herbal detox patches on the affected parts, various illnesses may be reduced or eliminated so that the body can function normally.

You can apply the patch according to foot reflexology areas. According to Asian energy medicine, the patch extracts "internal dampness and expels harmful waste from our bodies." That may reduce foot odors, discolorations, and germs. One Japanese company makes the Sole Patch, which comes in three varieties:

- Sole Patch—regular strength for everyday use (eight patches per box)
- Lavender Patch—contains lavender essential oil to aid the body to calm and relax; may help soothe the mind and promote restful sleep (six patches per box)
- Chili Patch—adds chili powder to make the patch warming and speed up the extraction process; do not use on broken, fragile, or irritated skin (eight patches per box)

Each box contains patches and stickers in a resealable plastic bag. The main ingredients are bamboo vinegar, chitosan, vitamin C, and dokudami leaf. Chitosan, a shellfish by-product, is very interesting, because current Chinese research in development is making antibacterial surfaces used in hospitals from chitosan. Chitosan is derived from chitin, the main fiber component of crustacean shells. It has powerful absorption abilities which, according to www .modernherbshop.com, "aid in the effectiveness of the patch by isolating fatty tissue and assisting in dispelling it out of the body."

Herbalists at Suigetsu Dojo, an active martial arts community in Long Island, New York, describe the action of the Sole Patch this way: "According to ancient Oriental knowledge, our human body has over 360 acupuncture points, with more than sixty acupuncture points found on the soles of the feet. Known as the 'second heart,' they are the reflective zones of our major internal organs. They are also potential homes for toxins. When the blood circulates to the soles, the Sole Patch can absorb toxins released from these acupuncture points. Even after only one night of body detoxification, there may be significant changes to the smell and color of the patch (from brown to grayish black) as it reflects the amount and degree of toxins that were extracted from the body. With continuous usage, there should be a visible reduction in the stain and odor of the patch."

For my money, a general detoxification program that stresses reducing yeast, mold, and fungus works a lot better than soaking feet in irritating vinegar and taking potentially harmful drug medicines for a fungal infection.

Sesame Oil Rejuvenation

Many of us spend a small fortune on skin creams and treatments, forgetting that whatever we apply topically eventually enters our blood stream and affects our nerves. It is wise to use the following rejuvenating skin treatment that is safe enough to eat. Mild sesame oil used for skin moisturizing and massage eases tensions, soothes wrinkles, and feels rejuvenating down to the bone. Sesame Seed Oil has been used as a healing oil for thousands of years. It is naturally antibacterial for common skin pathogens, such as staphylococcus and streptococcus, as well as common skin fungi, such as athlete's foot fungus. It is naturally antiviral. According to Youthing Strategies Inc., suppliers of pharmaceutical -grade sesame oil products in Branson, Missouri, sesame oil is a natural anti-inflammatory agent. In India, experiments showed that sesame oil was useful in unblocking arteries. In recent experiments in Holland by Ayurvedic physicians, the oil has been used in the treatment of several chronic disease processes, including hepatitis, diabetes, and migraines. In vitro, sesame seed oil has inhibited the growth of malignant melanoma and has inhibited replication of human colon cancer cells.

Research shows that sesame seed oil is a potent antioxidant. In the tissues beneath the skin, this oil will neutralize oxygen radicals. It penetrates into the skin quickly and enters the blood stream through the capillaries. Molecules of sesame seed oil maintain good cholesterol (HDL) and lower bad cholesterol (LDL). All in all, it is one of the best skin oils and culinary oils, used unheated, to support rejuvenation.

Light Therapy

Chapter 5 features light-emitting diode (LED) treatments for chronic pain. This chapter, covering skin issues, describes cosmetic light treatments. Enhancing circulation and reducing inflammation with LED light therapy may also prove useful for uncomfortable skin conditions such as purpura and shingles. That remains to be proven. According to a product description for Light-Therapy-LED, "Studies have shown light therapy can assist in repairing some forms of DNA." According to professional sources, cancer researchers have noted that a single red frequency combined with a topical cream kills certain types of skin cancer cells. Researchers also noted that it stimulated skin tissue to regenerate and improve the appearance of the skin. Circulation is increased, and fibro-blastic activity, collagen production, and healing are promoted. This effect has produced very positive results in the treatment of rosacea, antiaging skin treatments, and sun damage.

You may have experienced light therapy at a beauty shop or doctor's office. Certain wavelengths encourage a corrective skin response. Red LED lights consists of 650 nm (nanometer) wavelengths that heal and encourage natural collagen production, which helps the skin to repair itself. Blue LED lights repair damaged skin and minimize blemishes. The blue light has 470 nm wavelength, recommended over the 415 nm that improves acne. The blue light suppresses melatonin (a hormone that makes you feel sleepy) and is easy on the eyes. LED light therapy claims to improve sleep, boost energy, and enhance mood and well-being. Certainly on dark wintery days, more light is always welcome.

Directions warn not to use any other skin treatment with red and blue LED light therapy. Always wear protective eye goggles and only do one fifteen-minute session daily. Results are variable. Some users report improvement in skin texture and color, with a reduction of acne; others, little improvement. That may be because of differing skin texture, hue, and tone. Caution: avoid LED light therapy if one of the following conditions applies:

- Pregnancy—studies have not sufficiently assessed the risk to pregnant women and their babies; therefore it is not recommended.
- Patients with porphyria should avoid most forms of light therapy.
- Epilepsy—certain light frequencies can trigger an epileptic seizure.

- Thyroid condition—if you suffer from a thyroid condition or are on thyroid medication.
- If you are photo-allergic, or are taking any medication that causes light sensitivity, such as tetracycline.

High-tech therapy is becoming mainstream as our demand increases. I noticed recently an article in a woman's magazine that mentioned LED room lighting "in the bathroom of the future" so that home pain and beauty treatments can become as easy as flipping a switch.

Chapter Thirteen

Toothaches

I am called a dog because I fawn on those who give me any-thing, I yelp at those who refuse, and I set my teeth in rascals.

—Diogenes (Greek philosopher, 412 BC–323 BC)

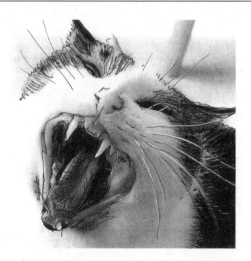

HAVE YOU SET YOUR TEETH IN ANY RASCALS LATELY? SOME COULD GIVE YOU A toothache. Diogenes believed we should live by the dictates of reason and went out of his way to disprove Plato's metaphysical sophisms. When Plato defined the human being as an animal, biped and featherless, Diogenes plucked a chicken, brought it into the lecture room, and announced, "Here is Plato's human being." Diogenes lit a lamp in broad daylight and said he was searching for a human being. I hope this chapter of simple, practical advice serves as a guiding light for avoiding tooth troubles. Common signs of aging include hair loss, wrinkled skin, and deeper problems of fragile bones and lost teeth. This chapter stresses a holistic rejuvenating approach to support your health and beauty.

The earliest recorded toothache was 275 million years ago for *Labidosaurus hamatus*, one of the first reptiles to move out of water and live on land. That move changed their diet and teeth. Permanent teeth meant bacterial infections and tooth decay and profoundly affected our evolution. We were in for it: regular dental checkups, toothaches, root canals, bridges, and Jurassic dental bills. In the 1930s, Mae West (American actress, 1893–1980) said, "Love conquers all things except poverty and a toothache."

Many annoying tooth and gum discomforts resulting from overwork, poor habits, and stress may be avoided with proper care. Unfortunately, few health professionals recommend foods and herbs that specifically protect teeth and gums. Most people acknowledge that for general health it is best to avoid smoking, junk foods, and harsh chemicals that damage teeth. However, this chapter stresses a unique but sound approach based on traditional Chinese medicine: teeth are like little bones. You will see that much of the same nutritional advice for building strong bones applies as well to teeth. This chapter also includes a shocker: what your dentist does not tell you and may not know.

Problem Signs

It is highly recommended that you visit the dentist every six months for a tooth cleaning and checkup. The following signs indicate potential problems, and you should inform your dentist if you see them.

- Tongue, inner cheek, and throat are red, puffy, or discolored white.
- Gums are swollen, red, soft, or bleeding.
- A tooth is injured or dislodged.
- A tooth or surrounding gums hurt.
- You have a tendency to grind your teeth.
- You have pain near the jaw joint.
- You have chronic headaches or TMJ pain.

Gum problems often occur from poor nutrition, chronic illness, certain medications, and blood loss, and eventually harm the teeth. If diet and absorption are faulty, teeth become loose or fall, develop decay, easily break, or become discolored. For that reason, my nutritional and herbal treatments benefit our *source* of vitality for teeth, gums, and bones, regulated by deep energy fields of the adrenal glands, blood, and bone marrow. The building matter of teeth and bones includes minerals absorbed by healthy bacteria in the colon.

It is interesting how the health of our teeth reflects qi energy. Have you ever developed tooth or gum trouble when you were exhausted, depressed, stressed, or overindulging in spicy foods, or after surgery or childbirth? Weakened immunity sets the stage for tooth and gum trouble.

Teeth, Gums, and Acupuncture Meridians

You may have seen charts showing points on the feet used in reflexology that correspond to areas of the body. Acupuncturists observe the tongue and twelve wrist pulses, and may treat acupuncture points on the nose, ears, or hands and feet in order to affect other troubled areas in the body. In the 1950s, a scientist began measuring electrical currents in acupuncture meridians. Electrodermal screening, originally called "electroacupuncture according to Voll" (EAV), was developed by Dr. Reinhold Voll, a German engineer, medical doctor, dental surgeon, homeopath, and acupuncturist. Based on therapy derived from Chinese acupuncture and modern electronics, Voll-machine testing became popular among a few holistic-minded dentists. Dr. Voll claimed that "Ninety percent of all chronic disease has an orientation in the mouth." Disease can be observed by changes in teeth and gums because acupuncture meridians pass through the mouth on the way to the brain. A dentist once told me that pulling a tooth harms meridian qi, and a root canal may weaken the body since bacteria may continue to grow at the site. A tooth and its root are located on a meridian pathway. Gum infections harm heart health because our blood and qi circulation work together to maintain health. Weak teeth, pale gums, and increased tooth breakage indicate poor absorption of vital nutrients.

Prevention: The Big Picture

The causes of tooth decay and breakage closely resemble bone loss because their building materials are the same. As you will see, adding the right foods and herbs to your diet can improve both problems. For clues to proper treatment for teeth and gums, let's look at bone loss as an epidemic problem.

Bone Loss and Your Teeth

Osteoporosis is the progressive thinning and weakening of bones that leads to *repeated* fractures and bone breaking with minimum force. If osteoporosis is a widespread problem globally, as many experts claim, there must also exist a major problem for our teeth. With osteoporosis, there are often no symptoms until you break a bone with a sneeze or lose a tooth biting into a bun. More importantly, after repeated fractures a person's risk of death increases. "We do not understand the reason yet, but for almost all osteoporosis fractures the person's risk of death doubles compared to that of a nonosteoporosis person of the same age and similar circumstances," said Professor John Allan Eisman, in an interview during January 2004. Dr. Eisman is Director, Bone and Mineral

Research Program, Garvan Institute of Medical Research, and Professor of Medicine, University of New South Wales, Sydney.

Risk Factors for Weak Bones and Teeth

According to Dr. Eisman, "The evidence based on an aging population indicates that there may be a 50 percent increase in the number of people with osteoporosis in India within ten years." Why? They drink milk in India! The cow is sacred. Herbal medicines are often taken with milk. The answer includes hormones, aging, bad habits, certain drugs, and allergies. A weak jawbone cannot support teeth, and because of reduced estrogen production after menopause, women tend to have more jawbone fractures. Estrogen slows the breaking down of bone matter, and around the onset of menopause, women lose bone mass rapidly for five to ten years. But for women who smoke, live a stressful life, or who have surgery resulting in early menopause, the signs of osteoporosis appear much earlier. Men are at risk of developing weak bones and teeth now as much as women because of smoking, a lack of daily exercise, and the use of steroids.

Another risk factor for weak bones is allergies. Though dairy products, which are high in calcium, are an important part of the diet, many people become lactose-intolerant because of bacterial infections and, I think, from antibiotics which cause stomach upset. There are excellent sources of calcium that do not contain dairy, including tofu, sesame seeds, and leafy green vegetables.

Medicines and Bone and Tooth Loss

I warn women clients and friends not to use bisphosphonates, drugs frequently prescribed for postmenopausal women to prevent bone loss. Common oral bisphosphonates are etidronate (Didronel), pamidronate (Aredia), alendronate (Fosamax), risedronate (Actonel), zoledronate (Zometa or Reclast), and ibandronate (Boniva). Numerous lawsuits have come to the attention of the general public after these drugs caused bone loss in the jaw. Dentists complained that teeth fell out or could not tolerate fillings because of an abnormally fragile jawbone in postmenopausal women using that category of medicine. More than that, bisphosphonates have caused cancers. In an analysis involving some eighty thousand patients tracked for more than seven years on average, individuals diagnosed with esophageal cancer were 1.93 times as likely to have received at least ten prescriptions for oral bisphosphonates compared with controls not having cancer, reported Dr. Jane Green of the University of Oxford in England. As of 2010, the Federal Drug Administration (FDA) has collected over sixty-eight case reports of esophageal cancer in patients taking bisphosphonates, half in the United States and the rest in Europe and Japan, but has not ordered label warnings.

Bisphosphonates cause dramatic changes in bone physiology. In women or men whose bone density T-score is lower than –2.5, or who already have a ver- tebral fracture, these medicines are prescribed to "reduce the incidence of frac- tures and improve the quality of life." It is no small problem. I once received an email from a man with osteoporosis. No one believed him, but he broke bones when he sneezed. Osteoporosis, a common problem for women, is becoming epidemic among men who live longer, smoke, and take steroids.

How can we avoid weak bones and teeth? Especially in youth but throughout life, it is important to have good physical activity; good intake of calcium from leafy green vegetables, sesame seeds, tahini, and tofu; enough exposure to sun- light for vitamin D; and no smoking or other harmful dietary habits. A person at risk of osteoporosis shows subtle signs due to poor mineral absorption. They include rounded shoulders; gum inflammation and loose teeth; chronic lower backache; weak nails, hair, or teeth; leg cramps; insomnia; and restless, anxious behavior. Female hormones do more than maintain a healthy production of estrogen. They reduce stress and increase loving, nurturing qualities. Do women with decreased estrogen frequently "set their teeth in rascals"?

An Ayurvedic Antiaging Approach

A holistic approach to teeth and bone strengthening does more than zero in on supplementing minerals such as calcium. Ayurvedic treatments are useful because they aim to achieve overall balance by supporting vitality and sexual hormones. They reduce stress and build immunity to illness and aging. Diet, select herbs, and elaborate healing practices are used to balance three humors: vata, pitta, and kapha. Simply stated, these three represent nervous energy, digestive energy, and our flesh and bone. The three humors must work together to ensure health. Vata tonics and especially adaptogens are important for reduc- ing such signs of aging. Hormone balance for men and women and good diges- tion (pitta) are necessary for maintaining bone metabolism. Having adequate *absorbable* calcium, magnesium, zinc and mixed trace minerals (kapha) pro- tects bone growth and strong teeth.

Diet

A wise diet for preventing bone and tooth loss includes complex carbohydrates, low-fat foods, reduced protein, and hypoallergenic calcium sources includ- ing dark green leafy vegetables such as broccoli, kale, and collards; yellow and orange vegetables, including pumpkin and carrots; beans (including soy if pro- cessed with calcium); low-fat milk or ghee (barring allergies); soft-boned fish; and shellfish. Also important are very ripe citrus fruits (providing vitamin C and natural sodium necessary for calcium absorption), kelp seaweed for magnesium, and mixed trace minerals supplements. Leafy vegetables and broccoli provide beta carotene.

Hypoallergenic Sources of Daily Calcium

- Chew a big handful of white sesame seeds every morning that gives you at least 1,200 milligrams of natural calcium. Dependency on calcium from dairy products may clog arteries, but white sesame seeds, rich in calcium, won't.
- Almond milk is tasty and light. Almond combined with goat's milk has a significant amount of calcium. Peel ten almonds that have been soaked overnight and blend them with a cup of warm goat's or soy milk. Pour them into a glass, adding a pinch of cardamom, saffron, and ginger. Drink it before breakfast and another time before bed.
- One tablespoon of black or white sesame seed powder, one-half teaspoon shatavari powder, with one-half teaspoon ginger powder and raw honey to taste, is good for the bones.

Avoid cola or soda drinks because they are high in phosphate, which directly interferes with calcium absorption. Overconsumption of processed food (refined grains and too few dark green leafy vegetables) is usually the culprit in magnesium deficiency.

Rejuvenation Tonics for Bones and Teeth

Ayurvedic rejuvenating tonic powders or pills are quite useful because they touch many bases for superior health while strengthening nerves, muscles, and bones. Shatavari (*Asparagus racemosus*) is an excellent source of female hormones that rejuvenates sexuality and female sexual tissue. Powdered ashwagandha root (*Withania somnifera*), bala (*Sida cordifolia*) and amla, a wild cherry (also known as amalaki, *Emblica officinalis*) can be taken in water with a dose of one-half teaspoon each daily. Also used are shatavari and vidari kanda (wild yam, *Ipomoea digitata*) mixed in equal parts, or just shatavari taken on a regular basis (one-half teaspoon twice daily) with warm milk. Vidari kanda root powder, a white yam, is a sweet, nutritive tonic that is a rejuvenative for vata and pitta. It increases kapha and therefore may slow digestion or add body weight when used to excess. Traditionally, it is used to nourish and rejuvenate the body and to support proper function of reproductive systems. The root contains beta-sitosterol, which has been shown to be effective for reducing prostate swelling discomforts and unhealthy cholesterol.

It promotes healthy muscle and nerve tissue and strengthens vata-constitution seniors who are weak, nervous, and thin with dry hair and very wrinkled skin. Recently, vidari has been proved to have antibiotic effects. Moistening, rejuvenating herbs such as shatavari and vidari kanda are said to reduce vata. They are sometimes called "vata-pacifying" herbs and may help to make up for estrogen in the metabolic cycle because they are dietary precursors of estrogen and progesterone.

The East Indian cherry amla, a great rejuvenator, nourishes the bones, strengthening the teeth and causing hair and nails to grow. One teaspoon of the powder in water twice a day is used as a general tonic. Triphala contains amla and can be used on a regular basis as a balancing, cleansing tonic for people of all ages. Triphala is used to balance all three humors, vata, pitta, and kapha, while it detoxifies and tones the digestive tract and supports healthy metabolism. See the section on triphala in chapter 1.

Avoid Stress

For building strong bones and teeth, it helps to prevent wear and tear on your nerves. Ayurvedic doctors recommend avoiding overwork, arguments, and excess empty chatter. A good excuse to avoid unpleasant people! Stay warm, eat warm nourishing foods, relax, practice patience, and do gentle yoga stretches to enhance flexibility.

A Tooth Health Maintenance Plan for Life

Make bone- and tooth-building herbs part of your overall health routine. Try adding some of the following to your diet:

- Green tea—prevents fatigue, cancer
- Tofu—source of calcium and protein
- One teaspoon daily of Amla for rejuvenatiaon
- Trifala pills with meals for digestion
- One half teaspoon each of powdered shatavari and ashwagandha in yogurt for bone and muscle strength
- One teaspoon of Tahini or two tablespoons sesame seeds—source of calcium
- Goat's milk and whey—source of minerals
- 2,000 IU of vitamin D3
- 2,000 milligrams of food-based calcium pills for strong bones

Simple Pain Relief at Home

Sometimes, for a number of reasons, a tooth or gum area may act up, causing pain. It might be from food stuck between the gums and teeth, a meridian imbalance, or from temporary bad habits. Is there something better to take for a simple temporary toothache than aspirin? Yes. A powerful antibacterial herb is more specific for preventing tooth decay.

The neem tree is highly valued in India. It grows quickly in tropical climates, including south Florida. The leaves are very bitter and act as an antibacterial, antiviral, and antifungal medicine. In India, housewives spread dried neem leaves among their linens to avoid mold and bugs. Yogis chew the bitter antimicrobial stem to avoid tooth decay. The brewed tea and oil are applied externally to eliminate skin parasites and infections.

Letha's Advice: Neem for Teeth and Gums

Brush your teeth with powdered neem leaf. Though it tastes bitter, it kills germs and strongly reduces inflammatory pain. You can swallow the juice from the powder in order to detoxify the digestive tract. I have used this treatment myself and it worked within a day to eliminate a pain flare-up of an impacted wisdom tooth. I felt the cooling action reach the meridians in my neck, face, and gums. If stomach cramps result, reduce the dose of neem powder or drink ginger tea.

Another recommended treatment that works quickly is to mix pure organic neem oil and turmeric powder and apply this with a cotton swab to the affected gum overnight. Using neem regularly, since it is a bitter detoxifying herb, tightens loose gums, stops bleeding, and reduces gum swelling and inflammatory pain. If you order the oil, read the label to make sure it is organic and suitable for internal use. Most labels read "for external use only." Neem is also widely used as a natural insecticide in gardening.

Naturally Healthy Toothpastes

Are there ready-made products that protect the health of teeth and gums? Decidedly, yes. Here are my favorites to date. They are easily available online and in a few specialty health shops. Good toothpastes do not have to be expensive. The simplest tooth cleanser that I prefer is powdered neem leaf, which is antibacterial, antiviral, antifungal, and does not have that "refreshing minty taste." You may prefer baking soda powder, an abrasive often added to whiten teeth. In Tim's Chinese herb shop and iron works, located on U.S. 1 in Homestead, Florida, my eye caught an attractive yellow envelope with Thai writing on it and a stamp that looked like your typical Thai grandmother. The powdered ingredients for Viset-Niyom Traditional Tooth Powder (since 1921) are white clay, calcium salts, and borneol. The powder, applied with a toothbrush or your finger—to massage sore gums, strengthen teeth, and reduce plaque, coffee, and nicotine stains—can also be used as a paste on skin blemishes.

Three other great brands of natural toothpastes are Silvafresh by Trimedica and Neem, Pomegranate Toothpaste made by Himalaya Herbal Healthcare and Natural Tea Tree Oil Toothpaste (ginger) made by Desert Essence.

Vicco Toothpaste and Tooth Powder

Vicco Pure Herbal Toothpaste is the original Ayurvedic toothpaste. Vicco cleans teeth, freshens the breath, and stimulates the gums. Vicco contains fine chalk and twenty pure herbal extracts long established by Ayurvedic herbal tradition to benefit teeth, mouth, and gums. Vicco Toothpaste is formulated to include herbs with a significant action on the gums. It contains no artificial ingredients, refined sweeteners, harsh abrasives, fluoride, saccharin, or parabens. Instead the naturally detoxifying ingredients include licorice root, almond, walnut, spices such as clove, betal nut, prickly ash, eucalyptus, and others.

Vicco Tooth Powder (also known as Vajradanti) is a famous Ayurvedic herbal combination which means "diamond teeth." I like this red herbal powder even better because it contains no chalk. It has the same ingredients as the toothpaste with additional deep cleansing and balancing triphala, as well as rice husk, sugar, alum, and salt. If you hate the taste of mint toothpaste, you might like this. It tastes and feels a bit like salty tree bark as it tightens and strengthens the gums and eliminates bad breath. After brushing with the toothpaste, you can brush with the powder and leave it in the mouth for five minutes before rinsing.

Bad Breath

Ayurvedic doctors recommend for prevention of halitosis and gum infection:

- Vitamin C–rich foods like oranges, kiwi, strawberries, guava, lemon, etc. One Ayurvedic clinic online recommends, "Chewing a piece of fresh coconut and one baby carrot every morning after brushing the teeth prevents bleeding."
- Gargling with one tablespoon unrefined sesame oil for ten to fifteen minutes every morning after brushing teeth. Do not swallow the oil; instead spit out and rinse your mouth with water.
- Protecting and cleansing the liver to prevent bleeding gums. (See the liver flush protocol in chapter 6.) Liver tonic herbs such as *Eclipta alba* and niruri are said to immediately stop bleeding gums.

> ## Letha's Advice: Nopalea for Inflammatory Pains, Swelling, and Infections
>
> Detoxifying the body and reducing inflammation help protect teeth and gums by protecting general health and circulation while reducing chronic pain and acidity. There are many cleansing products detailed in this book, but one of the best-tasting food supplements I can recommend is drinking one glass of water with one ounce of Nopalea concentrate once or twice daily. Nopalea, made from nopal cactus, fruit enzymes, grapeseed extract, concentrated fruit juices, and more, provides vitamins and minerals necessary for cleansing and maintaining digestion at optimum efficiency. Nopalea reduces toxins and inflammation throughout the body, which makes it helpful for correcting most inflammatory pains and imbalances covered in this book.

More Holistic Dental Products

Dr. Bill Wolfe, DDS, NMD, is a holistic dentist who practices in Santa Fe and Albuquerque, New Mexico, focusing on "biological dentistry," which includes the principles of electro-acupuncture, kinesiology, and homeopathy. Dr. Wolfe's products, sold online, include homeopathic pill remedies for toothache, gum infections, and detoxification from heavy metals. His toothpastes combine homeopathic ingredients in a base of aloe vera.

Toothache Homeopathic Medicine

Toothache is "for relief of minor toothaches" with the usual warning: "If symptoms persist, contact a health professional. Pregnant women should consult their health professional when using herbs and homeopathic remedies. The tablets are taken by dissolving them slowly under the tongue. For common symptoms, take one tablet three to four times daily. As required for relief, tablets may be taken as often as every five to fifteen minutes. Children ages two to six receive half the adult dosage.

The homeopathic ingredients are: arnica montana radix 4X, asafoetida 6X, belladonna 6X, coffee cruda 10X, hekla lava 12X, hypericum perforatum 4X, magnesia phosphorica 6X, and staphysagria 6X.

Infection Homeopathic Medicine

These tablets "for relief of minor jaw infections" are taken by dissolving slowly under the tongue. For common symptoms, take one tablet three to four times daily. As required for relief, tablets may be taken as often as every five to fifteen minutes. Children ages two to six receive half the adult dosage.

What Your Dentist May Not Tell You

Dr. Wolfe fills teeth with composites and ceramic and uses anesthesia that are tested for biocompatibility with the patient. Has your dentist asked you about your allergies to fillings, heavy metals, or medications? I was shocked to learn about unregulated stuff used in fillings, root canals, etc., all smashing together, creating energy fields in our mouths that may reduce vitality in the upper body. See www.drwolfe.com for a full list. For example, scrap amalgam (low-grade metal used to make fillings) that is removed by a dentist from a patient's mouth cannot be discarded in the trash. Otherwise the dentist is subject to a $10,000 fine by the Environmental Protection Agency! The scrap is considered a toxic waste to be removed by a hazardous waste company. Toxins are bound to affect the subtle energy fields (meridians) that pass through the mouth.

Besides mercury fillings, used by many dentists, there are problems with the constituents of resins in composites (white, tooth-colored fillings); nonprecious nickel used in crowns and root canal posts; and the composition of implants, etc. Our teeth and gums are part of the meridian system that affects the entire body. Dr. Wolfe told me, "The upper molars and lower bicuspids are stomach teeth, and the lower molars and the upper bicuspids are large intestine teeth." That means our digestion profoundly affects gums, teeth, and circulation along those meridians in the face and arms. The immune system has to deal with any foreign substance in the body. If circulation and vitality are threatened by scrap materials in our teeth, our immunity suffers. It would be ideal if you and your dentist could sit down and create a "dental menu" of materials to use, considering your allergies and immune system. Better yet, add the health foods and immune-building herbs from this chapter to avoid dental problems altogether.

Pain Prevention/Relief Supplies to Keep On Hand

WHAT SIMPLE HOME REMEDIES AND PAIN-RELIEF SUPPLIES DO YOU KEEP AT home or at the office? As you read through the book, you will want to enlarge this list, making it specific to your needs:

- ❏ Acidophilus capsules to help keep digestion and absorption healthy.
- ❏ Aloe vera juice or gel to drink, for heartburn, bad breath, PMS, and cramps
- ❏ Aloe vera gel to apply, for burns and cuts
- ❏ Cinnamon powder for enhanced circulation, hypothermia prevention/ treatment
- ❏ Ginger powder as tea for chronic inflammatory pain and stiffness
- ❏ Hawthorn berry capsules for heart weakness and irregularity, cholesterol
- ❏ Homeopathic silver antibiotic spray for skin and household surfaces
- ❏ Massage cream or oil with natural analgesic ingredients
- ❏ Mineral bath crystals or powdered kelp seaweed for the bath
- ❏ Neck pillow or neck/shoulder massager
- ❏ Neem powder for reducing teeth/gum inflammation
- ❏ Organic neem oil for skin infections and parasites
- ❏ Stevia sugar substitute
- ❏ Tea for skin burns and a daily beverage for general health
- ❏ Tea tree oil (organic) for fungus, bacteria, and virus germs, and diluted as a mouthwash.
- ❏ Tibetan goji berries, a nutritive tonic to enhance energy, immunity, and mood

❐ Toothpaste or powder made with natural herbal and/or homeopathic
   ingredients

❐ Triphala pills for digestion/absorption, internal cleansing, and energy
   balance

❐ Turmeric powder for antibiotic use, with aloe or neem

❐ White Flower analgesic oil or Kwan Loong pain-relieving oil for aches,
   strains, headaches, dizziness, and motion sickness

❐ Yunnan Paiyao capsules for injuries, bleeding, bruises, and surgery

Part Three

A Pain-Free Lifestyle

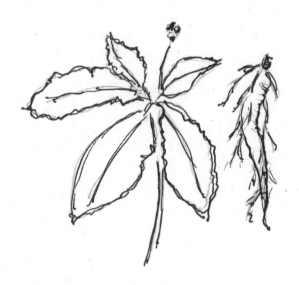

CHAPTER FOURTEEN

Emotional Trauma

Humor is emotional chaos remembered in tranquility.

—James Thurber (American humorist, author, and
cartoonist, 1894–1961)

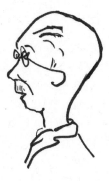

James Thurber

AS A CHILD JAMES THURBER WAS BLINDED IN ONE EYE WHEN HIS BROTHER
William shot him with an arrow while they were playing William Tell. Eventually
he became totally blind and developed a vivid imagination. We love his comic
character in "The Secret Life of Walter Mitty." Over forty years, Thurber wrote
short stories, plays that enjoyed success on Broadway, essays, autobiography,
children's books, and fables. His line-drawing cartoons of large women, bald
husbands, and philosophical dogs gave *The New Yorker* magazine its wry wit.

Drawing inspiration from James Thurber's life and works, the ideal solution
for emotional trauma is to recycle bad feelings and terrible memories into something positive. I hope this chapter helps you create the tranquility necessary for
creativity. It addresses long-term effects of chronic anxiety, anger, depression,
insomnia, and withdrawal symptoms. The body *feels* emotional trauma, and the

mind reacts to physical pain. For that reason, this and the following chapter, covering remedies for heart troubles and chest pain, are related. You may not be able to improve your living situation or repair your loss, but you can reduce the impact of negative emotions on body and mind. That work requires time, energy, and patience. But being human gives you a great advantage: you were created to triumph over adversity. You were meant to survive.

Your Earth Connection

Among life's great pleasures is our ability to enjoy a deep, vital connection to the earth. We may not think of it while sitting at the computer or driving along the freeway. But it is during quiet personal moments that we replenish vitality. If we connect with earth's elements—fire, earth, air, water, and the animal and vegetable world—we can find balance. I know a famous dancer, originally from the seashore, who spends two hours in a warm bathtub in order to rejuvenate and prepare for performance. Another friend, Larch Hanson (www.theseaweedman.com), has harvested Maine seaweed for forty years. He writes poetry to the sea and teaches apprentices to harvest its treasures.

To ease pain and tension, I soak in a tub, adding kelp powder. That green food soothes dry skin, and the oceanic aroma is entrancing. Water is my element. With it, I can wash away emotional pain, float, and create new ideas. Light is also my element. I grew up barefoot in the desert southwest. Now, with an LED lamp containing red and blue lights, I bask in sunshine on dark days. It helps me face a challenge.

Do you garden? Do you unwind in a sauna? What is your most comfortable retreat? That is your curing earth element. Do music or literature uplift your spirit? They are like air to enlarge consciousness. Laughter is fresh air. Watching a day of Marx Brothers movies may be what you need to chase grief. Gradually you will be able to improve energy by supporting your earth elements with foods and herbs from this book.

Another way to honor your love of fresh air, blue sky, and the tranquil sound of wind through the pines is yoga breathing. Sit quietly with both feet on the floor and hands cupping your navel. Breathe slowly, allowing your hands to feel warm and relaxed. Drop your shoulders and lift your head as though floating on a string. Inhale and exhale into the lower abdomen and allow your legs to melt into the floor. When you are relaxed, imagine a time and place in which you were content, at peace, and hopeful. If you cannot find that place within, imagine you are in a lovely spot enjoying sunshine. Feel the warmth relax tensions. Your inescapable connection with earth is internal and external. We are made of water, earth, and air. We absorb sunlight through our skin. Light energizes every cell in our body. Long ago, ancient philosophers charted our connection with the universe using those earth elements. Let's take a new look at the Chinese five elements (fire, earth, air or metal, water, and wood), their functions, associated organs, and what their health may inspire in us.

Fire: Circulation—heart, triple heater (an acupuncture energy system), small intestine—love, compassion, warm-hearted understanding of others, and the ability to see through a situation and get to the heart of the matter.

Earth: Digestion—stomach, spleen, pancreas—the ability to overcome suffering and create a new world with ideas, image, sound, or sensation.

Air: Breathing and detoxification—lungs, large intestine—expansion of horizons, flight of imagination, and purity of purpose.

Water: Adrenal energy—kidney, adrenal glands, water balance, hormones— the ability to feel at home and loved, and the courage to do great things.

Wood: A healing connection with plants and animals—liver, gallbladder, muscles, and tendons—joy of movement, travel, and creativity.

When we are calm, our hearts and respiration work at optimum levels. Digestion functions smoothly and we think clearly. But faced with a terrible situation, our bodies react as though escaping a predator. We are hardwired for survival.

Emotional Discomforts—Hot or Cold

When emotionally upset, do you feel hot and angry or chilled and empty? It may vary with the situation, but *feeling* the sensation of your emotions makes a difference for your best choice of remedies. Where do you experience your discomfort? Is it like being choked, slapped, or abandoned? Choose a treatment that reverses that feeling to support vitality and free creative thinking. Emotional turmoil glues us to a painful situation: we obsess, scold, or cower. A treatment that improves circulation is bound to unleash natural recuperative powers. Here are two easy home remedies: pearl is cooling and clove is heating.

Use them as needed, according to symptoms described on the following pages.

- When they have worked, stop using them.
- Herbs are not vitamins: they are catalysts for change. When overused beyond their need, they may lead to side effects.

Anger Is Hot

Anger transformed by compassion cuts to the quick, grasps a challenge, and takes action. Anger left to fester kills the one trapped in a sauna. Anger must be freed to flow, then cooled, and it can light your way to creativity. Asian herbal medicine uses liver cleansers that release bile such as artichoke, dandelion, milk thistle, and bupleurum to liberate energy and ideas choked by anger.

Pearls of Wisdom

One of the oldest and simplest remedies for nervous insomnia and inflammatory problems ranging from skin rash to stomach ulcers, anger, or hypertension comes from the sea. A pearl is made from years of pressure. A tiny grain of sand, an irritation in an oyster, produces a beautiful precious gem. Chinese herbal doctors recommend internal use of pure powdered pearl for children's fevers and adult acne. One main ingredient is calcium carbonate, but the relaxing energy of the gem itself is healing. Purified pearl powder is sold in Chinese herb shops in tiny tubes. Mix the contents of one tube of the powder with a teaspoon of yogurt and consume it at bedtime for a deep restful sleep. The remedy is cooling for inflammatory symptoms. (See a reddish tongue, fast pulse, and restlessness.) Anger and frustration can be hot or cold. When hot, we rage; when cold, we may plot revenge or weep. Your hot emotions can be cooled with bitter, alkaline tonics such as aloe vera. Drink the juice and spread some on your face and scalp to feel fresh as a desert landscape.

Sadness Is Cold and Damp

Sadness is part of the human condition because there is suffering in the world. It is normal and healthy to feel pain for the misfortune of others and to take action to cure our own hurts. Think of weeping as a way the body reduces excess water. It washes our eyes, lightens our chest with sighs, and opens doors in our vision to see more clearly. Tears are an important way of letting go of grief. When weeping is unproductive, when it cannot be stopped, then you need a remedy. See homeopathic pulsatilla in the chapter covering women's issues. Excess weeping can sometimes signal a hormone imbalance.

More than likely, ordinary internal cold symptoms or signs of adrenal fatigue such as shortness of breath, constant yawning, chills, frequent urination, and lower backache require a warming, stimulating treatment in order to avoid temporary physical discomforts turning into depression. The spice clove is a simple home remedy that can brighten and lift your qi and deepen a shallow breath. It is especially useful for wheezing asthma or tuberculosis, or exhaustion and despair. Add a pinch of clove powder to water as a tea. It clears breathing for someone who has watery phlegm, weak digestion, and water retention. If you have a reddish tongue or other inflammatory issues, clove may give you a headache and dizziness. It is too hot.

Comfort the Heart

Traditional Chinese medicine explained the mind/body connection long before modern psychology and psychotropic drugs were capable of affecting behavior. The ancient science that gave us acupuncture explains physical and emotional unity in terms of a spirit (in Chinese, *shen*) that influences our internal organs. For example, our heart contains a spirit (*jingshen*) that keeps our emotions stable and mind capable of functioning in the real world. Some heart tonic formulas contain herbs such as jujube red date, said to pacify the *shen*, that is, reduce anxiety, nightmares, and palpitations.

When the heart is upset, either from our emotional experience or unwise habits, we may have palpitations, irregularities, or chest pain. Chinese herbal remedies for heart health are very wisely formulated to encompass adrenal health and circulation. They are not your ordinary sedative mind drug. They enhance life force. One such herbal combination pill is called Ding Xin Wan. In the following chapter, you will learn about herbal formulas such as HeartCare or the herb arjuna that reduce cholesterol and protect the heart muscle. But Ding Xin Wan is used primarily for emotional discomforts and insomnia.

Do you use prescription medicines for your mood?

They often have side effects. For example, antidepressants and antianxiety drugs may increase body weight and weaken sexual vitality. Never stop taking medicines suddenly or without medical guidance. The result may be a "rebound" effect that increases the original symptoms. If you plan to add herbs to your health regime, with the guidance of your health professional, start with a small dose and continue with your regular medicines until they are no longer necessary.

Ding Xin Wan

Ding Xin Wan (also known as Tranquilex Tea Pill) is a Chinese patent remedy that combines herbs to support blood production and heart health. (Do not use this if you are pregnant or nursing.) The original Ding Xin Wan formula contained succinum (amber) used for insomnia, anxiety, forgetfulness, nervous seizures, and urinary retention; ophiopogonis tuber to cool and ground lung energy and reduce chronic nervous cough; along with unnamed "subsidiary substances" which may have included animal bone or other ingredients to reduce internal heat (inflammation). Today's formula no longer contains hard-to-find or endangered substances.

The ingredients include Oriental arborvitae (biota seed, bai zi ren), a moistening seed used to quiet palpitations and correct dry mouth and cough; poria, a diuretic included to prevent heart congestion; polygala root, a famous herb used by ancient sages for enhanced psychic visions, which is calming for insomnia and nightmares; jujube red date, a moistening and nourishing heart tonic. Other ingredients include the blood tonic dong quai, ginseng, and Chinese skullcap to calm anxiety and anger that may result from liver inflammation.

The formula is recommended for restlessness, anxiety, insomnia, palpitations, poor memory, difficulty concentration (poor mental function), and dry mouth from stress and mental fatigue. The usual dose is six pills two times a day. However, if you are exhausted from overwork, worry, or mental upset to the point of chronic insomnia, it may cause sleepiness. In that case, use it to refresh your mind and spirit with deep comfortable sleep. You might use it two hours after dinner and again before bed. The herbs react to your individual needs.

Calm Spirit

Calm Spirit pills, made by Health Concerns, are a modern update on the ancient Ding Xin Wan formula. They contain stress-reducing enzymes and taurine, which controls heart arrhythmia and hypertension aggravated by stress. Other enzymes, including amylase, CereCalase, protease, catalase, lipase, and glucoamylase, reduce free radicals produced by stress. Magnesium, a tranquilizer, is added to regulate the nervous system. Other ingredients used from the original Ding Xin Wan formula are biota seed, polygala root, jujube date, codonopsis root, ophiopogonis tuber, and amber.

Calm Spirit pills are recommended to support healthy heart tissue and calm the heart's *shen*, that is, reduce anxiety and inflammatory palpitations. The medicine moistens the intestine and is therefore helpful for constipation. If diarrhea develops, the dose should be reduced or treatment stopped. (Use with supervision or avoid it during pregnancy.)

Emotional Upset and Substance Withdrawal

Calm Spirit can be used along with another Health Concerns formula, Ease Plus, to improve nervousness, insomnia, emotional distress, migraine and other headaches, and to ease withdrawal from tobacco, drugs, medicines, or other addictions. Ease Plus treats gastric acidity, ulcers, hiccups, and chronic belching from "stuck liver qi" energy. Imagine holding in anger and anxiety until you feel your sides will burst. You may have jaundice, a yellowish color; nausea; liver pain in the right side of the ribs or chest; or metallic bad breath: That is stuck liver qi. Anyone can develop stuck liver qi from inherited liver weakness or illness, by eating too many fatty, greasy, and spicy foods, or from long-term unpleasant emotions, especially anger and frustration. It is surprising how much calmer and better you might feel by improving diet and using bitter and stimulating herbs to "move stuck liver qi." Ease Plus combines calcium carbonate to support the liver and muscles along with herbs to cleanse and tone sluggish liver such as bupleurum, ginseng, ginger, pinellia, skullcap, and rhubarb. Often, for chronic anger, a bitter laxative is a good tonic.

Letha's Advice: Mind Over Matter

Think of uncomfortable, unpleasant thoughts as though they are poisons to cleanse from the body. Religious traditions from the beginning of civilization have used prayer, cleansing practices, and spiritual teachings to excoriate sins, improve habits, and remove so-called evil thoughts and actions. Traditional Chinese medicine uses herbs to get digestion (liver qi) moving smoothly, because that frees our mind and spirit for insight and action. Studying acupuncture and herbal medicine at the Shanghai College and Hospital of Traditional Chinese Medicine, I learned how and why herbal formulas and acupuncture used for emotional balance work and witnessed their good effects in practice. For one thing, the patients, ranging in age from childhood to the elderly, were not routinely sedated with medical drugs that dulled their senses or minds. They came with physical and emotional symptoms and received a balancing acupuncture treatment that simultaneously improved digestion, breathing, and mental clarity.

Sometimes all you need is to get qi flowing smoothly again with a massage, a fragrant healing bath, or digestive herb tea. Aromatherapy has a subtle but powerful effect upon emotions. Lavender, geranium, and sage may feel especially strengthening. Essential oil of fennel is sweet but slightly bitter for cleansing. It is recommended for breast cancer. It helps ease tension. Add five drops of an essential oil to one teaspoon of a neutral carrier oil such as canola or soy oil and use it to gently cleanse the lymph system. Massage with light fingertip touch from the head downward toward the chest and from the feet upward toward the kidneys.

Violent Action

Imagine an angry spirit: The face is a grimace of pain, rage; a red blemished face or yellow jaundiced face from bile invading the blood instead of moving the bowels as a laxative. The demon breathes (bad breath) fire, has steam coming from a head of thinning hair, nervous fast movements, and quick, shrill, agitated speech. The appearance is the opposite of the cool, calm appearance that may result from cleansing and blood-nourishing herbs. Chronic inflammation from post-menopausal hot flashes, chronic fevers with night sweats, and other fever conditions may not necessarily be angry, but will benefit from the cooling, cleansing, balancing herbs and energy treatments in this chapter

The spirit that protects the liver is harmed by anger. Stuck liver qi, causing chest pain, a lump in the throat, or violent outbursts, may be soothed, along with acid-related rashes, headaches, and dizziness, by herbs that release bile flow. That's why a combination of Chinese herbs for anxiety or anger often contains bupleurum (chai hu) to increase bile flow and a laxative such as rhubarb to help dissolve uric acid stones. For daily use, bitter herbs that help dissolve stones, such as dandelion greens added to salads or taken as a capsule or dandelion root beverage, are helpful for the liver, for circulation in the chest and abdomen, and for pain reduction. How does cleansing the liver lead to resolution of anger? That is a karmic question that you must answer for yourself. Freeing bile with herbs cleanses the wastes of digestion, clears the mind, and readies us for creativity. It is creative thought and action that really heals anger.

A Cool Complexion and Mind

An herbal treatment I recommended for someone had amazing results that illustrate the vital connection of mind and body. The middle-aged man had been healthy and active, but after a terrible injury with his snowblower, he was left partially paralyzed and mute much of the time. He dropped off to sleep in public and sometimes did not finish sentences but instead nodded into a zombie-like state. Soon after the accident, he developed a terrible red, itchy eczema rash over most of his body. This added to his feeling of isolation and despair. When I examined his symptoms, his pulses raced and all his vital signs—tongue, complexion, etc.—were bright red. His energy seemed to be stuck in panic, the result of his near-death experience. He used no drugs. He showed interest neither in foods nor in the company around him.

Considering his internal heat signs, I chose a strongly cooling combination of herbs normally used for fever conditions; ear, nose, throat, and skin infections; and skin rash. They were Coptis Purge Fire Formula and Skin Balance Pills from Health Concerns. Coptis Purge Fire can be used for hives, strep throat, sinus infections, pelvic inflammatory disease, tooth abscess, nasal infections, chronic liver inflammation, migraines, urinary tract infections, and constipation from illness and fevers. Coptis, anemarrhena, gentiana, skullcap, forsythia, and phellodendron are the main anti-inflammatory herbs in Coptis Purge Fire Formula.

After a week of using the strongly anti-inflammatory herbs, the man's rash was greatly reduced and his mental clarity improved. He paid attention and was more present in public. His wife said that he regained his senses. It was as though physical and emotional trauma had burned his brain, which was now refreshed and beginning to heal. Here is another example of possible damage done by inflammation affecting the brain.

In February 2012, an article on MSNBC quoted Harvard professor of neurology Dr. Ole Isacson who suggested that brain inflammation, or "brain fever" resulting from the flu, may increase our risk of developing Alzheimer's and Parkinson's. He hoped that one day science would find a way to cool "brain fever." Though research is still necessary to prove the connection between inflammation affecting the brain and Alzheimer's, it pays for us to know about Asian "brain-cooling herbs" including *Coptis sinensis*. In fact, a Chinese herbal remedy that contains coptis is commonly used for many fever symptoms and is called Huang Lien Shang Ching Pien, recommended for colds, flu, headaches, strep throat, tonsillitis, conjunctivitis, eye stye, ear infection, or sinus infection. It can also be used for stomach and intestinal heat causing tooth infection, mouth ulcers, swollen infected gums, nosebleed, or constipation, and for skin infections and reactions including boil or redness and itching, and epidemic hemorrhagic conjunctivitis. Hopefully herbs and modern science may work closer together to solve our deep and lasting problems. A very old wise herbalist I knew, Dr. Bernard Jensen, always advised people to keep a cool head. "Never let your brain get too hot," he would say. That advice is part of our language and culture. We trust someone with a cool head during a crisis. Now you can protect your brain, mind and emotions with healing herbs.

Depression: A Dark, Sticky Place

With chronic depression, there can be either hot or cold signs. In either case, the treatment is aimed to strengthen and stabilize digestion, our emotional and digestive center. Then we can effectively process our food as well as our life.

Xiao Yao Wan and Herbal Substitutes

Xiao Yao Wan is a Chinese patent remedy available with several names (Relaxed Wanderer, Relaxx Extract, and others). It is a digestive remedy recommended for anxiety, depression, PMS, stuck liver qi, hiatal hernia (a condition in which a portion of the stomach protrudes upward into the chest through an opening in the diaphragm), chronic burping, jaundice, and other digestive and emotional upsets. It regulates digestion. The ingredients are ginger, mint, bupleurum, tang kuei, atractylodes, peony, and fu ling, a diuretic. It makes our emotional and digestive centers work better and feel comfortable. When depressed, do you feel stuck, tight, jammed, cramped or empty of vitality? Your body is reacting to your mood. When we use herbs such as those in Xiao Yao Wan to regulate circulation and improve the functioning of internal organs, we feel more comfortable and safe, and we can react more calmly to stress.

The dose is dependent on the severity and type of symptoms. For someone with a pale tongue and shortness of breath from chronic anxiety or a choking feeling in the chest, the dose might be as much as ten pills of Xiao Yao Wan twice or three times daily until the tongue regains a normal pink color. For someone with a red, dry tongue and chronic anxiety or for a smoker, the dose may be six pills twice daily, taken with up to one-fourth cup of (alkaline, laxative) aloe vera juice to cool heat symptoms like cramps, bad breath, or skin blemishes, or angry PMS. Possible substitutes include Quiet Digestion pills by Health Concerns or a homemade tea made with green tea, fresh ginger, mint, and lemongrass.

Postpartum Depression

It is understandable that you may feel emptied, weakened, and washed out after carrying a child full-term or after an abortion. That amounts to what Chinese herbalists call "collapsed qi." The symptoms are shortness of breath, diarrhea, or urinary incontinence. You may feel exhausted, anxious, and depressed or stuck in a crying jag. You may crave sweets and have a backache, dizziness, or cloudy thinking. You may be spotting blood and feeling pain or have deep uncontrolled chills. That sort of emotional and physical collapse is very common among mothers.

The ingredients in Postpartum Pills by Health Concerns give us an indication of correct herbal treatment. That formula contains warming herbs such as Chinese ginseng and blood tonics such as tang kuei, ho shou wu (*Polygonum multiflorum*), and ligusticum. It contains drying fortifying herbs such as citrus peel and energy- and immunity-stimulating astragalus. It contains salvia root (dan shen) to help normalize heart action and protect against damaged blood vessels. The aim of the formula is to help women regain the strength and balance they need to feel confident and comfortable. Seek medical attention if heavy bleeding after childbirth continues. Do not use Postpartum Pills if you have the following inflammatory symptoms: night sweats, hot soles and palms, chronic thirst, dry mouth, and fast wiry pulse.

Letha's Advice: Imagine a Clear Day

As an experiment, practice this calming qigong practice for fifteen minutes daily for a week. Sit comfortably or lie flat at a quiet time and place where you will not be disturbed. Breathe slowly into the lower abdomen. Let it rise when you inhale and relax as you exhale. Breathe through your nose quietly. There is no need for sound. Surround yourself with a psychic barrier of light and protection that extends far beyond and above you.

Slowly inhale into each part of your body, recognizing its uniqueness. Inhale into your hair and as you exhale, mentally tell your hair to relax. Then repeat this until your hair seems to melt. Move down through your body through head, face, neck, arms, hands, fingers, chest, upper back, middle and lower back, abdomen, pelvis, sexual area, legs, and feet. Each time you inhale, accept the vitality of the pure air of wellness. As you exhale, eliminate everything and everyone in your life. Empty yourself completely and relax. Breathe in a steady, slow rhythm until you feel at ease.

Imagine a clear, sunny day in a place of perfect peace. Let the glow of light refresh you. Imagine a garden of beautiful flowers and trees in your abdomen. There may be fruits, incense, music, or other pleasures that you choose to fill your center. Stay there in that tranquil place for as long as you like. Each part of your body is relaxed and refreshed.

If you remember unpleasant feelings or feel physical pain as you relax muscle tension anywhere in the body, put the feelings aside. Let them become separate from you. Let them become "chaos remembered in tranquility." A memory need not stay with you. The fact that it is a memory already makes it different from the original experience. Tears are a form of detoxification. Your breathing and visualization can transform the negative into something positive over time.

If you practice this qigong exercise as directed for fifteen minutes daily, after a short while your blood pressure, circulation, and emotions can become regulated. Nerve-related pains can be reduced and mental clarity will seem easier. Sleep may also improve. A relaxation technique such as this helps to put every aspect of health in place, fills every cell with healing oxygen, and eases muscle tensions that choke vitality. Depression happens when we feel powerless, trapped or cut off from our essential well-being. Creating a healing space within ourself is the beginning of freedom from pain and suffering.

Other Useful Chinese Herbal Formulas

Clear Phlegm

Do you feel spacey, out of focus, and dulled by depression and worries? The impact of our emotions, dietary choices, and fatigue may create an imbalance damaging for body and mind. In traditional Asian medicine phlegm, a humor, refers to the ill effects of low vitality and poor nutritional absorption leading to a heavy, dull, stuck feeling and a variety of symptoms including joint swelling, digestive bloating, stabbing pain, cloudy thinking, chronic fatigue, and depression. People who overindulge in sweets and oily foods, who are obese, or who have a hormone imbalance or heart issue leading to water retention, or congestion illnesses such as asthma, are prone to have more problems with phlegm. Phlegm is also increased by damp cold weather that weakens vitality. Have you noticed that you feel blue and achy during a spell of rainy weather and dark skies? You can use herbs to brighten your energy and mood.

Clear Phlegm pills made by Health Concerns are recommended for phlegm (mucus and congestion) disorders, including profuse foamy white sputum, nausea, vomiting, dizziness, palpitations, insomnia, restlessness, timidity or hyperactivity, attention deficit disorder, chronic tracheitis, bronchitis, emphysema, and mental instability. According to traditional Chinese medicine, a kind of physical and mental sluggishness, gallbladder congestion, abdominal pain from fullness, numbness of limbs, stroke, and dulled senses can result when water retention and phlegm (*she*) collects in the digestive and/or heart center.

Clear Phlegm can be used long-term to clear problem energy from the heart (palpitations and hypertension), liver (anger/anxiety/frustration), lungs (cough or slight thirst), and stomach (bloating, nausea, etc.). For people with serious inflammation, it can be combined with Coptis Purge Fire Formula.

Power Mushrooms

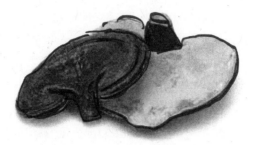

Are you depressed and/or irritable from chronic inflammatory pain, chronic fatigue, or an autoimmune illness? Medicinal mushrooms are edible fungi such as shiitake, reishi, and fu ling or cordyceps are immune-balancing. They are useful for autoimmune illnesses such as certain forms of arthritis, multiple sclerosis, and some cases of chronic fatigue. They are extremely nourishing and can be useful for inflammatory conditions. Power Mushroom pills are an easy way to add mushrooms to a health routine. Otherwise, reishi can be slow-cooked for several hours and consumed as a tea daily. Shiitake can be cooked with pasta, rice, or eggs. In each case mushrooms must be thoroughly cooked in order to potentiate their health benefits and to kill possible harmful bacteria.

Mushroom allergy symptoms include rash and choking. If you enjoy culinary mushrooms, you can use medicinal ones unless you have candida yeast. In the case of a yeast infection, see my dietary suggestions summarized on page 171.

Ease 2

Do you hold your tension and negative emotions in your neck, shoulders, upper back, or gut? Do hours of sitting at work or driving make you irritable, anxious, and aching? Health Concerns makes Ease 2 pills for relaxing muscular tension, especially in the neck, shoulders, and upper back, headaches, gastrointestinal disorders such as irritable bowel syndrome (IBS), and body aches. It might be useful for alternating loose or constipated stools, food allergies, abdominal tenderness and bloating, and belching. It contains bupleurum, pinellia, ginger, and skullcap to help regulate digestive energy. Cinnamon is added to enhance circulation. Although this type of formula is used, more strictly speaking, for digestive complaints, problems such as IBS certainly have an emotional correlative. As a general Chinese herbal antistress treatment, Health Concerns recommends combining several of their formulas that impact digestion and mood. Combine Calm Spirit with Ease 2, two tablets of each three times daily for depression/

anxiety with diarrhea or loose stools. For normal bowel movements, use Calm Spirit with Ease Plus pills.

I prefer describing and recommending Health Concerns products for several reasons. Their Chinese herbal ingredients are safe, tested, and made according to health-food store standards. They are made and regulated in California and can be sold in health-food stores. Based on successful Chinese patent remedies, they have been updated to address modern needs and people. Their names are easier for Western readers to remember than, for example, Xiao Yao Wan. In my teaching and writing I describe an herbal product and its ingredients in order to explain how and why the herbal combination works. An experienced Chinese herbal practitioner is the best guide to herbal use. However, if you study the herbs in combination, you begin to understand the dynamics of the treatment. For depression: lighten your load by clearing breathing and fortifying energy and courage.

A Diet for Emotional Balance

Avoid heavy, rich foods when energy is depleted or your mood is low, because difficult foods demand strong digestion. Avoid overstimulating, spicy foods when in a temper. Such practical advice is useful but hard to remember in daily life. Is there a dietary plan, a lifestyle, for maintaining emotional balance? For the answer, we look to ancient sources of wellness, because their aim was to bring the individual person into harmony with his or her surroundings while maintaining the healthy integrity of body, mind, and spirit.

Ayurveda provides a dietary path to enhanced mental function and a calm spirit. Sattvic foods and herbs are a vital part of a yogic lifestyle, because they provide access to higher consciousness. For those of us who are not yogis, they may help with troubled relationships, intense mental work, creative arts, and meditation. They may be used to improve energy and memory. Sattvic foods are rich in *prana*, also known as life force in Ayurvedic medicine. Prana, like air and nourishment from foods, fills the center of us in the chakras and gives inspiration and conscious intellect. Fresh, wholesome foods prepared with love increase their sattvic or spiritual quality.

The ancient Ayurvedic notion of sattvic foods is simple. They are vegetarian foods that are grown organically on rich fertile soil, foods that are attractive and harvested at the correct time of year. They should be fresh, natural, whole foods. Chinese herbalists might consider prana to be similar to qi. Some foods are full of qi and others dead and denatured. Sattvic foods should be grown without pesticides, herbicides, chemical fertilizers, hormones, irradiation, or anything unnatural. Modern use of refinement processes and chemical additives, besides actually adding substances to our foods, depletes foods of their prana or qi.

For mental clarity it is best to avoid foods that dull the mind (called tamasic foods) and those that overstimulate and increase anxiety (called rajasic foods).

Tamasic Foods that Dull the Mind:

- Meat, poultry, fish, eggs, alcohol, intoxicants, and drugs; tobacco, onions, garlic, fermented foods, vinegar, stale leftover food, contaminated or overripe substances
- Foods that are overprocessed, no longer fresh, and/or difficult to digest
- Foods that are prepared unconsciously or while angry or in a negative mood
- Food in excess

Rajasic Foods that Overstimulate:

- Foods that are very hot, bitter, sour, dry, or salty
- Sharp spices or strong herbs
- Stimulants like coffee and tea
- Meat of animals and fish, eggs, salt, and chocolate
- Eating in a hurry

If you have a demanding work schedule or are an endurance athlete, it may be helpful to consume a wise combination of both Sattvic (vegetarian) and Rajasic (stimulating) foods.

Sattvic Foods

Sattvic means pure essence. Sattvic is considered the purest diet for a consciously spiritual and healthy life. It nourishes the body and maintains it in a peaceful state. Ayurveda considers it the best diet for physical strength, a good mind, radiant health, and longevity. And it calms and purifies the mind, enabling us to function at our maximum potential. If we could retreat to a mountaintop and meditate, we would not have to be depressed at all. How can we benefit from an ancient tradition in which yogis are supported by a devoted public? How can we go to work and to the mountain at the same time? Add some of these foods to your diet and give yourself a little quiet time daily to refresh your spirit.

A sattvic diet consists of light, soothing, easily digested foods such as sprouted whole grains, fresh fruit, land and sea vegetables, pure unsweetened fruit juices, nut and seed milk and cheese, legumes, nuts, seeds, sprouted seeds, honey, and herb teas. Sattvic foods do not agitate the stomach and are consumed in moderate portions. Here is just a partial list of foods you can consume on a sattvic diet.

- **Fruits**: apples, kiwi, prunes, apricots, loquat, tangerines, bananas, lychee, pomegranate, cantaloupe, mango, papaya, cherries, melons, nectarines, cranberries, honeydew, oranges, grapefruits, watermelon, pineapples, grapes, peaches, plums, guava, pears, persimmons
- **Vegetables**: artichokes, eggplant, lettuce, beets, mustard, greens, asparagus, daikon, onions, endive, fennel, maitake, parsnips, bok choy, peas, broccoli, green beans, potatoes, brussels sprouts, kale, radishes, cabbage, leeks, lima beans, shallots, carrots, celery, spinach, cauliflower, chard, chanterelles, sprouts, corn, squash, shiitake, mushrooms, watercress, turnips, yams
- **Sprouted Whole Grains**: amaranth, barley, buckwheat, bulgur, millet, quinoa, Basmati rice, brown rice, wild rice
- **Oils**: olive, safflower, sesame, sunflower, garbanzo, lentil, mung
- **Herbs and Spices**: asafoetida, coriander, basil, cumin, nutmeg, black pepper, fennel seed, parsley, cardamom, fenugreek, turmeric, cinnamon, cloves, ginger
- **Nuts and Seeds**: almonds, Brazil nuts, pumpkin seeds, sunflower seeds, walnuts
- **Milks and Cheese**: seed milk, hemp milk, almond or other nut milk, oat or soy milk
- **Sweeteners Used Conservatively**: cane juice, raw honey, stevia, fruit juices, maple syrup

It takes time for the effects of dietary changes to manifest on the mind. Changing your diet may not impact your psychology overnight, but in a period of months can affect it significantly.

Tibetan Herbs for Mind and Spirit Expansion

Many people who have turned away from their childhood religious training or who never had the benefit of a spiritual tradition feel cut off from a deeper level of personal healing. They may feel neglected or abused by medical testing, fearful of risky treatments, or generally dissatisfied with health-care opportunities offered them.

Each day, I receive health inquiries on the Internet. I can answer in general, but unfortunately, I cannot easily give direct diagnosis and follow-up of treatments. But there are clinics that can. One such oasis of healing is the Tanaduk Clinic of Tibetan Medicine on Orcas Island, near Seattle, Washington, and online. Tanaduk Clinic offers private consultations, Tibetan herbs, diet and lifestyle advice, and Buddhist prayers and healing ceremonies for individual patients. Here is how it works: when requesting an appointment for consultation, a person is asked to send a brief medical history including age, weight, height, diet history, and other habits.

Patients who cannot go to the clinic can have a phone or email consultation. After reviewing the information and consultation, a healing protocol is designed by the physician and sent to you. Some people have come to expect miracles from Tibetan medicine because the Tibetans have touched the hearts of so many. But Tibetan medicine, like other alternative medicines, requires participation from the patient.

One basic tenet of Tibetan philosophy is that we can improve our life horizons by helping others. Removing obstacles to healing is a good start. Obstacles can be psychological, physical, or both, but whatever the obstacle, it can be recognized and removed. Where the issues are psychological, it may be necessary to revise subconscious scripts. On the physical side, diet and lifestyle regimes often need to be revised, healing internal organ energy. According to Amchi (Dr.) Thubten Lekshe, Doctor of Tibetan medicine, "In nearly every instance, once the obstacle is addressed, healing proceeds swiftly, and failure to eliminate the obstacle diminishes the effectiveness of whatever treatment is used."

What are your personal obstacles to health and happiness? Practice this experiment regularly. Sit quietly for twenty minutes imagining that you give gifts of food to the hungry, money to the poor, and medicines to the sick, and make a gift of your best work and your favorite art to others in order to end their suffering. See an animal trapped in a cage and free it. See those who are suffering become happy and well. How do you feel after doing this? Where and how do you feel more comfort and ease in your body? How do you feel emotionally? You have isolated and improved the obstacle that you must address with a healing regime.

Tibetan Precious Pills

There are several Tibetan pills that help support longevity. For example, Nagpo Gutup Pill is made of nine substances, contains many blessings, and from the point of view of Tibetan medicine, "It has the potency of prolonging life, protects against illness, and makes us more happy."

Letha's Advice: Happy Birthday

I take Tibetan Precious pills consecutively for three days before my birthday, not to overcome trauma, but to add the pleasure of balance and longevity to my life. Some people prefer to use the healing power of Tibetan medicine during the full moon or on holy occasions. When taking Tibetan pills, we are advised to avoid meats, eggs, spices, alcohol, cold showers, and sex. (In other words, follow a sattvic diet.) Open the pill covered with cloth in darkness, exposing the pill to neither light nor heat. Place it in a porcelain cup and fill the cup with hot water, allowing it to steep for several hours. When ready, take the pill, repeating a prayer. Then sit quietly or rest in bed, keeping comfortably warm for an hour or more. You may find the answers to your questions and new directions.

Happiness of Mind

This is a traditional Tibetan compound widely recommended for a wide range of imbalances such as depression, stress, and mood complaints. These range from mild, moderate, and even severe depression to seasonal affective disorder (SAD) and "the blues." It produces results in most people in just a few days, often in hours. It can be used to manage stress, anxiety, and depression on a daily basis; many people find their overall quality of life increases. When things get overwhelming, reset with Happiness of Mind. The pill brings support to the kidneys, liver, blood, and overall circulation. This formula is said to be especially supportive to meditation practitioners and for anyone who uses his or her mind with intensity. Use one to two pills once a day in the morning or evening with hot water.

Among other benefits, the ingredients are grounding (nutmeg); cleansing (triphala); soothing and nourishing (bamboo); cooling and balancing for harsh emotions (sandalwood); beneficial for circulation (safflower); and stimulating and clarifying for breathing and the mind (clove). With better mental and emotional clarity, physical vitality, and eased circulation, there is less pain and a better chance to develop creativity.

Pain vs. Creativity

Why do I stress creativity when curing emotional trauma? Pain and negative tendencies such as jealousy, anger, envy, and grief are sticking places that prevent happiness and emotional growth. They stop creativity. Freeing creativity is like correcting the effects of bad circulation that strangles and starves us from inside out. If you can draw, write, sing, dance, or describe your pain, you have begun to heal it.

The famous, influential woman explorer of Tibet, Alexandra David-Néel, walked over the Himalayas to Lhasa, Tibet, with her adopted son Lama Yongden.

She had studied with her guru in a cave, learning esoteric practices, including telepathy and how to stay warm in subzero weather. She said, "Pain, you are but a word." David-Néel was born French, sang opera as a girl, lived many years in Asia, and, upon the advice of the thirteenth Dalai Lama, learned to speak Tibetan. She wrote over thirty books, introducing Buddhism to an avid Western audience. To survive harsh conditions and constant dangers of traveling incognito in China and forbidden Tibet during the 1920s, she had learned a very basic belief in Tibetan Buddhism: *Change the way you think about something, and it changes.* The pathway of pain changes direction when you name it. It becomes something nonphysical. It is not experienced as real in the same way, and it can stop bothering you.

There have been times when painkillers have failed to work for me. I could neither sleep nor relax from the acute pain of a damaged spinal disc. I got out of bed and very slowly did a qigong exercise, the soaring crane, lifting my arms above my head as I inhaled and gracefully sweeping my wings downward with my arms again at my sides when exhaling. I flew for miles, bringing oxygen into my weary body, and became the crane.

I hope this chapter has helped you to look at your emotional pain in a new way. We have taken a trip together, passing through several Asian healing traditions. Their gems have healed generations. Travel, imagination, and creativity are part of my gypsy spirit. I love to share them with you and wish you the best for your recovery.

CHAPTER FIFTEEN

Heart Troubles and Chest Pains

Every heart attack is a broken heart attack.

—Wilhelm Reich (Austrian-American psychoanalyst, 1897–1957)

I WAS AT THE BEGINNING OF MY NATURAL HEALTH PRACTICE MANY YEARS AGO when a young woman named Angela asked me to give a massage to her uncle Julio, who had recently suffered a heart attack. I rarely left Manhattan to see clients, but she pleaded, "He is my favorite uncle, a romantic figure, the playboy of the family. Now he lives at home with my mother, who is driving him crazy. Please! You have to help him." In Queens, Angela led me to a frail-looking man lying on a small bed in the hallway of their brick house. She watched from the doorway. He rose on one elbow to greet me. His unshaven face was drawn and shriveled, his hair uncombed. On a table next to his bed were a red rose in a vase and a framed photo of a young man dressed in evening clothes. From the other room, a big woman yelled that he should not move. Julio spoke to me in whispers with labored breath. I sensed he was in terrible pain.

His pulse was hard to find, his tongue white. His dark eyes never left my face as he self-consciously rearranged his bedclothes. I couldn't stop looking at the young man in the photo and *wondering...* It must be him. As he spoke, I felt a deep sense of loss come over me. Julio's business had failed, and soon after that he had his heart attack. He lost everything, his home, work, and his identity as a handsome, vital man. He was too weak for massage, but I recommended that he take capsules of hawthorn berry to strengthen his heart. When it was time for me to leave, I felt a heavy weight on my chest and tightness in my throat. He very slowly rose to his feet. I tenderly put my arms around him and he lightly kissed my cheek; a youthful sexual energy swept through us, then passed away.

I wish I had known then what I know now. There are wonderful Asian herbs such as Chinese dan shen (*Salvia miltiorrhiza*) and the Ayurvedic herbal combination HeartCare that regulate cholesterol and heart rhythms to protect the heart. They might have prevented and treated Julio's physical and emotional pain. Because nature's remedies support the integrity of our organs and energy without taking over the work of the body, they strengthen our vitality and who we are. This chapter covers ways Eastern and Western medicine treat heart problems and looks at the advantages of each approach.

In a nutshell: do not wait until you develop heart symptoms. Heart attack is sudden, often painful stoppage of blood flow in the heart's blood vessels. It can result from plaque, a blood clot, an arrhythmia, or as a result of illness. Heart failure, often gradual or with no apparent warning, occurs when heart muscles stop working due to a blockage, lack of oxygen, or other causes. Diabetes is a factor. Get regular medical checkups. You can use dietary and herbal advice from this chapter for prevention of heart troubles or along with your prescribed heart medicines. Exercise regularly. Lifestyle is very important for heart health. Heart trouble may develop from overweight and lack of exercise. But infections, injury, emotional trauma, and genetic causes also weaken the heart.

Prevention: A Daily Necessity

Prevention is key because so much of what troubles the heart is impacted by digestion, adrenal vitality, and stress reduction. Reducing body fat and dietary fats and sugars helps lower harmful cholesterol that becomes plaque. Gradually increasing exercise can improve circulation and stamina. People over age forty, smokers, or those who have a challenging lifestyle require special herbs to protect the heart. Medical testing is quite useful for measuring existing disease. But medications come with side effects and drug dependence. For example, statins are frequently prescribed cholesterol-reducing drugs. Statins exhaust the cells of the enzyme that makes cells work: CoQ10. When that nutrient is gone, cells die. CoQ10 is most abundant in muscle cells and brain cells. That may be one reason why people taking statin medications complain of fatigue, muscle aches and pains, plus mental fogginess and inability to think clearly.

Note: You can combine Asian heart herbs with heart and other medicines because the body accepts herbs as food. However, stop all blood-thinning medicines, foods, and herbs at least two weeks before surgery.

Interconnected Energy: Asian and Western Views

Ancient Chinese medicine recognizes the heart as the "emperor" of body and mind. Heart qi and spirit (*shen*) decide our actions, emotions, and ultimately our health and well-being. But it neither begins nor ends there. In traditional Chinese medicine, the heart, often described by Western medicine as a muscle or a pump, is protected by a chain of events, including muscle strength and the smooth flow of qi promoted by the wood element, which in turn regulates liver function. The water element, which controls kidney and adrenal qi, energizes the wood element and protects the heart, the fire element. Water nourishes wood; wood increases fire. There is an elegantly simple, ancient explanation of the link between the adrenal cortex and pituitary master gland known as the hypothalamic-pituitary-adrenal (HPA) axis. We cannot have a strong heart without adrenal vitality. Adrenal weakness impacts the mind, memory, and behavior. Adrenal strength protects the heart.

Said another way, the HPA axis is a complex set of direct influences and feedback interactions among the hypothalamus, the pituitary gland located below the hypothalamus, and the adrenal glands located on top of the kidneys. The hypothalamus organizes and controls complex emotions and motivational states, including hunger, appetite, and food intake, and everything to do with the concept of pleasure including satisfaction, comfort, and creative activities. The pituitary gland and the adrenal glands (endocrine glands) secrete hormones (chemical messengers) into the blood system and impact the entire body. The HPA axis interactions control our reactions to stress and regulate body processes such as digestion, the immune system, mood and emotions, sexuality, and energy storage and expenditure. The HPA axis is where, in modern medical terms, mind meets body. Recent research suggests that adrenal stress hormones may interfere with memory retrieval. But much more than memory is impacted by adrenal stress.

Asian Herbal Formulas for Heart Health: How They Work

Heart health—a strong, steady heartbeat—is possible with adrenal vitality. For that reason, most traditional Asian (Chinese and Ayurvedic) herbal formulas that protect the heart reduce cholesterol, regulate heartbeat, and improve the elasticity of blood vessels. They contain herbal tonics for the adrenal energy and circulation (qi and yang). Calming, nourishing, blood-enhancing (yin) herbs are added to reduce stress affecting heart tissue. We have said that health is balance. Nowhere is this more evident than with heart health.

A heart attack is dramatic. A blocked blood vessel, from a blood clot or collapsed blood vessel, can cause severe pain or a sudden blackout. However, heart failure (also known as congestive heart failure) may be slow, creeping exhaustion, shortness of breath, and a backup of blood flow into the heart. There may be swollen ankles with or without chest pain. In both cases, reducing harmful cholesterol (plaque) and inflammation are key components of heart health. Pulmonary hypertension may accompany heart trouble. When blood vessels leading to the lungs become congested with plaque or collapse, then the heart must work much harder and eventually stops. Heart problems are often diagnosed with an echocardiogram.

Peripheral arterial disease (PAD) occurs when blood vessels in the body are blocked with plaque and harm circulation in the arms or legs. Other PAD symptoms include foot numbness and tingling, cold extremities, and skin discolorations or leg and foot sores that do not heal. Leg, buttocks, and foot pain increases from walking or exercise and subsides with rest. Your doctor can test for PAD by taking your blood pressure at the arm and ankle. Smokers, people with diabetes, and women more often develop PAD. PAD greatly increases risk of heart attack and stroke.

Most heart attacks are caused by a blood clot that blocks one of the coronary arteries. They bring blood and oxygen to the heart. If the blood flow (call it qi) is blocked, the heart starves for oxygen, and heart cells die. In atherosclerosis (hardening of the arteries), plaque, made up of cholesterol and impurities, builds up in the walls of coronary arteries. Heart attacks can result from several conditions:

- Plaque slowly builds up, blocking coronary arteries. During exercise the heart becomes oxygen-starved.
- The plaque develops cracks or tears and blood platelets stick to them, forming a blood clot (thrombus). A heart attack can occur if this blood clot blocks the passage of blood to the heart. This is the most common cause of heart attack.
- Occasionally, sudden, significant emotional or physical stress, including an illness, can trigger a heart attack.

Who Is at Risk of Heart Attack?

According to the numbers, high-risk people are over sixty-five, especially people with diabetes or high blood pressure, or those who have a family history of coronary artery disease, smoke, eat too much fat, have high LDL ("bad") cholesterol, and have chronic kidney disease. I include women as well as men, though statistically men tend to have more heart attacks. That will change in women who take on responsibility as the head of a household, are after menopause, or smoke. Do you get the picture? They have chronic stress, are overweight and weak from junk foods, and in pain from smoking and not exercising. They sit at work and on the weekend decide to go hunting and drag a deer to the car, cut down a tree, take a long hike, rearrange the furniture, have a big argument, or in some other way shock the body.

Symptoms Often Ignored in Women

Chest pain is a major symptom of heart attack, but pain may move from the chest to arms, shoulder, neck, teeth, jaw, belly area, or back. According to many medical sources, heart trouble is often not diagnosed in women. They may fail to pay attention to shoulder or leg pain. Severe or mild pain can feel like a tight band around the chest; bad indigestion; heaviness or squeezing pressure on the chest. The pain usually lasts longer than twenty minutes. Other symptoms may include coughing, fainting, anxiety, shortness of breath, dizziness, extreme sweating, and palpitations. Some people (the elderly, people with diabetes, and women) may have little or no chest pain. A "silent heart attack" has no symptoms. Symptoms may also go away and come back.

Symptoms in TCM and Ayurveda: Blocked Energy Flow

Chest pain and blocked blood vessels, either from chronic or acute lifestyle abuse, are viewed as blocked qi. In order to avoid pain and physical damage of blood vessels, qi (or in Ayurveda, prana) energy must be made free-flowing. This is accomplished with long-term use of herbs that dissolve plaque. They include herbs that are astringent and stimulating to dissolve masses such as clots and stones. Other herbs fortify the integrity of healthy blood vessels (reduce hardening of the arteries), and still others promote energy and blood flow through the heart and blood vessels. A heart health formula includes tonics that impact not only the heart but other organs necessary for smooth qi. The herbs aid digestion and elimination of fat and impurities that make plaque. They enhance circulation and regulate adrenal energy. The overall aim is to create or restore normal circulation, lower blood pressure, and regulate heart action.

What to Do During a Heart Attack

A heart attack is a medical emergency. Do not try to drive yourself to the hospital. **Do not delay getting help,** because life-threatening irregular heartbeats are the leading cause of death in the first few hours of a heart attack. These arrhythmias may be treated with medications or electrical defibrillation by the ambulance medical team. The team will also give you oxygen, even if your blood oxygen levels are normal, so that your body tissues have easy access to oxygen and your heart doesn't have to work as hard. Because it is vital to increase oxygen for the heart as soon as possible, it is wise to use the following natural remedy, a famous Chinese "heart-reliever" pill called Suxiao jiuxin wan.

Herbal Treatment for Chest Pain and Heart Attack

While waiting for an ambulance to take you to the hospital, you can take a dose of Chinese over-the-counter herbs, Suxiao jiuxin wan, tiny pills that work like nitroglycerin to open blocked blood vessels and help resolve chest pain. Some people take a small dose of these herbal pills daily as part of their heart trouble prevention program.

Suxiao Jiuxin Wan

Suxiao jiuxin wan (also known as Quick-Acting Heart Reliever pill) is commonly used in China. An older, overweight friend who had developed chronic heart failure symptoms before using Asian herbs regularly takes a small dose (four to five pills) of Suxiao jiuxin wan in order to walk with ease in New York's streets polluted with ozone. He walked into a Chinese-run laundry in Manhattan, and the women behind the counter smiled at him, saying, "You use Chinese medicine." She smelled the faint aroma of camphor (like Vicks VapoRub) from Suxiao jiuxin wan on my friend's breath. That's how commonly that medicine is used by Chinese people. Fifteen clinical trials involving 1,776 people were reported for Suxiao jiuxin wan.

Chinese suxiao jiuxin wan (pills) for angina pectoris and heart attack: Keep the small ceramic bottle of pills at your bedside, in your wallet, or purse.

The conclusion of the trials was, "Suxiao jiuxin wan appears to be effective in the treatment of angina pectoris, and no serious side effects were identified." Another study cited at the website for University of Maryland Medical Center states: "Suxiao jiuxin wan improved ECG measurements and reduced symptoms and frequency of acute angina attacks compared with nitroglycerin." The Chinese are slow to run strict clinical trials on herbs that have been in common use for hundreds of years. However, more research is being carried out on Asian herbs at NIH and at universities.

The small pill that tastes like medicinal camphor, its main ingredient, is commonly used for chest pain and prevention of blood-vessel blockage. The camphor (also known as borneolum) dilates blood vessels. The other ingredient, chuanxiong (*Ligusticum chuanxiong*), stimulates heart action to sweep blood vessels clean. According to TCM, the small pill that is dissolved slowly in the mouth or under the tongue, "promotes qi and circulation. Relieves pain, like headaches, abdominal ache, chest pain, muscle pain, boils, difficulty in menses (painful period), amenorrhea (no period). It corrects blood stasis." It feels cooling for your throat and sinus. It is relaxing and improves breathing. It may lower blood pressure and ease circulation in the head, neck, and chest.

If you take this sort of natural nitroglycerin pill regularly, do not take it with food, but wait, if possible, to take it between meals. But it may be taken at any time for severe chest pain. The dose for prevention is four to six small pills under the tongue three times daily. For acute heart attack, take ten to fifteen pills once or twice as needed. This pill is also useful for sex. According to the manufacturer, other effects of Suxiao jiuxin wan include:

- Dilates coronary arteries, improves blood flow to heart muscles, lowers oxygen consumption of heart muscles
- Improves blood flow to the brain and limbs, lowers resistance of the peripheral blood vessels
- Resists radiation
- Antibiotic effect
- Anticoagulation of platelets
- Helps resist effects of lack of vitamin E

Chinese Dan Shen

Dan shen (*Salvia miltiorrhiza*, salvia root) reduces cholesterol, supports the integrity of blood vessels to help prevent hardening of the arteries, and regulates the heartbeat to avoid arrhythmia and palpitations. In China, a liquid form of the herb is injected to quickly eliminate harmful cholesterol. In the West, we can order dan shen powder or find the pills in Chinese herb shops or online. Dan shen does not work quickly like Suxiao jiuxin wan, but gradually reduces plaque buildup and reduces heart stress. It is safe and pleasant to use. It is suitable for weak or elderly people and can be used long-term. The powder can be added to tea or soup. Mix one-fourth teaspoon of dan shen powder to water to make a cup of herbal tea or follow directions on the label. According to Chinese medical sources, dan shen has the following actions:

- Gets rid of clot blood, pain
- Invigorates blood circulation to break up blood stasis
- Reduces menstrual pain and regulates the period in case of amenorrhea (lack of period)

- Reduces tumors
- Treats and prevents angina
- Reduces inflammatory pain
- Reduces restlessness, insomnia, irritability
- Reduces swollen spleen and pain in digestive system

Dan shen is antithrombotic, antihypertonic (lowering blood pressure), antimicrobial, antipyretic (lowering inflammation and fever), and hepatoprotective (protects the liver); it inhibits fibrinogen and aids in the reabsorption of fibrous plaques in the liver; it is sedative and modulates cancer growth and metastases.

For long-term use and prevention of heart troubles, add the powder to water or tea; or use Dan Shen Wan pills.

A Common Threat for Computer Addicts

Heart failure, often called chronic heart failure, is an example of weak qi affecting the heart muscles. The heart is not strong enough to pump blood so that blood backs up into the heart again. Or a blood vessel blocked with plaque or a damaged blood vessel stops the flow of blood and qi. Sometimes there is no chest pain, only extreme fatigue and shortness of breath, especially when climbing stairs. Here is an example that may seem very familiar.

Sam, in his seventies, is an overweight lawyer who sat most of the day, except to occasionally walk to a pastry shop. He did not smoke and always took a shot of whiskey with dinner to reduce stress. Gradually his face became puffy and bloated. Bags of water formed under his eyes. He needed three pillows when sleeping and complained that he could not breathe well at night or when walking. He thought he might have asthma. He gained weight, especially in the middle, felt exhausted, and finally went for a medical exam.

A golden rule for heart health and longevity: the larger the waistline, the shorter the lifeline.

Sam's echocardiogram showed that his heart was working at only half capacity. He had heart failure. The cardiologist flatly gave him at most five years to live and told him that if he did not use the prescribed medications he could easily die sooner. Could such a diagnosis become a self-fulfilling prophecy? Many tests were made. The doctor suspected that Sam had had a severe shock, illness, or infection that led to heart failure. But all tests were negative. There was no blockage of blood vessels, no previous infection or trauma. Sam had weak qi made worse by a stagnant lifestyle—no exercise and excess sweets and fats in his diet. A TCM analysis of his problem would find low digestive, breathing, and kidney/adrenal qi. His tongue was bloated with water like most of his body. His pulse was halting (stagnant).

Sam told the cardiologist that his illness came from sitting and working for years under pressure. Many of us could say the same. The high dose ACE-inhibitor drug recommended for Sam made his legs fill with water like elephant legs. He immediately quit the medicine and consulted with me for herbs. I recommended a combination of herbs that included both Western and Eastern herbs described in this chapter. Within a year, Sam looked and felt much better. A year after his initial echocardiogram, his heart reading was normal. The herbs worked! Today Sam controls high blood pressure with a low-dose diuretic and ACE-inhibitor combination. And to protect his heart, he takes the herbs I recommended. His blood pressure is normal and heart health improving. He still needs to lose weight and exercise more. But he religiously takes his Chinese and East Indian herbs.

Ayurvedic Herbs to Prevent Heart Troubles, Hypertension, and Cholesterol

In traditional India, health and well-being are the rewards of a wise, disciplined life and a loving heart. The Ayurvedic approach to heart care is elaborated to include a cleansing, light diet of fruits and vegetables and traditional lifestyle practices such as periodic deep cleansing and fasting, yoga, meditation, and good works. But I will only cover a simple herbal regimen that may easily be added to any wellness program.

Arjuna, Guggulu, and HeartCare

In Vedic literature, Arjuna, a noble warrior, is the devoted disciple of Sri Krishna, the god of love. Arjuna tree bark is also the most important Ayurvedic astringent herbal tonic for a healthy heart. It protects against heart weakness and heart failure and reduces harmful cholesterol. Ayurvedic tradition recognizes that a strong heart protects against fatigue, chronic pain, and depression.

Arjuna: Regulates Heartbeat and Reduces Cholesterol

Arjuna tree bark (*Terminalia arjuna*) is a cardioprotective botanical used in Ayurveda since 2500 BC. It has remarkable cardioprotective, heart-muscle strengthening properties. Here are good reasons to take 250 milligrams of arjuna with meals once or twice daily.

- Arjuna bark powder is rich in saponins, natural antioxidants (flavonoids), gallic acid, ellagic acid, oligomeric proanthocyanidins, phytosterols, and minerals including calcium, magnesium, zinc, and copper.
- Regular use of arjuna improves the pumping activity of the heart, which makes it very useful for heart weakness and congestive heart failure.
- Arjuna improves cardiac muscle strength.
- Arjuna decreases LDL cholesterol levels. Arjuna's ability to suppress the blood's absorption of lipids indicates that it has cholesterol-regulating properties. Its principle constituents are beta-sitosterol, ellagic acid, and arjunic acid.
- Arjuna bark is rich in Co-enzyme Q-10, which prevents risk of heart attacks.
- Arjuna also has tonic and diuretic effects that benefit cirrhosis of the liver.
- It induces a drug-dependent decrease in blood pressure and heart rate.
- The bark of arjuna is useful as an anti-ischemic and cardioprotective agent in hypertension and in ischemic heart disease, especially in disturbed cardiac rhythm, angina, or myocardial infarction.
- Arjuna helps maintain a healthy heart and reduces the effects of stress and nervousness.
- Arjuna enhances prostaglandins and lowers risk of coronary heart trouble.
- Arjuna can relieve symptomatic complaints of essential hypertension such as giddiness, insomnia, lassitude, headache, and the inability to concentrate.

In a study on the efficacy of the bark powder in treating congestive cardiac failure (CCF), over 40 percent of the cases showed marked improvement. CCF due to congenital anomaly of heart and valve disease was also brought under control. Four out of nine cases of CCF due to chronic bronchitis were also relieved by the treatment.

Therapeutic Dosage: Arjuna is sold in health-food store capsules at Vitamin Shoppe and online. Arjuna pills and powder are available in Indian groceries and online. For prevention the recommended dose is two capsules of 500 milligrams each daily. You might add one-fourth teaspoon of arjuna powder to your morning pot of tea. It is astringent, which means it will make your mouth pucker like a strong red wine. Here is a simple recipe.

Recipe for Heart Health

Here is a simple recipe for a drink to take with you to the gym or on your daily walk. Diuretics are the first course of action against hypertension. Cranberry and apple are cleansing and alkaline. Hawthorn berry strengthens the heart muscle and regulates cholesterol.

Ingredients:
1–2 tablespoons cranberry apple concentrate
1–2 capsules hawthorn berry
1–2 capsules arjuna
2 cups or more water
stevia to taste

Combine all ingredients and mix well.

Guggulu: Clears Phlegm, Fat, and Cholesterol

Guggulu, a relative of myrrh, is the perfect tree resin, a deep-acting cleanser, suited to overcoming the effects of our polluted and stagnant lifestyle. Guggul is a small tree or shrub. Guggulu is excreted by the mucous membranes of the body, which stimulates and disinfects their secretions. It also contains guggulsterones Z and E, guggulsterols I–V, two diterpenoids, and a terpene hydrocarbon named cembrane A.

The gum resin shows pharmacological properties, uses, and clinical application. It is astringent, expectorant, aphrodisiac, demulcent, carminative, alterative, antispasmodic, and emmenagogic (makes the period possible). Ayurvedic doctors praise its use for infertility, arthritis, leprosy, impotence, sterility, liver disorders, and hemiplegic numbness and paralysis. It has hypolipidemic and thyroid-stimulating properties. It is useful in atherosclerosis, psoriasis, and cardiac ischemia. It is used against obesity. Guggulipid is hypocholesteremic. Guggulu helps regulate the lipid metabolism, showing excellent results in weight control and body fat reduction. It modulates your lipid profile. The hypocholesteremic activity of guggulipid in guggulu is used in hyperlipidemia and obesity.

Are you overweight? Do you have excess mucus congestion, asthma, fibroids or fatty cysts, swollen joints, lethargy, or depression, especially during humid weather? Guggulu is a great cleanser to detoxify body and mind.

Therapeutic dosage: as a dietary supplement, adults take one vegetarian capsule three times daily with food, or as directed by a health-care professional. Clinical strength dosage: as a dietary supplement, adults take two vegetarian capsules three times daily with food, or as directed by a health-care professional.

If you are wondering when to fit these heart herbs into your daily schedule, here is a suggestion: Take heart-conditioning herbs, mixed minerals, and tea together before or during breakfast or at a 10:00 a.m. break. Tea, fruit, or a simple acid food, not a big meal, makes absorption of minerals easy. The heart runs on electricity driven by minerals such as potassium, calcium, and magnesium. Since heart troubles show up more often during morning hours, build your defense with regular use of herbs with light, easily digested foods, and tea.

You can add capsules of guggulu along with arjuna to protect your heart. Or take one of the following combinations.

HeartCare and Hart Care Capsules

Two Ayurvedic heart remedies have almost the same name, which can be confusing. Either combination can help reduce risk of heart attack and heart failure. HeartCare is made by Himalaya Herb company. In India it is called Abana. The complex formula contains many herbs that reduce stress, build stamina, and support heart health. Among them are major tonics: arjuna, ashwagandha, amla, eclipta, and shilajit. Also added are herbs to ease circulation such as cyprus and gotu kola, and stimulants such as ginger, cardamom, and clove. It is an overall heart tonic that can and should be used long-term for prevention and treatment. The recommended dose for reducing high cholesterol is three pills twice daily until cholesterol level is safe, and then you can reduce to twice daily. For heart weakness you may also add three capsules twice daily of hawthorn, a Western heart tonic herb that grows wild in the United States. Hawthorn berry strengthens the heart muscle and regulates heartbeat while it reduces cholesterol.

Hart Care Capsules, made by Goodcare Pharma Ltd., part of Baidyanath Bhawan company in India, contain a proprietary blend with two additional herbs, arjuna and guggulu. Both are the same low price and most likely contain most of the same herbs for heart health. The dose is two capsules twice daily.

Arjuna, Guggulu, Hawthorn, and HeartCare for Heart Strength

The recommended dose for HeartCare is to take three pills twice daily until cholesterol level is safe; then you can reduce to twice daily. For heart weakness, you may also add three capsules twice daily of hawthorn berry. For people with chronic heart failure, overweight, and/or arthritis that feels heavy with swollen painful joints and poor digestion and absorption, I recommend HeartCare, hawthorn, and guggulu capsules. An overweight client of mine followed that program and improved his echocardiogram dramatically. Within a year, his echocardiogram became much closer to normal, an increase from thirty to forty-five. His cardiologist, Dr. Alan Kono, MD, FACC, Director of the Congestive Heart Failure Clinic at Dartmouth Hitchcock Medical Center in New Hampshire, was pleased but not amazed. Originally from Hawaii, the heart specialist said he appreciated the value of Asian herbs. The doctor prescribed heart medicines to lower the patient's hypertension, advised a low-sodium diet and exercise, and said he should continue with the herbs and other health protocol, which was working well. The patient said the heart herbs helped him to exercise, which in turn improved his circulation and reduced joint pain.

Heart Health and Alcohol

Many current studies recommend a daily drink of alcohol for relaxation and general heart health. However, that needs refining. Dr. Kono once told me, "Alcohol may be helpful to reduce tension and may even improve our chances of avoiding heart attack. However, alcohol is *poison* for the chronic heart patient." It may relax the heart muscles too much. Alcohol does not help prevent breast cancer or ulcers. So use discretion.

Diet for Circulation Pain, Cholesterol, Fat, and Triglycerides

Triglycerides are the scientific name for the chemical formulation of animal and vegetable fats. Research shows high triglyceride levels (a.k.a. fatty liver) as an important indicator of stroke risk. Since triglycerides are stored in body fat, here is my simple diet advice: cut fruit juices with water to reduce sugar. Cut out soft cheeses made with high butter fat, and eat breakable cheeses and saturated fat foods with salad. Slim (cleanse) the liver with bitter herbs like dandelion and artichoke extract.

Add these important foods for heart health. According to medical sources, they are sources of healthy fats that replace damaging ones from meat and dairy products. A few easy recipes follow. You can easily expand on them.

- Olive oil on bread and pasta with herbs—sage, rosemary, oregano, thyme
- Fatty fish: salmon, tuna—steamed or broiled without butter
- Red wine
- Black beans
- Walnuts, walnut oil dressing; almonds; flaxseed
- Soy: edamame, tofu for the protein
- Sweet potato
- Orange

- Cherries (they contain an antioxidant that protects blood vessels)
- Swiss chard for blood pressure
- Blueberries
- Carrots
- Barley, oats, and oatmeal
- Low-fat yogurt
- Black coffee and tea
- Chili pepper (helps control blood sugar)

A Columbia University study found that having high levels of "good" cholesterol may help prevent Alzheimer's disease later in life. People in the study who had the greatest levels of high-density lipoprotein, or HDL, were 60 percent less likely than those with the lowest levels to develop Alzheimer's disease over four years. HDL, often called the "good" cholesterol, is one component of total cholesterol and is the exception to doctors' recommendations to keep overall levels low. "Take care of your cholesterol; because of that, you can lower the risk of Alzheimer's disease," said Dr. Christiane Reitz, MD, PhD, an assistant professor of neurology at Columbia University's Taub Institute in New York, in a 2011 telephone interview. "Based on our study, even at the age of sixty-five, the higher the good cholesterol, the lower your risk of developing Alzheimer's disease."

Shiso Leaves

Japanese shiso leaves are a good source of healthy omega-3 oil. Try adding it to salads, green tea, and soups.

Sources of HDL

Low HDL cholesterol has been linked to heart disease. The higher the HDL level, the less LDL, or "bad" cholesterol, that accumulates on artery walls, blocking nourishment from reaching vital organs and causing inflammation to the artery linings. HDL has many virtuous effects on the heart and blood vessels. HDL positively affects platelet function that contributes to clotting. Dietary choices profoundly affect HDL production. Unless heredity is an issue, a plant-based, whole-foods diet is shown to reduce the risk of stroke and heart attack.

Avoid greasy animal meats and full-fat dairy products that undermine otherwise healthy arteries and vital organs. HDL has antioxidant, anti-inflammatory, and anticlotting effects. Saturated animal fats blunt these protective effects of HDL cholesterol. Cutting down on the portion size and the consumption of highly marbled meats is vital to successfully increasing HDL. It's important to become familiar with dangerous foods and eating behaviors that inhibit HDL's job, or the effort will produce temporary results.

Eat fish oil found in tuna, lake trout, sardines, salmon, krill, and mackerel. It contains omega-6 and omega-3 fatty acids that are effective food sources that increase HDL. Nuts and seeds are also sources of omega-3, 6, and 9. The American Heart Association recommends eating fatty cold-water fish at least two times a week. Clinical testing reveals that eicosapentaenoic acid (EPA) and docosahexaenoic acid (DHA) found in fish oil help reduce risk factors for heart disease, including high LDL cholesterol. There is strong evidence that these substances can help prevent and treat atherosclerosis by inhibiting the development of artery-clogging plaque and blood clots. Flax oil is another quality source for essential fatty acids. They all benefit HDL integrity.

Consume organic whole grain foods, beans, cucumber, garlic, onion, apples, prunes, pears, and other high-fiber foods to cleanse arteries and organs from accumulated fat and plaque, thus fortifying HDL presence. Eating a variety of vegetables and fruits that contain powerful antioxidants is crucial in increasing appropriate HDL levels. Omega-6 can also be found in many common vegetable cooking oils such as soybean oil, sunflower oil, canola oil, and corn oil, but not olive oil. Drinking organic green tea daily may also help the body cleanse itself. Cardiologists remind that patience and vigilance are required. It's taken a lifetime for plaque to build up to a perilous level. It will not disappear overnight. Here are some basic menus to help you get started.

Basic Heart Health Menus

Breakfast 1

- Orange juice or unsweetened cranberry or cherry juice concentrate with water
- Whole-grain oat and barley cereal with almond or soy milk
- Coffee

Breakfast 2

- One cup plain low-fat yogurt, adding black cherry concentrate
- Orange slices, very ripe
- Coffee

Lunch or Dinner 1

- Vegetable soup with cloud ear fungus and herbs
- Steamed salmon with pineapple, red pepper, and red onion
- Bitter salad greens with endive and watercress, olive oil, cayenne
- Tuocha tea (also known as pu-erh tea) from Yunnan (known to reduce cholesterol)

Lunch or Dinner 2

- Black bean soup, adding a little red wine or black tea; walnut or olive oil, bay leaf, thyme, and sage
- Baked sweet potato
- Steamed asparagus (optional)
- Whole grain peasant bread with olive oil and leaf herbs: oregano, thyme, rosemary
- A mixed green salad

Lunch or Dinner 3

- Edamame
- Cold hijiki seaweed and cloud ear fungus salad; walnut lemon dressing
- Raw block of firm tofu, cut in cubes, adding one teaspoon low-sodium soy sauce, one sliced scallion, sesame seeds, and balsamic vinegar
- Tuocha or pu-erh tea

Afternoon Snack or Dessert

- Fresh fruit
- Coffee or tea

Following a Heart Attack

Some people after suffering a heart episode walk on eggshells; some continue habits as before. I heard of an elderly man who had multiple heart attacks over the years. Once in the emergency room during a cardio test, he ate a ham sandwich and coffee offered to him by a nurse. Genetics may have a role to play, but hopefully, most people will experience heart trouble as a wake-up call. Lifestyle changes, including diet and exercise, reduce pain, depression, and aging. A heart-healthy diet and lifestyle can improve memory and mental clarity. Weight loss and improved circulation, you will see, also improve your sex life.

Sex and Heart Patients

In most cases, doctors advise heart patients to resume exercise and gentle sexual practices when ready, often within weeks or months of the heart episode. Sex, after all, is nice exercise for the heart. To feel adequate and safe, we need sexual tonics. Asian herbal tonics for sexual potency support circulation, production of sexual fluids and sexual hormones, and heart health. An excellent example is sold in American health-food stores and online.

Python Extra

Named after a big snake, according to men who use it, the herbal pill made by Vitamin Shoppe makes their sexual parts big and strong. The first ingredient, usually the main ingredient in a formula, is a heart herb, rhodiola (arctic root), a form of ginseng. Chinese herbals call it hong jing tian. The root is respected as treatment for poor memory and heart weakness. That in itself shows the important connection between heart health—circulation—and sexual potency. The formula contains other ginsengs, gingko to enhance peripheral blood circulation (where it is needed), and stimulants, including 100 milligrams of guarana, herbal caffeine. The formula is balanced and strong enough to treat impotence when used wisely as directed.

It comes with warnings: affecting hormones can increase facial hair in women, hair loss in men (increased testosterone), acne, and aggressiveness. It can increase heartbeat and should be avoided by people with prostate swelling or cancer, unchecked heart disease, or low good cholesterol. Otherwise, the recommended dose is two tablets daily with a meal. I would suggest starting slowly with half the recommended dose to see if it can be tolerated as a long-term tonic. To have the desired effects, use should be regular even with a low dose.

Women can use certain herbs that are precursors to testosterone, since we also make it. Without testosterone, girls could not enter puberty. Python Extra can strengthen muscles in lower back and legs and lift your mood. However, overuse of herbal testosterone can result in fibroids as well as female facial hair. Women using Python Extra should use half the recommended dose, use it temporarily, and watch for signs of menstrual discomfort or irritability, and reduce the dose accordingly or stop taking it.

> ## Letha's Advice: Circulation, Suxiao jiuxin wan, and Sex
>
> Something fast-acting is Suxiao juixin wan. I described these Chinese heart-reliever pills earlier in the chapter as a treatment for angina and heart attack. They are not intended as a sexual tonic, but do enhance circulation. Borneol dilates blood vessels, and ligusticum stimulates heart action to help remove "blood stasis." It feels cooling to the throat and sinus cavities, yet stimulating in order to improve breathing and reduce chest pain. The drug Viagra also dilates blood vessels, increasing sexual potency for men with poor circulation. After one or two suxiao jiuxin wan pills are totally dissolved in the mouth, your saliva still has some of the healing effects. The pills can also be dissolved in a few drops of water. When applied externally to skin, the momentarily uncomfortable sensation feels burning/cooling/stimulating. By increasing local circulation, it may produce more intense enjoyment.

Heart Trouble and Cold Weather

A report in the December 13, 2004, issue of *Circulation: Journal of the American Heart Association* found that the rate of heart disease–related deaths rose sharply between December 25 and January 7 each year. In fact, the death rate peaked on Christmas Day and New Year's Day. Does that say something about the holidays? Heart stress is also increased by cold weather. Chinese herbalists know that cold weather "challenges the kidneys," which means it tends to cool down adrenal vitality. Cold weather and iced drinks can impair circulation and increase urination. Scientists also believe that weather can affect hormones. During the winter months, "there is a change in the ratio of daylight hours to dark hours, which changes the hormonal balance, and the hormones involved, such as cortisol, can lower the threshold for a cardiovascular event," explains Stephen P. Glasser, MD, a professor of preventive medicine at the University of Alabama at Birmingham School of Medicine.

Cold temperatures cause arteries to tighten, restricting blood flow and reducing the oxygen supply to the heart, all of which can set the stage for a heart attack. "In cold weather, there is more oxygen demand by the heart because it is working harder to do the work and maintain body heat," Glasser says. Studies show that heart attacks and heart disease complications occur more frequently in the morning hours.

Western research suggests that the early-morning rise in blood pressure or "a.m. surge" that occurs in most people may dramatically increase the risk of having a heart attack or stroke. "In the winter, people tend to exert themselves or do yard work in the morning because it gets dark earlier," Glasser says. "This shift of activities to morning hours adds to the normal circadian variation in mornings—further increasing heart rate, blood pressure, and the hormones that lower the threshold for a cardiovascular event."

Here is another area where there is an overlap of Eastern and Western theories on heart health. Chinese doctors and Chinese martial artists trained in Chinese medical tradition can predict when internal organs are weakest because the flow of qi in them is reduced. The heart is weakest around 9:00 a.m. to 11:00 a.m. because blood and qi flow to the heart are reduced then.

Letha's Advice: Cinnamon for Circulation and Diabetes

Take your heart herbs and supplements early, before or during breakfast, and do not overdo exercise in the morning. A regular fifteen-minute walk is better for the heart than shoveling snow once a year. After returning inside to a warm house, prevent/treat hypothermia by drinking a warm cup of water, adding one-fourth teaspoon of cinnamon powder to sweat out a chill before it happens. Cinnamon also improves diabetes, a big factor in heart disease. Take from one-fourth teaspoon to one teaspoon daily for diabetes. It increases insulin uptake. Cinnamon is very heating and stimulating for circulation. It improves aches that result from exposure to cold weather. It may even improve the health of blood vessels, but that is yet to be proved.

CHAPTER SIXTEEN

Your Nerves

Great events make me quiet and calm; it is only trifles that irritate my nerves.

—Queen Victoria (1819–1901)

DO YOU AVOID DRAFTS AND AIR-CONDITIONING? DO LOUD VOICES AND AUTO-mobile traffic sounds irritate you? Do blasts of pain shoot through your body? Is it hard to sit still without wiggling your legs or tapping your fingers? Do you feel your clothing is an aggravating weight against sensitive skin? Some people think it weird to be hypersensitive, but the nervous system can sometimes overreact as though eliciting an autoimmune response. At those times, our nerves torture body and mind. Certain people seem always crabby and nervous. They may have addictions or chronic pain and depression. But anyone of any age may suffer from nerve pains increased by stimulants such as caffeine, overwork, chronic fatigue, and illness. This chapter offers relief from nerve-wracking annoyances that can wear us down and cause irritability, nerve pain, and depression.

You must build vitality to prevent chronic and acute nerve pains. The herbs described here help you to tolerate anxious situations, inclement weather, and aggravations. Foods and herbs that protect and nourish the nerves are helpful for everyone, because it is always better to implement positive lifestyle changes whenever possible and avoid prescription drugs. For example, a study published in August 2011 in *Stroke: Journal of the American Heart Association* reports that women with a history of depression have a 29 percent greater risk of having a stroke than nondepressed women, and those who take antidepressants, particularly selective serotonin reuptake inhibitors, or SSRIs (such as Prozac or Zoloft), face a 39 percent higher risk. It is not clear to me whether stroke is more prevalent in women because of the *causes* for depression, such as lifestyle habits, poverty, emotional problems, illness, or because of the *medications*, especially brain chemical–modifying drugs. In any case, it is safer to deal with mental and emotional health issues naturally.

For one reason or another, we may become highly sensitive to our environment. Today, there is a medical name for it. Complex regional pain syndrome (CRPS), also called reflex sympathetic dystrophy syndrome (RSD), is a chronic neurological disease affecting an estimated one and a half to more than six million Americans. RSD is a malfunction of the nervous system and the immune system as they respond to tissue damage from trauma, such as an accidental injury or medical procedure. Even a minor injury, such as a sprain or deep bruise, might trigger RSD, causing nerves to misfire, sending constant pain signals to the brain. Other common symptoms are complexion and nail changes such as swollen skin, excess sweating, or sensations of hot or cold in the area of injury or pain. Women tend to develop RSD more often than men, but so far no hormonal connection has been made. It is rarely seen in children.

No standard test is used to diagnosis RSD, although a patient history and blood tests may be recommended. There is no recognized cure for it, but physicians may prescribe sedative drugs, nerve blocks, or antidepressant medicines. It seems to me that sort of treatment is too drastic and too late. Why depress vitality in an attempt to sedate pain? Besides, the side effects of antidepressant drugs are famous. They often increase body weight and sexual dysfunction. Some of those medications deplete essential fatty acid reserves, so supplementation with omega essential fatty acids (EFAs) is very important. EFA deficiency is associated with attention deficit disorder, depression, and bipolar disorder. So EFA deficiency leads to depression, and medications for depression lead to a severe EFA deficiency. Antidepressants also deplete CoQ-10 (required for the life of every cell), vitamin B6, and vitamin E, three nutrients long associated with autism, Alzheimer's disease, and depression.

Recognition of your nerve pain triggers and prevention of stress are key because our nerves are constantly stimulated by computer use, microwaves or other waves, cell phones, not to mention injuries and work and family stress.

Nervines vs. Tonics

Nervines are a category of herbs that improve the nervous system. Herbal medicine recommends nerve-stabilizing tonics for migraines, nerve pains (neuralgia), anxiety, and insomnia. Some may prove useful for chronic nerve pain or RSD. However, many people are so depleted that they need a stimulating tonic more than a nervine that works as a sedative. They are too exhausted to sleep, think clearly, and feel adequate energy to prevent and overcome stressful situations. They are nervous wrecks. Tonics, especially adaptogens, help us to function better during the day and sleep better at night because they regulate energy, circulation, and blood production. You may need to use a vitality tonic from chapter 17 for up to several weeks before fully benefiting from the nerve-regulating herbs presented here. This chapter can help you identify the source of your nervous pain and irritations. The herbs described below provide support for vitality, circulation, and emotional balance as well as treatment for nerve pain. We begin with prevention.

First: Avoid Nerve Pain

Our nervous systems are communication networks that warn us against enemies, protect us from inclement weather and injury, and tell us when to quit working. But given adequate cause, our nerves easily overreact. Below are listed common nerve irritants. You may need to moderate or avoid them in order to recover. You may need to compensate by using nourishing tonics and nervines to reduce pain while continuing useful stimulants such as coffee and tea.

Avoid nervous triggers that increase irritability, insomnia, and nerve pain:

- Caffeine (nerve stimulant in coffee, chocolate, and some over-the-counter painkiller pills)
- Cigarettes (dehydrating)
- Late night work or play, lack of sleep
- Excess talk, useless chatter, and loud music
- Alcohol, more than one to two glasses of wine or two ounces (slightly more than one shot) of liquor daily, or if allergic
- Herbal stimulants such as guarana and yohimbe
- Dehydration from sweating or foods (fluids nourish muscles, joints, and nerves)
- Acne medications known to increase anxiety (Accutane)

Nerve Tonics vs. Sedatives

It is worth repeating: a tonic helps body and mind to work better by allowing us to adapt to stress, normalize body functions, and get proper nourishment. Tonics are extremely helpful for rejuvenation, immunity, and mood. Many nerve tonics are Asian herbs because a main emphasis for those cultures has traditionally been to increase intelligence, maturity, and enlightenment that hopefully accompany wise living and aging. We will revisit herbal tonics in the following chapter. For now, let's consider remedies that enhance nerve stability and reduce nerve pain.

Because of my training in traditional Asian medicine, I recommend *individualized* nerve remedies. I emphasize the difference between a nervine (nerve tonic, nerve-stabilizing herb), a stimulating tonic, and a sedative because they work differently. They can cause problems if misused. Herbs sold over-the-counter for nervousness or insomnia, such as hops and passionflower, are certainly relaxing and pleasing. Those herbs are sedative. However, because they affect circulation, the heart, and mood, I do not recommend them for people with heart trouble, obesity, depression, or other medical problems related to low vitality. An herbal problem arises when someone with low adrenal vitality, low blood pressure, or mental exhaustion becomes trapped in a hyperactive state such as anxiety or insomnia. Adding a sedative to an already exhausted condition only increases risk of illness, such as heart failure or bipolar depression. I have provided some helpful guidelines below.

Avoid Sedatives If You:

- suffer from obesity
- have heart failure or irregular heartbeat
- have asthmatic wheezing or emphysema
- have depression or suicidal thoughts
- are using psychiatric drugs
- have recently had surgery or given birth

Ground rules for using nervine remedies:

- Choose your remedy carefully to treat chronic symptoms, never acute illness such as colds and flu.
- Do not overuse an herb so that you become too sleepy or relaxed to function effectively.
- Try the lowest recommended dose first, and then increase gradually as needed so your body becomes accustomed to the treatment.
- Do not mix sleep remedies with meals, prescription medicines, or sedative herbs.

Targeted Nerve-Enhancing and Stabilizing Herbs

The following are trusted aids to natural relaxation, improved sleep, memory, and concentration for most people. They are not sedatives but work to enhance wellness. Use an herb intended to treat the nervous system between meals; otherwise it may interfere with digestion. You might use one remedy for up to a week or more to test the results. Do not mix several remedies unless in a prepared combination remedy. If you have a weakened condition, consult your natural health expert before using herbs or foods that may act as a stimulant or sedative. If you are pregnant, have chronic fatigue, chronic diarrhea, chills, shortness of breath, chest pains, heart trouble, or depression, avoid using sedating remedies. You need to address such symptoms specifically with appropriate chapters and under the supervision of expert medical care. Here are a few easily available healing balms and teas that anyone can use to ease nerve pain resulting from injury, overuse of muscles, or stress.

> ## Letha's Advice: Teas to Settle Your Nerves and Improve Sleep
> Herbal teas are sometimes sold as single herbs or in combination teas. Brew one tea bag or one-half teaspoon of dried herb for three to five minutes in hot water. These are considered safe for nearly everyone, but when necessary I have added cautions based on traditional Asian medical diagnosis.

Vervain tea is recommended for nervous tension and anxiety; it is a liver-calming remedy with a pleasant lemony flavor. It is a popular after-dinner beverage in Europe.

Hops capsules or tea are recommended for restless insomnia and anxiety. Avoid them if you have low vitality, heart trouble, or chronic depression.

Passionflower is sometimes found in herbal sedative pills for insomnia-related problems like anxiety, overburden, and nervous fatigue. In England it is considered as a great tranquilizer with no negative effects. However, do not use it with obesity, chronic depression, or heart failure.

Valerian is a central nervous system (CNS) depressant for treating insomnia, stress, menstrual cramps, and panic. It is considered one of the best herbal tranquilizers because it does not have dangerous side effects similar to artificial sedatives prescribed by doctors. It comes in capsules and makes a strong earthy-flavored tea. However, avoid it if you have wheezing asthma, asthenia, chills, numb extremities, heart trouble, or chronic diarrhea.

Prunella vulgaris tea can be used for anxiety, itchy skin/herpes, thyroid inflammation, and nervous insomnia. It is detoxifying, cooling, and calming.

Skullcap is a CNS depressant, useful for fever, anxiety, insomnia, and hot flashes; skullcap was originally used as a treatment for rabies because of its tranquilizing effect on the central nervous system. Clinical studies have demonstrated skullcap's ability to improve blood flow in the brain, inhibit muscle spasms, and act as a sedative. Some alternative health practitioners use skullcap to treat symptoms of attention deficit hyperactivity disorder (ADHD). Skullcap is used in the treatment of a wide range of nervous conditions including epilepsy, insomnia, hysteria, anxiety, delirium tremens, and withdrawal from barbiturates and tranquilizers.

Caution: A medicinal infusion of skullcap is used to promote menstruation; it should not be given to pregnant women since it can induce a miscarriage. The infusion is also used in the treatment of throat infections. The skullcap infusion is given for nervous headaches, neuralgia, and headache arising from incessant coughing or pain, inducing sleep when necessary, without any unpleasant symptoms following. If you have never used skullcap or are very sensitive to herbs, start by adding three to five drops of the liquid extract to a cup of water and observe the results. You may feel more relaxed.

If you feel your heart thumping at your temples when tired, if you have low blood pressure and backache, you more likely need an adrenal-supportive herb instead of skullcap for recovery from illness or fatigue. For example, ashwagandha promotes muscle strength. Dan shen regulates heart action and strengthens weak heart muscles.

Relaxing Treatments: Hot and Cold

A nice warm bath does a lot to soothe nervous tension. You might add drops of valerian (warming) extract to the water as Victorian ladies did. Or for hot flashes and fever conditions, add cooling, bitter skullcap extract. Massage the herbal extract into your temples while soaking in a relaxing tub.

Ayurveda makes numerous massage oils to balance body and mind. A soothing massage oil can be applied with gentle strokes from the head and hands toward the heart and from the feet toward the kidneys in order to promote circulation and lymph cleansing. The ingredients used for the massage oil vary according to the condition treated. Cooling oils such as coconut and olive treat inflammation. Sesame oil is traditionally used for aging, dry skin, chills and aches made worse from cold weather, and chronic anxiety. When using an antistress oil, apply it and allow it to penetrate for half an hour; then remove it in a warm bath or shower. Overuse can feel overly sedating or stimulating for some people.

A Soothing Rub for Muscle Pain

If your nerves are on edge or stuck in high gear, any touch, even the feeling of your own breath on your arm, may feel irritating. That is not the time to apply a strong warming, stimulating, or cooling rub or get a deep massage. But there is one gentle healing balm that I have found to be very helpful: it is Xtra Mint Muscle Rub made by Common Sense Farm. Xtra Mint Muscle Rub is formulated to bring relief to aches and pains in muscles and joints. It is a very concentrated product. I recommend this for nerve pain because the ingredients are balanced to reduce irritation. Mint relaxes smooth muscles, menthol is cooling, while clove and nutmeg are warming and stimulating.

Letha's Advice: Avoid Hidden Stimulants in Cosmetics

People with chronic nerve pain should avoid harsh ingredients in lotions, shampoo, hair spray, perfumes, or other daily body treatment products. For example, avoid soaps and complexion products that contain alcohol if possible, because alcohol makes veins more fragile and therefore may increase visible capillaries and bruises. Although medical specialties do not recognize the connection between cosmetic ingredients and anxiety, I suspect that chronic nerve pain, even bearable nerve pain, is aggravated by noise, odors, chemical stimulants, etc., and that nerve-related pain makes us more sensitive to irritants.

In general, it helps to recognize that most of us are addicted to stress, stimulants of one kind or another, and life situations or relationships that may eventually lead to anxiety, chronic pain, and fatigue. Life is not under our control. But we can reduce the negative effects on our nerves, energy, and immunity by applying rejuvenating remedies covered in this chapter and the following chapter covering tonics. Even if our problems are purely emotional or resulting from a damaging relationship or work situation, easing physical discomfort greatly improves our vitality and mood. Calm reflection, a deeper breath, and physical comfort from balanced energy can help you to find a better way of life.

CHAPTER SEVENTEEN

Tonics

---

*What most persons consider as virtue, after the age of forty is
simply a loss of energy.*

—Voltaire (French writer, 1694–1778)

THE FOLLOWING ASIAN HEALING GEMS ARE IMPORTANT TONICS AVAILABLE IN
many American health-food stores, in Asian herb shops, and everywhere
online: ashwagandha, gotu kola, Saraswati churna, Siberian ginseng, and tien
ma. They enhance overall wellness, improve mental and physical performance,
moderate nervous problems, and reduce various types of pain to improve quality of life. Why, in a book about pain treatments, should we bother with herbs
that improve memory and the mind? Why not simply kill pain with a sedative
or deaden it with an injection to quickly eliminate the problem? We are given
the opportunity to use every experience, even pain, as a vehicle for learning and
self-improvement. Our lives become rich and our understanding deep if we trust
in nature and improve overall health. Our pain is part of a growing process.

The nervous system and muscles are key for performance. Muscles hold our
skeleton upright and allow smooth, easy flow of blood to lubricate ligaments,
joints, and nerves. The heart is also a complex muscle system that must function smoothly to prevent pain and illness. Ashwagandha, an Asian panacea
sometimes called "Indian ginseng," feeds our nerves and brain as it strengthens
muscles. Who can doubt the mind/body connection using this healing trea-
sure? Chronic backache, low vitality, and poor memory from adrenal weakness are draining and depressing. Ashwagandha helps you regain strength to
reverse pain, muscle weakness, and numbness resulting from overexertion and
improves paralysis diseases such as multiple sclerosis.

Ashwagandha: Adaptogen, Tonic for Muscles and Nervous System

Do you have:

- An aching lower back
- Nerve pain, muscle weakness
- Weak legs, numbness, or paralysis
- Mental and physical exhaustion
- Nervous insomnia and restlessness
- Poor memory and concentration
- Low sexual vitality

Ashwagandha (*Withania somnifera*, winter cherry), a vine in the tomato family, is one of the most famous Ayurvedic rejuvenative plants used in many herbal formulas. Ashwagandha helps maintain proper nourishment of the tissues, particularly muscle and bone, while supporting the adrenal glands and reproductive system. Used by men and women, it acts to calm the mind and promote restful sleep. Ashwagandha, an adaptogen, promotes our ability to resist stress. It prevents or minimizes imbalances that lead to disease, whether from poor diet, lack of sleep, mental or physical strain, or chemical toxins in the environment. It is especially beneficial in stress-related arthritis, hypertension, diabetes, and general debility, or recovery from illness and surgery. It has also shown impressive results when used as a stimulant for the immune system.

Uses

Use ashwagandha to prevent and/or treat stress, overwork, muscle weakness, congestive heart problems, sexual debility, low immunity to illness, including colds, flu, and allergies, and for cancer prevention. Cancer, like repetitive nerve pain, may be viewed as an autoimmune disease. The body overreacts with cell production with cancers and pain production with RSD. Both require regulating foods and herbs, and lifestyle changes. Since ashwagandha prevents/treats fatigue, muscle aches, and stress, it can improve pain while it helps prevent cancer cells. That alone reduces anxiety for many people.

> **Letha's Advice: Muscle and Bone Tonic**
>
> I like to use ashwagandha powder along with an equal dose of shata-vari powder (wild Indian asparagus, a moistening tonic herb) to build muscle strength, and stop muscle and nerve trembling and weakness from exercise, sports, dancing, or overuse of caffeine. I might take one-fourth teaspoon of each herbal powder in a little goat's milk or water at night as an overall rejuvenating/sexual enhancement treatment, espe-cially useful during fall and winter months. Reduced daytime sunshine impairs our calcium absorption and may increase pain and bone loss in the long bones of the legs.

At my website, www.asianhealthsecrets.com, a number of my readers who are weak or underweight have asked whether ashwagandha can help them to gain weight. Although it does not increase weight, it increases stamina. For reversing vata problems such as a frail constitution in elderly persons or chronic arthritis, sexual debility, and nerve pain in thin people, I recommend using one-half teaspoon each of ashwagandha and vidari kanda powder (*Ipomoea digitata*), a hormone-balancing yam, in water once daily. See vidari and the recommended diet for reversing bone loss beginning on page 193.

Dosage: Start with one-fourth teaspoon of ashwagandha powder in water once or twice daily or take one to two capsules of 500 milligrams ashwagandha daily with meals. Increase if needed.

What Can I Expect?

If you are exhausted and insomniac, ashwagandha may help you to sleep better (act as a sedative) before it increases energy. It is balancing for both issues. In India, ashwagandha is given in the final trimester to expectant mothers to reduce lower back pain and to shorten delivery time.

As a sexual tonic, use ashwagandha with an equal amount of shatavari, vidari kanda, or with shilajit capsules. These tonics are not aphrodisiac but increase stamina, sexual hormones, and sexual comfort. Vidari and shatavari, moisten-ing nourishing tonics, increase semen for men. Shatavari (wild asparagus) sup-plies female hormones and rejuvenates fragile vaginal tissue for postmenopausal women. Vidari increases lactation and menstruation. It gradually soothes and rejuvenates dry, aging skin and supports healthy muscles and bones.

Side Effects or Warnings

None.

Gotu Kola: Adaptogen, Tonic for Nerves, Brain, and Circulation

Do you have:

- Poor memory
- Stress-related complexion and hair problems
- Weak veins
- Poor circulation or excess bruising in the legs
- Chronic anxiety and nerve sensitivity

Look at the Indian God Shiva, lord of the dance, destroyer of the ego, and promoter of positive change. The famous cosmic dancer destroys and creates again the world, through his dances of *Lasya* (beauty, happiness, and grace) and *Tandava* (vigorous action). He dances surrounded by a ring of fire, revealing the cycles of death, birth, and rebirth. Under his feet he dominates the demon of ignorance. He has long, beautifully thick hair, a graceful body, and a calm expression. His wisdom encompasses the bravery of the tiger and gentleness of the cow. His intelligence has the subtlety of the nagas, snakes that live underwater and know secret truths. He feels no stress! The Ayurvedic rejuvenation herb brahmi (gotu kola) is sometimes called "the semen of Shiva."

Gotu kola (*Centella asiatica*) balances all systems in the body. Ayurvedic physicians say it balances the three humors: vata, pitta, and kapha. As such, it impacts respectively nerve communication, inflammation, and problems associated with water retention and slow metabolism. Gotu kola is most known to enhance and rejuvenate memory, improving the nervous system, and is said to be the most important rejuvenative herb in Ayurvedic medicine. It is the main revitalizing herb for the nerves and brain cells, recommended for increasing intelligence and strengthening the immune system and the adrenal glands. Because it improves circulation, it is also said to be helpful for stress-related hair loss and complexion issues. Caution: since gotu kola regulates the nervous system, it can have varying effects on energy depending upon your condition. Some people find the herb to be stimulating; others sedating. See the dosage information that follows.

According to University of Maryland Medical Center, gotu kola has been used for thousands of years in India, China, and Indonesia to heal wounds, improve mental clarity, and treat skin conditions such as leprosy and psoriasis. Chinese herbalists have called it "the fountain of life." One ancient Chinese herbalist is said to have lived for more than two hundred years as a result of using gotu kola. Historically, gotu kola has been used to treat syphilis, hepatitis, stomach ulcers, mental fatigue, epilepsy, diarrhea, fever, and asthma. Today, American and European herbalists use gotu kola most often to treat chronic venous insufficiency (a condition where blood pools in the legs). It is also used in ointments to treat psoriasis and help heal minor wounds.

Gotu Kola and Anxiety

Triterpenoids (the compounds found in gotu kola) seem to decrease anxiety and increase mental functions. One study found that people who took gotu kola were less likely to be startled by a new noise than those who took a placebo. Since they believed that the "startle noise" response may be an indicator of anxiety, researchers theorize that gotu kola might help reduce anxiety symptoms. But the dose used in this study was very high, so it's impossible to say how gotu kola might be used to treat anxiety. If a low dose of gotu kola feels calming, it may be easing your anxiety. Taking a bigger dose does not necessarily work better and may in fact increase mental functions, which for some people feels like anxiety.

Dosage: To make gotu kola tea, add one-fourth teaspoon of dried gotu kola leaf to one cup of boiling water and steep for ten minutes, one to two times daily. Standardized extracts should contain 40 percent asiaticoside. Websites selling gotu kola capsules recommend taking 1,000–4,000 milligrams up to three times daily. That dose may be useful for athletes who want to stimulate leg circulation. I think that is way too high to begin. Nervous, sensitive people, and people over sixty-five, will find that gotu kola taken at such a high dose *increases* nerve sensitivity, that it acts as a stimulant, not a nerve depressant. If you want to use gotu kola but are unsure how it may affect you, start with one capsule of 475–500 milligrams between meals once or twice daily for a couple of days. Increase very gradually as needed, up to five or six capsules daily and not after eight o'clock in the evening. It can increase wakefulness and creative thought. Capsules containing 175 milligrams each of gotu kola (*Centella asiatica*) and Siberian ginseng (*Eleutherococcus senticosus*) are useful for stress-related nervousness, insomnia, and pain.

Do not mix or use gotu kola along with irritating or inflammatory herbs or foods such as garlic, onions, cayenne, peppers, or alcohol. Wait at least two hours after using caffeine or inflammatory herbs before using gotu kola.

Letha's Advice: Sleep Rejuvenation Treatments

Rest is so important for pain prevention and healing. However, it is often difficult to get past work, worry, and fatigue in order to sleep soundly all night. Here are ways to relax brain stress: apply a little Xtra Mint Muscle Rub to temples, in front of your ears along the jawline, at the hairline in back of your neck, and along the top of the shoulders. You might also use a drop of essential oil of mint or other cooling, calming oil, or take one or two gotu kola capsules during the evening. Try taking a warm bath, adding powdered goat's milk, or massage your feet, applying a drop of sesame oil to the sole. Practice relaxed deep breathing. If these remedies do not bring sleep, rest quietly in a comfortably warm, dark room that is free of noise or other disturbances. Eliminating stimuli can sometimes feel as restful as sleep.

A calming bedtime treatment is especially useful for arthritis and chronic joint and muscle pain that prevent sleep. Take a warm seaweed bath, adding kelp powder and Epsom salts to bath water. Rinse and dry. Massage Banyan Botanicals Joint Balm on to the bottom of feet, hands, knees, and painful joints and wear clean cotton socks to bed. Add one-fourth teaspoon each powdered ashwagandha and vidari kanda powder to a cup of warm water before bed.

What Can I Expect?

Some gotu kola products suggest very high dosages, but test for allergies before using a dose higher than 500 milligrams. If you develop any of the following side effects adjust the dosage or stop using gotu kola.

Cautions

Gotu kola has been used in some studies that lasted up to one year. However, in some people, gotu kola may affect the liver. It's best not to use gotu kola for more than six weeks without talking to your herbal doctor. You may need to take a two-week break before taking the herb again. According to medical sources, people with liver disease or who take medications that affect the liver should not take gotu kola. ·

Asiaticoside, a major component of gotu kola, has also been associated with tumor growth in mice. Anyone with a history of precancerous or cancerous skin lesions—such as squamous cell, basal cell skin cancer, or melanoma—should not use gotu kola. Gotu kola is not recommended for children. People older than sixty-five should take gotu kola at a lower-than-standard dose. Your health-care provider can help you determine the right dose for you, which can be increased slowly over time.

Side effects of gotu kola are rare but may include skin allergy (with external use), headache, stomach upset, nausea, dizziness, and extreme drowsiness. These side effects tend to occur with high doses of gotu kola.

Saraswati Churna: Tonic for Memory and Nerve System Regulation

Do you have:

- Mental fatigue, poor memory
- Poor digestion
- Nervous anxiety, feelings of being "ungrounded"
- Irregular sleep patterns

Saraswati, the beautiful Indian goddess of culture, learning, language, and the arts, plays the veena, a graceful string instrument made from a jackwood or khadira tree. The Vedas (ancient teachings) are believed to have sprung from her head. She is serene and radiates intelligence. Saraswati churna, an herbal tonic combination (*churna* means "powder"), is the perfect remedy for drowsy gray days of rain, seasonal depression, low vitality, poor memory and concentration, and nervous exhaustion. The spicy-tasting herbal remedy, made by Baidyanath or Vadik in India and sold in East Indian groceries, is recommended for improving the health of the nervous system, memory, and concentration. It is said to relieve anxiety, worry, stress, fear, and sleeplessness, and improve immunity, which is perfect for all.

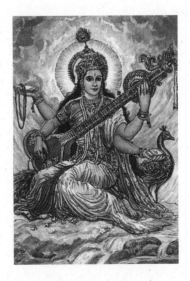

Saraswati, Indian goddess of culture, learning, language, and the arts

Saraswati churna ingredients:

- Ashwagandha, the wonderful rejuvenating tonic for firm muscles that reduces lower back pain and improves memory and sleep for mentally and physically exhausted persons
- Cumin, a digestive spice
- Caraway seeds, a digestive spice
- Ginger and black pepper, digestive spices
- *Piper longum*, a spicy, rejuvenating pepper pod
- *Acorus calamus*, a form of sweet flag used for flavor and to quiet the mind
- *Convolvulus pluricaulis* (bindweed; in Sanskrit, shankhapushpi), used in mental stimulation and rejuvenation therapy

Isn't it interesting how by enhancing digestion with warming, grounding spices we can think clearly and reduce stress! Digestion is a center for processing thought and emotions. Strong digestion, kidney/adrenal vitality (ashwagandha), and a calm mind (calamus) are a reservoir of courage. One study shows shankhapushpi to have antiulcer effects due to the augmentation of mucin secretion and glycoproteins. Another study shows that shankhapushpi may be helpful in improving symptoms of hyperthyroidism by reducing the activity of a liver enzyme. The whole herb is used medicinally with cumin and milk for fever, nervous debility, and memory loss. Shankhapushpi is a brain tonic, a psycho-stimulant and tranquilizer. It is reported to reduce mental tension. The ethanolic extract of the plant reduces total serum cholesterol, triglycerides, phospholipids, and nonesterified fatty acid.

Dosage: The usual dose is one-half to one teaspoon of the powder in a cup of warm water or milk twice daily. Caution: since caraway is drying, and pepper and ginger are pungent digestive herbs, avoid this remedy if you have stomach ulcers or acid stomach. It may feel too warming. (You can cool acid indigestion and help prevent GERD by drinking aloe vera juice or gel.) The peppers in Saraswati churna feel warming, grounding, and soothing for digestion. If after taking the remedy for several days, you develop signs of inflammation, such as burning joints or dry mouth, use a lower dose.

Saraswati churna is balancing because it supports adrenal and nervous system health for prevention and treatment of burnout. It is digestive for people who stay awake and nervous trying to figure out their lives, and it is soothing and rejuvenating for the mind. I tried it and was soothed to a calmer state and eventually a deeper sleep. The brain becomes frayed from city life. Saraswati offers a brain balm.

Eleuthero: Tonic for Nerve Sensitivity

Do you have:

- Pain resulting from cold or inclement weather, stimulants, or anxiety
- An autoimmune illness or poor immunity due to illness or stress
- Exposure to environmental poisons
- Cancer risk and cancer treatments
- Diabetes

The Russian Olympic swim team and many other athletes have used eleuthero (a.k.a. *Eleutherococcus senticosus*, Siberian ginseng) to help them tolerate cold water. Exposure to cold and wind tightens muscles, causing pain and stiffness. Eleuthero is an adaptogen, which means it helps us adapt to various kinds of stress. Its properties are antitoxic, antiradiation, immunoprotective, and immunoregulatory. I have also found taking 500 milligrams of Siberian ginseng very helpful for relieving nerve pain resulting from overuse of caffeine. It may also be useful at work to prevent stress injury from computer use. This herb, not a real ginseng, helps normalize the body by reducing nerve sensitivity. Experts agree: Eleuthero (Siberian ginseng) could be used under any circumstance where there is the need to normalize any physiological, biochemical, or immunological defects.

In cancer therapy, the immune defenses are weakened, and eleuthero offers a better tolerance to such treatments. It is also possible that it may offer prophylaxis against the development of cancer. The glycans, eleutherans A, B, C, D, E, F, and G, have hypoglycemic effects; therefore, Siberian ginseng could be used in diabetes. It delays exhaustion by allowing efficient release of stress hormones. Have you seen the ads on television for a dietary supplement that prevents belly fat? That extra layer of fat is the body's natural response to a stress such as starvation. The trouble is most of us are not starved, just stressed. Eleuthero has immunoprotective effects against breast, stomach, oral, skin, and ovarian cancers. But caution should be used when it is used with other medications, since it inhibits certain drug-metabolizing enzymes and may prevent the biotransformation of other medications to less toxic compounds (i.e., it may make chemotherapy less toxic).

Use this adaptogen if you feel fragile, overworked, and prone to illness during cold weather, emotional upset, or to prevent and treat nerve pains or migraines brought on by stress, overwork, and insomnia.

Dosage: Try a smaller dose first, such as one 250-milligram capsule daily for a few days to feel the results. Overuse may be stimulating. There are no known contraindications.

Tien Ma: Nerve Stabilizer for Pains, and Numbness

Do you have:

- Hypertension dizziness and headache, migraine, or neuralgia
- Vertigo
- Nervous exhaustion
- Numb extremities

Chinese tien ma (*Gastrodia elata*) is the tuber of a perennial alpine plant with a large central root and twelve smaller tubers on the side. The fresh tubers are used as food, and the dried tubers are used as medicine. It is a superior herb, well recognized by Chinese herbal doctors as the most effective remedy for headaches, vertigo, and other neuralgic afflictions caused by inflammations of the liver. In Chinese traditional medicine, the liver energy extends beyond the liver organ beneath the right side of the ribs. Liver qi begins at a point between the large and second toe of each foot; the meridian's path moves upward to the inner calf and thigh, through the uterus, the chest, the nipples, the neck, to the eyes and brain. Inflammation or troubled circulation along this pathway can provoke pain, cramps, dizziness, a tight throat, anxiety, chest tension, lumpy breasts, anger, and vision problems.

Tien ma is a nervine considered warming, sweet, and pungent. It is used for calming nervous exhaustion, headache, neuralgia, vertigo, and dizziness. It alleviates pain for migraine, numbness of extremities, and general fatigue. Sliced dried tien ma may be consumed as a tea or cooked for twenty minutes with sliced tang kuei to make a bland soup to help prevent and treat nervous exhaustion and migraines.

Chinese Patent Remedies Containing Tien Ma

Tien ma is combined with other herbs to treat a variety of nervous conditions, including hair loss. Here are two Chinese patent remedy herbal combinations that contain tien ma.

Tien Ma Tou Tong Wan

The translation is Gastrodia Root Combination, made by Guang Dong Yi Kang Pharmaceutical Co., Ltd., in Guang Zhou, China. Tien Ma Tou Tong Wan is recommended as especially effective for dizziness, headache pains, and numbness in the extremities. Other uses include treatment for hypertension, paralysis after stroke, neurasthenia, insomnia, mental depression, white hair, and hair loss from stress and blood deficiency.

Dosage: Take six pills, three times a day with warm water.

Tien Ma Mi Huan Su

Another Chinese patent remedy containing tien ma is Tien Ma Mi Huan Su, manufactured by Wuzhou RFX Company, China. This dietary supplement is designed to normalize blood pressure and sedate liver yang (dizziness and headache). It promotes healthy circulation.

This Chinese herbal pill "tonifies liver yin and blood," which means it supports the liver tissue and enzymes. It calms liver fire and wind (inflammation), and invigorates the blood circulation. It is used to relieve symptoms of hypertension including headache and dizziness, as well as numbness or tingling in limbs, and insomnia due to liver yang (overactivity, inflammation).

Dosage: As a dietary supplement, take three capsules two to three times a day as desired.

Tasty Tonics

The use of Asian herbal tonics improves life in so many ways that it seems odd they have become popular and easily available in the West only within the last twenty or so years. Perhaps our emphasis on killing germs and waging war against disease and pain has limited our appreciation of pleasure, wellness, and enlightenment.

To work effectively without side effects, tonics must be suited to individual needs. In this book you have learned ways to identify your needs for cooling and warming herbs, energizing or relaxing herbs, and so on. Tonics don't have to be a bitter pill to swallow or a dried root to be boiled overnight. There are some very tasty tonics you can enjoy as a pleasurable energy pickup. Here are two Chinese herbal favorites.

Extractum Astragali

For overwork and chronic fatigue, this tonic is suited for people who are weak or recovering from illness. They may have tired legs, an aching back, and low immunity to allergies or colds and flu. Extractum Astragali is a liquid extract made with astragalus (huang qi) and honey. Astragalus boosts energy and T-cell production. It is useful for cancer prevention and for HIV. As your endurance improves from the tonic, you will feel less pain.

Young Yum Pills

This one should be renamed "yum yum" pills. It is a moist Chinese herbal gumdrop you chew or add to water. It is made by Wai Yeun Tong in Hong Kong. Recommended for women's health and beauty and using an exclusive formula for over one hundred years, it contains important qi and blood tonics for long-term use. Ingredients are:

- Astragalus and *Radix codonopsis pilosulae* to improve circulation and vital energy
- *Radix rehmanniae preparata* and *Radix asparagi* to replenish essential body fluids
- *Radix angelicae sinensis* and *Radix paeoniae alba* to enhance blood production and circulation
- *Fructus ziziphi jujubae* and *Rhizoma dioscoreae* to strengthen digestion and blood production
- *Fructus lycii* and *Cortex cinnamomi* to nourish and replenish the liver and kidney

The manufacturer describes its functions: "To enhance basic vitality, nourish internal organs, and promote physical equilibrium in the entire body; maintain a capacity for well-being; regulate blood circulation and energy, improve general health, vitality, and resistance to fatigue, dizziness, abnormal sweating, chills, and low immunity to colds." Chronic chills are the key words here: if you tend to wear extra clothing to avoid being cold or developing nerve pains, chew one to two of these herbal balls daily until you feel stronger, which will be soon. Then continue as needed with one per day. It is a *warming* energizing tonic. Others include ashwagandha and Chinese ginseng.

On the other hand, if your pain is inflammatory, if you tend to run hot and dry—i.e., if you have chronic thirst, fevers, night sweats, red swollen joints, or burning nerve pains—neutral or cooling, moistening tonics will work better for you. They include gotu kola and raw tienchi ginseng, which reduces cholesterol and bruising and swelling pain. Choose the remedy suited to your needs and you will feel immediately better and live longer.

Make Your Own Tonic

I add tonic herbs to cooking whenever possible. As fall approaches, I seek warmer Ayurvedic herbs to strengthen muscles and bones and support vitality and willpower. The recipe varies with my current herbal enthusiasm. Lately I have been mixing one cup each of sesame seed powder and walnut pieces, one teaspoon each of powdered ashwagandha and shatavari, a dash of kelp powder, and honey to make a thick paste that I roll into balls. Sometimes I make no-bake brownies. The dry ingredients include one cup each of uncooked instant oat-meal, flaxseed meal, dark roast mate tea powder, unsweetened cocoa powder, unsweetened shredded coconut, puffed rice, a pinch of spirulina powder, and a teaspoon of a tonic herbal powder such as ashwagandha. I moisten it with a cup or more of strong black tea. I like the chocolate to remain bitter. Or I may sweeten with a little vanilla extract. I add a few teaspoons of flaxseed or other healthy oil to give it body and mix in nuts and raisins for flavor. The paste is thick and sticky. After refrigerating it for a few hours, it can be cut into squares. No salt, sugar, chemicals, or baking.

What Aggravates My Pain?

CHECK WHAT APPLIES MORE OFTEN FOR YOU. THIS IS NOT AN EXHAUSTIVE LIST but does cover some basic pain triggers. There are no correct or incorrect answers. Track what factors increase your pain and then use the key to guide you to the chapters that will provide specific remedies.

Weather conditions irritate my pain:

- ❏ Cold, damp weather increases my pain.
- ❏ Hot weather irritates me.
- ❏ I always feel an approaching storm or change in barometric pressure.
- ❏ Temperature or weather conditions that suddenly change affect my pain.

Foods affect my pain:

- ❏ Hot spicy foods increase my joint pain.
- ❏ Cold or raw foods and iced drinks are uncomfortable.
- ❏ Fattening, oily, or rich foods make me feel logy.
- ❏ I am overweight.
- ❏ I love dairy foods, ice cream, and soft cheese, but they increase weight and congestion.
- ❏ Tomatoes, peppers, and eggplant cause problems for me.
- ❏ I have acid reflux.
- ❏ I have chronic diarrhea or cramps and irregular elimination.
- ❏ Caffeine (coffee, black tea, chocolate) increases my nerve pain.
- ❏ I have diabetes.

I have circulation issues:

❒   I get pains in the chest, shoulder, arm, abdomen, or back, from stress or anytime.
❒   I get leg cramps.
❒   I have PMS and/or menstrual pain.
❒   I easily bruise when injured or even without injury.
❒   My legs fill up with fluid or I have varicose veins.
❒   I am taking heart or blood pressure medicines.
❒   My cuts, bruises, or wounds heal slowly.
❒   My muscles hurt or are stiff from overwork or computer use.

I have emotional or nervous issues:

❒   Anger makes my blood boil; then I hurt or feel stiff.
❒   I am taking mood-enhancing medication (antidepressants).
❒   I use painkiller drugs daily.
❒   When I feel sad or anxious, I feel pain more intensely.
❒   I have a lot to worry about.
❒   Insomnia increases my pain.

Here is the key to items that you chose, along with suggested chapters.

Section One: Weather Conditions

Outdoor temperature, humidity, and climate changes such as an approaching storm often affect joint and muscle pain. That is because as the barometric pressure drops, a relative vacuum is created around joints, and they swell in reaction. Cold, damp weather may increase nerve pain because muscles react by becoming stiff as though to create a barrier against the climate. Arthritis and rheumatism feel worse from weather changes. See Part One, especially the chapters devoted to arthritis and sciatica.

Hot temperatures, like spicy foods, may increase sweating, dehydration, and inflammatory pain, including headaches, gout, and skin rashes. See the diet in chapter 1 in order to avoid acidic (inflammatory) pain-trigger foods and appropriate chapters for local pains: chapter 2 for headache and chapter 5 for arthritis. Reducing rich, congesting foods also improves the heart and circulation.

Section Two: Foods

Many foods trigger pain depending upon allergies, age, and our physical and emotional condition. In general, if spicy and acidic foods irritate, your pain is inflammatory. To avoid further inflammation, see chapter 1 in order to avoid pain-trigger foods. Being overweight places additional stress on damaged joints and tired muscles. Weight issues are also involved with normal menstruation and fertility (chapter 7). Overweight and high cholesterol increase our risk of heart trouble (chapter 15), stroke, and certain cancers. Fortunately, avoiding pain-trigger foods, especially meats, cheese, sweets, soda drinks, and alcohol, improves weight loss and diabetes. A healthy low-fat, high-fiber diet such as the reduction diet (presented in chapter 1) may reduce fatty cysts and worse problems, even cancers. Caffeine is an obvious nerve irritant. Also see chapter 10 covering computer-related stress injuries to protect against nerve pains.

Section Three: Circulation

Chronic heart problems signaled by vague chest, arm, shoulder, or back pains may be improved by a wise diet and certain heart-regulating herbs. Leg cramps may result from simple dehydration (not drinking enough water) or from high cholesterol or vein blockage. Other factors may be cold feet. Try wearing socks to bed if your feet get cold. That may prevent leg cramps. Otherwise, heart-care advice in chapter 15 and massage and electro-stimulation treatments for injury found in Part Two can help. For female pain issues and repetitive stress injury pain, see respectively chapters 7, 9, and 10. Weak veins and leg circulation can be improved with gotu kola (chapter 17 covering tonics). Slow-healing wounds may be due to poor diet and lifestyle habits resulting in PAD (see chapter 15). However, a Chinese patent remedy quickly speeds healing for traumatic physical injuries and surgery. See chapter 8, covering home and field injuries, for information on Yunnan Paiyao, a Chinese herbal emergency treatment in a capsule.

Section Four: Emotional Problems

In order to heal properly, we need to feel comfortable with ourselves. Depression, anxiety, fear, and hysteria interfere with basic necessary healing functions such as breathing, circulation, and elimination of poisons. Useful chapters to help bring about normal health include chapter 14, covering treatments for overcoming the ill effects of traumatic and depressing situations, chapter 16 on RSD and nerve-related pain, and chapter 17 covering tonics.

CHAPTER EIGHTEEN

The Future of Pain Medicine

The distinction between the past, present, and future is only a stubbornly persistent illusion.

—Albert Einstein (1879–1955)

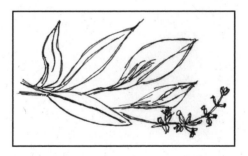

Sage

WE STILL KNOW SURPRISINGLY LITTLE ABOUT THE EVOLUTION OF DISEASE AT the cellular level. The word *cell* comes from the Latin *cellula*, meaning a small room. Recently, we have come to realize those rooms are full of important "junk." The human body's approximately one hundred trillion cells, each a unit of life, contain water and extremely complex genetic material—DNA and many types of RNA "messengers." During the spring 2011 meeting of the American Association for Cancer Research in Orlando, Florida, a new biological dimension of cell workings was described by Dr. Pier Paolo Pandolfi, professor of medicine and pathology at Harvard Medical School. Up to now we have considered only 2 percent of the cell genome as viable. The rest of our DNA was considered "junk" that is nonfunctional material. Under the new paradigm of cellular life, that "junk" becomes a necessary part of communication. Something even more shocking is that 90 percent of the protein-encoding cells in our body are *microbes*. So we have DNA and numerous subcategories of RNA molecules and microbes, some influenced by the environment, all communicating with each other in order to create our illness and wellness.

Imagine the chaos that would occur if someone blindfolded dropped a bomb into this delicate mess of hypersensitive, interlocking communication systems. It would stop the signals and redirect traffic in the cells. This example is useful for our understanding of painkiller drugs. Despite a limited knowledge of the channels of communication that control pain, most people try to stun or override their pain with sedative drugs and surgical treatments.

We may feel the effects of cell communication as pain and disease, but we are unable to simplify the chatter. However, long ago Chinese doctors described illness carried by "evil winds." Later the "winds" were redefined as microbes. We have finally come back to the idea of winds or channels that communicate within the netherworld of the cell. That ancient paradigm is still at work today. Asian medical foods, herbs, and health practices keep one of the largest, healthiest, and wealthiest populations on earth alive, well, and pain free. Hopefully, the development of new pain therapies will be inspired by important work done abroad where funding for research is free from political and religious prejudice. As you will see, China leads the way in stem-cell research and treatments. Stem-cell transplant treatments now exist at Wujing General Hospital in Beijing for stroke and brain and spinal cord damage. Stem cells have been used to repair scar tissue resulting from heart surgery. Countries such as India and Thailand aim to capture the foreign surgery market by offering up-to-date, safe treatments for a mere fraction of the usual cost. But first, here are additional low-cost home treatments that can help you to deal with everyday pain.

Light-Emitting Diode (LED) Lights

You may have heard of LED red and blue lights used in beauty shops to increase collagen production and thereby reduce wrinkles and skin discolorations. However, light-emitting diode (LED) light therapy is also used to treat muscle pain and joint stiffness, symptoms typically associated with arthritis. NASA research inspired the use of LED lights that penetrate deep into muscle tissue for treatment of chronic pain and stiffness and improving circulation. LED therapy is used on the NASA Space Station and by the U.S. submarine fleet for pain relief and wound healing. The Food and Drug Administration (FDA) has approved LED light therapy for the treatment of minor pain and stiffness and specifically for use by arthritis sufferers. The LED system transmits light waves at a speed of 880 nm into deep muscle tissue, stimulating DNA production and normal cell growth and function, which can be altered by the effects of chronic pain and arthritis. Manufacturers have created useful LED light products with a wide range of prices. The less-expensive LED systems are handheld wands or lights, and more expensive ones are free-standing units that can be strapped to the body. Be sure the product description says it is used for pain, because red and blue LED lights are also used for treating acne and healing wounds.

Laser Treatments

A number of acupuncture doctors have used cold lasers instead of needles for quite a while. Laser acupuncture is not always taught in traditional Chinese medical schools, but lasers are sold to acupuncturists and others who treat people and animals with this safe, painless method. With simple instructions you too can stimulate acupuncture points, reduce muscle spasms, and move qi as nature intended. Never point a laser light at the heart, eyes, or Adam's apple. I have described modified laser treatments for reducing pain from sciatica, knee injuries, tennis elbow, and carpal tunnel syndrome in this book.

Medical Injections

Injections of irritants and acids used in prolotherapy in order to prompt the production of cartilage at a joint or to tighten loose ligaments are considered nouveau treatments. Up to now, alternative-minded orthopedic doctors have opted for injecting patients with steroids or other painkilling drugs. Some have injected a chemical to deaden nerve pain by, in effect, killing the nerve. I consider that the same old medical painkiller approach delivered a different way.

PRP Injections

Platelet-rich plasma (PRP) injections, the new frontier in injection therapy, use the patient's own blood platelets to repair damage and speed healing from injury and surgery. At my website, I began a running commentary on my PRP and stem-cell injections used to treat severe osteoarthritis of both hip joints. Below is the first article I wrote on the day following an injection into each hip joint of my own blood platelets and stem cells taken from tummy fat and bone marrow. Other articles describing the procedure and my recovery can be found in the section called "Flesh and Bone" of my website.

PRP and Dr. Alan Lazar in Plantation, Florida

I first heard of Dr. Alan Lazar, MD, FACS, board-certified orthopedic surgeon, on the Internet. Meeting him in his office in Plantation, Florida, I immediately was impressed. He was very friendly and funny, a mensch. I thought, "What a generous man: he sees people in pain all day and tries to make them laugh." Originally from Brooklyn, Dr. Lazar has been practicing in South Florida for more than thirty years and is also the expert medical consultant on regenerative injection therapy for Appalachian State University athletics in Boone, North Carolina. Since 1992, Dr. Lazar has served as Clinical Assistant Professor, Department of Surgery, at Nova Southeastern University's Health Sciences College of Osteopathic Medicine. He is certified in age management (antiaging) medicine by Cenegenics.

Dr. Lazar's book, *Beyond the Knife: Alternatives to Surgery*, carefully details his procedure of medical injections used to relieve pain and repair damaged tissue such as torn tendons, ligaments, cartilage destroyed by osteoarthritis, and bone fractures. Read it before you consider surgery. Hopefully more doctors will be inspired to use autologous treatments (taken from your own blood) to speed healing during and after surgery. Dr. Lazar has brought pain relief for thousands and improved performance for some famous sports stars and entire college teams of young athletes. However, his treatment is appropriate for people of all ages. Before my first PRP injection I was in the doctor's waiting room and spoke to a plumber who had been out of work for a year following what he called "three botched knee surgeries." All his insurance money was used up. He came to Dr. Lazar for a treatment and within two months he was back at work and pain-free for nearly a year.

Dr. Lazar specializes in arthroscopic surgery, reconstructive surgery, orthopedic surgery, sports medicine, and ultrasound-guided injections for PRP and stem-cell treatments. He offers a wide range of holistic therapies, nonsurgical and minimally invasive surgical therapies and procedures for orthopedic injuries and osteoarthritis.

Platelet-rich plasma (PRP) is an in-office procedure in which the doctor removes a minimal amount of a patient's blood, stem cells, and fat and injects the combined fluid into an injured area or an arthritic joint. This platelet regeneration therapy procedure concentrates the platelets in the patient's blood. The bioactive tissue growth factors are released when the platelets are injected into the injured area. These factors are known to stimulate the healing cascade in musculoskeletal injuries and arthritis. Medical researchers report remarkable results using PRP in the treatment of common injuries, including tendinitis, the regeneration of cartilage in osteoarthritis of the thumbs, knees, and hips, and in nonsurgical repair of rotator cuff tears. Published studies show restoration and smoothing of roughened cartilage, improved range of motion, and resolution of pain in osteoarthritis of hips, knees, and shoulders. Many other conditions respond to PRP, including injuries to the back, neck, jaw, elbows, shoulders, hands, hips, knees, ankles, and feet.

My PRP and Stem-Cell Treatments in Plantation, Florida

Before I began PRP and stem-cell treatments, I sometimes stopped when walking, unable to move because my hip joints were jammed bone on bone. Over the course of a year, I had six PRP treatments from Dr. Lazar, including two bone marrow stem-cell injections, one done in a hospital, the other in his office surgery. Although PRP injections have been used for over thirty years during surgery on the battlefield and in some hospitals in order to speed healing and reduce pain and swelling, the treatment is considered experimental in America and is approved by neither Medicare nor insurance companies. This is very unfortunate because it is a safe, effective pain treatment. Our body does not reject our own blood platelets. Because stem cells are neutral, they can transform into whatever cells are needed at the injection site—muscle, cartilage, or ligaments, for example.

My injections eased my pain and increased mobility in my damaged hip joints. I could walk up stairs with ease. I have not used pain medicines at all since the treatments. The injections could not repair damage done over a lifetime to my femur, the top part of the thighbone that is replaced with joint replacement surgery, but some new cartilage showed up by the fifth treatment, visible with ultrasound. That cushioned my walk.

There was still work to be done. One leg is slightly shorter than the other, made worse by the osteoarthritis damage to my joints. As a result, my pelvis, like that of many women, is tilted. Joint damage resulted over time from the leg-length difference. That had to be corrected with a lift placed in the shoe. Many surgeons performing total hip joint replacement do not consider the problem of pelvic tilt, but only measure for correct leg length. The problem with that is pelvic pain and sciatica may continue from pinched nerves resulting from the tipped (uneven) pelvis. I still use my natural remedies to increase comfort, especially homeopathic dulcamara on rainy days when joints feel swollen. The final solution will come when we can put into place treatments that permanently replace lost cartilage and damaged bone and prevent further injury. We are working in that direction.

Medical PRP and stem-cell treatments are becoming more available from sports medicine doctors treating traumatic injuries. Hopefully, if treated early enough, they may someday replace risky, expensive joint replacement surgery. Maybe someday we, as the Chinese and other forward-looking scientists hope, will be able to grow new bones, joints, and organs, and will repair damage done with our own tissue.

Another treatment option on the horizon is sci-fi becoming real. Nanotechnology, the use of tiny computers and guided injections into blood vessels and damaged organs, will become part of medical practice. Someday there will be safe, efficient gene-delivery mechanisms using nanotechnology and bacterial bio-robots in order to render disease harmless. Dr. Lazar writes in *Beyond the Knife*, "Over the next couple of years, it is widely anticipated that nanotechnology, nanomedicine, and genetic therapy will continue to evolve and expand, resulting in many more *Beyond the Knife* treatment modalities. I can hardly wait."

Stem-Cell Treatments in China

Wujing General Hospital for Chinese People's Armed Police Forces was founded in Beijing in 1949. Located adjacent to the Olympic basketball stadium and forty minutes from the airport, it is one of China's high-level government and military hospitals, featuring integrated health-care services. It has fifty-five clinical departments and two hundred medical experts. The hospital promotes scientific research, medical treatments, and education as a top medical center. The website for the Department of Stem Cell Transplantation at Wujing General Hospital is www.sinostemcells.com. The department formed in 2003 is one of the first stem-cell clinics in the world. Since then they have treated more than 2,500 patients for various diseases. The website has research articles and information on treatments done at the hospital for cerebral palsy, spinal injury, Parkinson's, brain injury, stroke, diabetes, and others. Medical consultations are encouraged and offered online. Examples of the wonderful innovative treatments offered at Wujing General are cited at their website. They treat, among other traumatic injuries, spinal cord injuries. Here is how doctors at Wujing General Hospital describe the treatment of spinal cord injuries.

Stem-Cell Treatment for Spinal Cord Injury

When injury occurs to the spinal cord, the connections between the brain and the body are hampered or broken, which results in some level of impairment and a certain degree of paralysis. Symptoms may include movement disability, loss of sensation, impaired control of urination and defecation, cramps, pain, and depression. Conventional treatments for spinal cord injury are focused on prevention of secondary damage and providing rehabilitation.

How Stem Cells Help Spinal Cord Injury

The advancement of stem-cell treatments in China offers a novel treatment option for spinal cord injury. Stem-cell therapy can support the natural regeneration processes of the body by stimulating the repair of damaged tissues. It goes beyond symptomatic treatment and may potentially help you to improve or regain some of the impaired functions. Cell death occurs when cells are injured. However, these dead cells are surrounded by damaged and healthy cells. Stem cells have the potential to stimulate the healing of these injured cells by the secretion of cytokines, such as nerve growth factor, to promote the body's self-repair mechanisms.

At Wujing General Hospital, stem cells are injected by an innovative procedure known as a CT-guided intraspinal injection technique, and this is supplemented by further stem-cell transplantation via lumbar punctures or IV injections. The hospital pioneered the CT-guided intraspinal stem-cell transplantation surgical procedure, which is a landmark in the field of stem-cell therapy for spinal cord injury. To date, CT-guided intraspinal stem-cell transplantation is only available at that hospital in China. CT guidance enables the neurosurgeon to target the stem cells precisely, administering the stem cells inside healthy spinal cord tissue adjacent to the lesion. This technique avoids open surgery of the spine. Thus pain, risks, and healing time are all minimized.

The objective of the treatment is to repair the injured cell area around the lesion. This will lead to improved symptoms, mainly in physique and movements. The majority of patients show improvements right after the first or second transplant. They are going to continue improving for about six months to one year, when the final results settle. For spinal cord injury patients, the achieved results are permanent. Typical benefits of stem-cell transplantations for spinal cord injury have been observed to be the following:

- Decreased feelings of pain and cramps
- Decreased muscle tension
- Increased ability to control urination, bowel movements, and sphincter function
- Improved blood circulation
- Increased sexual function
- Increased strength of the limb muscles, including muscle tone
- Improved limb motor function
- Decreased muscle atrophy
- Corrected orthostatic hypotension
- Normalized perspiration dysfunction (especially with higher-level cervical spinal cord injury)
- Normalized skin temperature

According to Wujing General Hospital's website, "Children and young adults tend to react better. As time passes, effectiveness declines. However, some patients in their thirties have had positive results. Patients injured at the cervical level tend to respond much better, although their symptoms are more severe.

This may be due to better blood circulation at the cervical level. Incomplete spinal cord injuries have a higher success rate. Patients in the early chronic stage have better results. Patients discharged from hospital continue to see improvements over an extended period (usually six months)." For additional data, visit the section of Wujing Hospital's website covering stem-cell treatment data for spinal cord injury.

Years ago, one of the saddest moments in my professional health practice occurred when I received an email from a boy in his twenties. He had crashed his motorcycle into a wall and was paralyzed from the neck down. He typed by holding a pencil in his teeth. He asked for my advice. At a loss, I recommended that he receive energy work such as massage or Reiki treatments to improve his circulation and mood, not knowing that one day spinal cord injuries might be healed.

CHAPTER NINETEEN

New and Controversial Treatments

Any actor who doesn't dare to make an enemy should get out of the business. Who is your enemy? Anyone who interferes with your work.

—Bette Davis (actress, 1908–1989)

OPIOID PAIN DRUGS PRESENT A GUT-WRENCHING HEALTH CONTROVERSY WITH international consequences. Do prescription pain drugs make our lives better or worse? Ask yourself, "What is an addiction *for me*?" You might answer the way Bette Davis did. An addiction slows your game, stops your work. When does a painkiller become an addiction? When is a physician a drug-pusher? Pain-drug advocates complain, "How much do people in pain have to suffer before they can get a prescription painkiller?" The opposite side argues for stricter control of pain drugs. They have lost loved ones to pain-drug addiction. Meanwhile, the official status of addictive painkillers remains a problem for the Drug Enforcement Administration and Food and Drug Administration. After twelve years of debate, they are still studying whether to move hydrocodone-containing medicines, opiates widely used for pain, from the wide-open Schedule III category drug into the more restrictive Schedule II category. Schedule III drug prescriptions can be renewed six times, but Schedule II drugs are kept under lock and key. Prescription painkillers, widely sold on the black market, are fueling the new American drug war.

In 2001, the cost of chronic pain treatments in the United States was estimated at $40 billion annually. By 2011, the cost rose to $635 billion annually (Reuters). Yet, according to a 2011 report by the Institute of Medicine, 116

Americans suffer from chronic pain, "many of whom are inadequately treated by the medical system." The World Health Organization (WHO) and the Joint Commission on Accreditation of Healthcare Organizations (JCAHO) have both issued statements on the far-reaching effects of pain and the incapacity it causes. Their consensus is that persistent pain is a major public health problem accounting for untold suffering and lost productivity around the world. The problem posed by the pro-drug side may be summed up this way: Excessive concerns about addiction and the side effects of pain medicines often result in reluctance to prescribe appropriate analgesics, with the consequence that patients suffer needlessly from pain.

The antidrug advocates are equally emphatic. Today hydrocodone, a painkiller relative of OxyContin, is considered the nation's second most abused drug, linked to murders, celebrity overdoses, and a rising tide of violent pharmacy robberies. Nationally, emergency room visits related to nonmedical hydrocodone use have quadrupled since 2000—from 19,221 to 86,258 in 2009. In September 2011, pharmacists across Florida began keeping an online database of patients who bought prescription painkillers. While states have focused largely on narcotic painkiller addiction, experts say that benzodiazepines, the class of sedatives that includes Xanax, are also widely abused, often with grim consequences. A *New York Times* article from September 2011 states, "The Centers for Disease Control and Prevention last year reported an 89 percent increase in emergency room visits nationwide related to nonmedical benzodiazepine use between 2004 and 2008. And...the combination of opiate painkillers and benzodiazepines, especially Xanax, is common in fatal overdoses." According to a 2011 article in the Florida *Sun Sentinel*: "In 2009, about 223,700 controlled substance prescriptions written in Florida were filled by pharmacists in Alabama, Louisiana, North Carolina, Arizona and Vermont."

Abuse of prescription medicines is only part of the drug controversy. An old familiar pleasure drug is now being promoted by some as an effective painkiller. Consider which is worse for you: drugs or the weed.

Marijuana

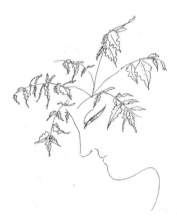

Medical marijuana is available by doctor's prescription in sixteen states and the District of Columbia for treating severe chronic pain such as arthritis, nausea and loss of appetite resulting from cancer chemotherapy, HIV, cancer pain, multiple sclerosis, Crohn's disease, and other conditions approved by individual states. There exists an FDA-accepted medical marijuana pill, but the future of medical marijuana is anyone's guess. Completely aside from the current political and economic debate over its use, I wanted to find out how marijuana actually works to curb pain—in other words, what mechanism makes marijuana turn off pain centers in the brain and whether a nonaddictive form can be developed. The information available on marijuana use depends on the point of view. From the National Institute on Drug Abuse, in a report posted in 2010, we learn:

> The main active chemical in marijuana is delta-9-tetrahydrocannabinol, or THC for short. When someone smokes marijuana, THC rapidly passes from the lungs into the bloodstream, which carries the chemical to the brain and other organs through-out the body. THC acts upon specific sites in the brain, called cannabinoid receptors, kicking off a series of cellular reactions that ultimately lead to the high associated with smoking marijuana… The highest density of cannabinoid receptors are found in parts of the brain that influence pleasure, memory, thinking, concentrating, sensory and time perception, and coordinated movement.

Not surprisingly, marijuana use can cause distorted perceptions, impaired coordination, difficulty with thinking and problem-solving, and problems with learning and memory. Research has shown that, in chronic users, marijuana's adverse impact on learning and memory can last for days or weeks after the acute effects of the drug wear off. As a result, someone who smokes marijuana every day may be functioning at a suboptimal intellectual level all of the time. Research into the effects of long-term cannabis use on the structure of the brain has yielded inconsistent results.

By contrast, a report from WebMD (find the link below in Further Reading), states, "No brain damage was reported for even heavy marijuana users." The popular social network community offered no help. Searching the Internet I found emotional tirades in favor of and against marijuana's use. The most intelligent articles were by medical and research teams—thousands of them—covering pro and con results for medical marijuana and pain. A separate report on the medical marijuana pill can be found at www.alternet.org.

I quote from the www.alternet.org article:

> A pill known as Marinol has been legal and approved by the Food and Drug Administration for use with a prescription anywhere in America since 1985. Its active ingredient? Dronabinol, better known as THC, the primary psychoactive element of the cannabis plant. "Marinol provides standardized THC concentrations, does not contain the other four hundred uncharacterized substances found in smoked marijuana, such as carcinogens or fungal spores, and is not associated with the quick high of smoked marijuana," said Neil Hirsch, a spokesman for Marinol manufacturer Solvay Pharmaceuticals. But Marinol is not the same thing as traditional, smokable marijuana. It is a less complex substance lacking both some of the good components found in traditional marijuana (such as cannabidiol, which has been found to have antiseizure effects) and the bad or not-yet-fully-understood components (among them potential carcinogens) that can also come with marijuana.

Researchers from the Department of Medicine, Minneapolis VA Medical Center, in Minnesota report that marijuana affects the brain by different means than opiates. "Cannabinoids act synergistically with opioids and act as opioid-sparing agents, allowing lower doses and fewer side effects from opioid therapy. Thus, rational use of cannabis-based medications deserves serious consideration to alleviate the suffering of patients due to severe pain."

The personal choice each marijuana user has to make is a trade-off. The risks are possible side effects, including long-term dizzy thinking, memory loss, and cancer, in return for enhanced comfort and the ability to eat without nausea. I have recommended digestive remedies, including the Chinese patent remedy

Xiao Yao Wan, that have proved very helpful for controlling chemotherapy related nausea and light-headedness. Hopefully, a completely safe marijuana pill is in the works.

Emotional Freedom Technique (EFT)

Emotional freedom technique was developed "for the personal release of emotional trauma and its detrimental physical, psychological, and spiritual effects" by Gary Craig, an engineer from California. He claims it is based on the five-thousand-year-old healing tradition of acupuncture and addresses the underlying causes of pain and illness, which are emotional trauma from injury, negative experiences such as post-traumatic stress disorder or rape, and illness. The method involves a person tapping with his/her fingertips certain points on the head, trunk, and fingers while thinking about the painful problem, voicing the problem, and vocally affirming self-love and acceptance. For example, someone might say, "I am really scared of (the problem) or very angry at (someone), but despite that I totally love and accept myself."

The EFT method taps acupuncture points, but no attempt at diagnosis is made. The results are judged subjectively by the user. The total lack of diagnosis of specific energy imbalance in organ systems and meridians, which is at the heart of traditional Chinese medicine, and the lack of careful treatment of meridians and points by engaging qi, would make a Chinese acupuncturist shrug. However, many people swear by this simple self-help method. I think there is nothing wrong with auto-suggestion, and I am a firm believer in acupuncture treatments with or without needles. EFT combines the two and "gives it to the people" with a fast, practical method for easing emotional distress. Does it work for everyone? Do the results last? I cannot answer. You have to try it for yourself.

It may take time to adequately uncover emotional sources of your problem. For example, you may have chronic headaches complicated by traumatic past experiences that limit wellness. EFT seems a practical way to accomplish a sort of "emotional trauma housecleaning." All sorts of issues may arise that never surfaced before. In that way, EFT may be useful as a meditation technique for self-discovery. It has been recommended for relieving everyday stress from a job or relationship. However, using the tapping method to relieve deeply intertwined physical/psychological issues seems problematic. For one thing, deep problems may awaken new pain as they resurface. That seems to me a good time to facilitate treatment with natural remedies to speed recovery. EFT allows you to observe how you feel about a situation. By tapping, breathing deeply, relaxing, and *accepting your feelings* no matter how difficult or painful, the situation may take on a new light. In effect, you are accepting yourself as worthy of your love and healing energy.

Herbs and Tapping

Herbal teas can facilitate many self-help practices. If during or after the session of tapping the emotion of grief surfaces, or if you have a weak heart, an irregular heartbeat or chest pains, a useful herb is dan shen, which regulates heart action and strengthens a weak heart. See the chapter on heart health for additional advice. If the emotions of anger, frustration, or depression surface, if you have burping or abdominal cramps, then a balancing digestive remedy such as Xiao Yao Wan is useful to ground and support the emotional center and digestive energy. You might take dan shen and Xiao Yao Wan pills together as needed for a period of time as you process your emotional changes and seek enhanced equilibrium. The herbal remedies work gradually to enhance both physical and emotional comfort.

Here is how my friend, Dr. Chrys, a chiropractor trained in yoga, nutrition, and Eastern spiritual practices, describes her EFT practice:

> Before you tap, check to see where your pain is, what its intensity is, whether it has a shape, color, or texture, and write it down. Drink some water to hydrate your body and allow the energy to flow more easily. Start by telling the story of what is bothering you, as if you were talking to a friend, as you tap along the points. For example, "my hips hurt, they have bothered me for so long, I have to modify my life to avoid the pain, etc." As you begin to tap, your emotions and/or discomfort may increase. This is normal and it is a sign that energy is moving in your body. Keep tapping and eventually your discomfort will subside.

You can find numerous videos by EFT users and several by Gary Craig describing the method on YouTube. He, ever the engineer in methodology, describes the brain's reaction to threat, fear, pain, etc., and advises following his manual in the sequence written before trying the method. My friend Dr. Chrys, who herself recovered from depression after a serious accident, uses both hands, a bilateral approach when tapping meridian points because, as she says sweetly in her video on YouTube, "I need all the help I can get."

That, in a word, is the approach I have used in writing this book: giving you all the help I can by sharing insights, techniques, and products offered by the best sources of natural pain relief. I trust that reading this you will discover and enjoy the methods you need to heal and fully accept yourself. Pain is a signal that life force is trapped. It may be trapped by an outdated, nonproductive emotion or memory, sunk in an area of weakness or poor vital nourishment, or bruised in a place of injury. Moving that pain out of your body frees your mind and spirit to heal your life.

Conclusion

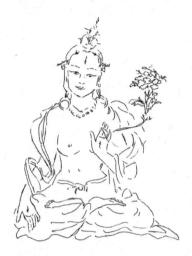

I BEGAN WRITING THIS CONCLUSION IN SEPTEMBER 2011, AFTER THE WORST natural disaster in Vermont's recent history. We summer in Vermont. Normally at this time of year, tourists from around the world arrive to enjoy "leaf season" as forest green turns to vibrant yellow, gold, and red foliage. But tropical storm Irene washed away over 250 roads that had been built in a valley along streams that no one expected to overflow. Flood waters swamped bridges and houses and left entire communities trapped like islands. Many households were without power, but Vermonters responded in typically cheerful and helpful fashion. Some walked to work, while others shared food with strangers. With groceries in limited supply, I cooked what I had on hand and as always, used herbs as medicine. While completing the final edit of *Naturally Pain Free* in Florida during February 2012, I was diagnosed with MRSA, a new, dangerous strain of staph infection after a bug bite became infected. The recovery was slow and required medication, but herbs helped to ease the pain. The lesson in this is to prepare for the unexpected.

As world health problems increase, our resources are shrinking. Climate change threatens to repeat such storms, raise ocean water temperatures to breed harmful bacteria, and cause havoc with the winds. At the same time the government resources in the area of healthcare are being cut back, America's most unpopular Congress ever is threatening to turn a deaf ear and blind eye toward suffering, illness, and aging. You and I are forced to defend our health as we do life and liberty. Natural home remedies are no longer an option but a necessity. Pain is a problem we all face during our lifetimes. Make prevention of pain and illness a daily pleasure and improve vitality for yourself and family.

Much of my professional work with natural pain treatments took place over the ten years preceding this book. I learned that pain left untreated takes on a life of its own, reducing activities, enthusiasm, and social contact. Living with chronic pain diminishes our perceptions and reflexes so that we accomplish less, live life less fully. We need not accept such barriers. My training in Asian healing modalities opened doors to treatments ranging from traditional herbs and acupuncture to cutting-edge medical procedures using our blood platelets and stem cells. I found that natural pain treatments accomplish much more than any sedative. Sedating pain does not eliminate its origins; it only dulls the senses.

Naturally Pain Free is a broad-reaching book that covers many sorts of pain problems, healing approaches, and affordable remedies. It is important to understand, from a holistic perspective, that by enhancing one aspect of health, we improve quality of life. For example, by improving the comfort and function of joints and muscles with select Asian herbal tonics, we simultaneously improve circulation, heart health, sexual vitality, mental clarity, and mood. We enhance both mental and physical health. Effectively dealing with acute and chronic pain is part of a healthy, enjoyable lifestyle. Difficult work, travel, and new challenges may increase our chance of experiencing pain. Temporary manageable pain often signals a growing process. How we deal with it makes all the difference in our health and well-being.

Here is something that may surprise you: eliminating your pain is not the final answer. Our bodies change and our pains change. What works for you today may give you another sort of pain tomorrow. Painkillers work for a time until your pain changes. Then you need to stop, look, and listen to your body. Have your tongue and complexion changed? Are you short of breath? Do you have chills or feel feverish? Do you feel depressed, weak, or irritable? These are the sorts of questions you might ask yourself, the feelings you might notice that indicate the underlying conditions of your pain have changed. This is important because, by ignoring the body's subtle communication, you may continue to use an inappropriate food or herbal treatment as a painkiller pill. Your body could remain out of balance. Our ultimate goal is to restore body and mind to the state of wellness we had before the injury, accident, or pain that we now suffer. It is to create comfort. You will find that preventing and treating pain can enhance communication in a loving home environment. What is more comforting than a delicious tea, a soothing herbal bath, or a skillful back rub? I will be happy if *Naturally Pain Free* enhances the health and vitality of you and your family.

Further Reading and Resources

Recommended Natural Product Sources

Chapter 1
Trifala (AKA Triphala), guggul: Ayurvedic Herbs Direct

Chapter 2
Chrysanthemum flower tea, organic: Pretty Wood Tea Company
Percussion massager: HoMedics

Chapter 3
Ashwagandha: Vitamin Shoppe
Shilajit: Swanson Superior Herbs
Seaweed: Maine Seaweed Company, www.theseaweedman.com

Chapter 4
Mobility 2: Health Concerns
Specific Lumbaglin Chinese patent remedy: Asiachi

Chapter 5
JointCare, arjuna, guggul, Śhilajit: Ayurvedic Herbs Direct
Vine Essence Pill: Chinese Natural Herbs
Maca powder: My Natural Market

Chapter 6
Gymnema sylvestre capsules, organic tea tree oil: Puritan Pride
Xiao Yao Wan pills: East Earth Trade Winds

Chapter 7

Black cherry concentrate, aloe vera juice: Vitamin Shoppe
Tibetan goji berries and *Tibetan Precious Pills*: www.gojiberry.com
Neem products: Neem Tree Farms

Chapter 8

Chinese pain and injury treatments, liniments, patches: Modern Herb Shop
Chinese remedies for pet injuries and pain: East Earth Trade Winds

Chapter 9

Yucca capsules, homeopathic arnica products: Vitamin Shoppe
Guan Jie Yan Wan: Chinese Herbs Direct
Cold Laser and Diode Light therapy equipment: www.lhasaoms.com

Chapter 10

Tens, muscles stimulators, cold lasers for acupuncture: www.lhasaoms.com

Chapter 11

Colloidal silver products: Colloids for Life LLC
Yunnan paiyao capsules, tienchi powder: East Earth Trade Winds

Chapter 12

Detoxifying Foot Patch: Modern herb shop
Trisnake pills, Skin Balance: Lin Sisters Herb Shop

Chapter 13

Neem and pomegranate toothpaste: Himalaya Herbal Healthcare
Silvafresh: Trimedica
Ayurvedic oils and beauty products: Diamond Way Ayurveda

Chapter 14

Chinese patent remedies, Anmien Pien, Ding Xin Wan: East Earth Trade Winds
Calm Spirit, Ease 2, Ease Plus: Health Concerns

Chapter 15

Dan shen powder, tienchi powder, arjuna, guggul: Herbal Provider
Python Extra pills: Vitamin Shoppe

Chapter 16
Skullcap: Vitamin Shoppe
Pure cleansing products: Common Sense Farms

Chapter 17
Ashwagandha, vidari kanda powder, gotu kola: Banyan Botanicals
Saraswati churna: Ayurvedic Herbs Direct
Extractum astragali: East Earth Trade Winds

Chapter 18
LED lights for pain: Light Relief

Chapter 19
States where medical marijuana is legal: www.medicalmarijuana.procon.org

Recommended Articles and Videos from www.asianhealthsecrets.com

Chapter 1
"Flamenco Vivo!"
"What are Triglycerides? – Qué son los triglicéridos?"
"Angry Pain"
"Posturology"

Chapter 2
"Headaches & TMJ"

Chapter 3
"Autumn Colors – Colores de otoño"
"Bone/Joint/Ligament Natural Remedies"

Chapter 4
"Sciatica"
"Nopalea!"

Chapter 5
"Pain Treatments"

Chapter 6
"Pickle Mania!"
"Heart Health Pickles"

Chapter 7
"Personal Renewal"
"Weight Loss for Cancer-Prevention"
"Osteoporosis: Men and Women"
"Women's Spices"

Chapter 8
"After injury increase energy – nach einer Verletzung steigerung der Energie"

Chapter 9
"Marathon knees – proteger vos genoux"

Chapter 10
"Stress Injuries including carpal tunnel syndrome"
"Computer pains"

Chapter 11
"MRSA: One UK Hospital Story"
"Pet MRSA"
"Beijing 'Fog'"

Chapter 12
"Women's Wisdom #1"
"A New Face"

Chapter 13
"Strong Teeth/Gums"

Chapter 14
"Heart Energy"

Chapter 15
"Protect your heart"
"Earthquake/Tsunami: Text this message"

Chapter 16
"Coffee/Depression Study"
"Tea and Oranges for Stroke"

Chapter 17
"Ashwagandha a wonderful tonic"
"Sexual Spritz: Why numb pleasure?"

Chapter 18
"My PRP stem cell injections"
"Beyond the knife: Alternatives to surgery"
"Telomere: Fountain of Youth"
"Stem Cell International Conference Events"

Chapter 19
"Medical Marijuana Update"

Acknowledgments

I THANK AUTHOR AND HISTORIAN MICHAEL FOSTER FOR NAMING THIS BOOK and giving me the loving emotional and financial support to continue my work. I thank my family in Albuquerque, especially my mother, Letha Elizabeth Hadady, for her lovely book illustrations of ink drawings and her constant encouragement; my sister Michelle for her love; and my brother, Dr. Eric Scott Hadady, DC, for his health treatments. The medical professionals I have interviewed for *Naturally Pain Free* have offered important guidance and current information on effective pain treatments. Among them are Dr. Alan Lazar, MD, FACS, and Dr. Iris de Jesus, DC, in Florida; Dr. Matthew Gammons, MD, specializing in sports medicine, Maureen Gibeault, PT, Director, Vermont Sports Medicine Center, in Killington, and Drs. Patrick and Raymond Cooley, DC, and Cheri and Bryan Bush from Natural Rehab in Rutland, Vermont; Dr. Alan Kono, MD, FACC, Director of the Congestive Heart Failure Clinic at Dartmouth Hitchcock Medical Center in New Hampshire; Dr. Gerald Ginsberg, MD, FACS, Director of Plastic Surgery at New York Downtown Hospital, Dr. Erik Walter Steiner, OMD, Dr. Chrys, DC, Dr. Diane Gioia-Bargonetti, ND, CTN, Sharon Smith, qigong master, and Christopher Phillips, CCH, RSHom (NA) and physical therapy experts Holly Haupt and Jon Guadalupe, in New York; Suzanna Marcus, holistic healer and author in Israel; and doctors from Wujing General Hospital's Stem-Cell Transplant Department in Beijing, China.

I warmly thank my herbalists and dear friends Frank and Susan Lin at Lin Sisters Herb Shop and acupuncturist Dr. Lili Wu in New York. I thank Andrew Gaeddert, CEO and herbalist of Health Concerns in California; Dr. Thubten Lekshe, Doctor of Tibetan medicine and Director of Tanaduk Clinic on Orcas Island, Seattle; and Sabuti Dharmananda, Director of Institute for Traditional Medicine, Oregon, for their contributions to Asian-American herbalism and for their help in my research.

I thank the following professionals in charge of health information programs for giving me the opportunity to teach and meet many enthusiastic clients and readers. They include Karen Fuller at Dorot Senior Center, Erdem Ozden from Continuum Health Partners Group, Beth Israel Medical Center, Aracely Brown at New York Open Center, author/radio personality Gary Null, and filmmaker/ director Scott C. Hoyt in New York. New York major media professionals who have enthusiastically encouraged my work include author and natural health advocate Montel Williams and CBS television executive Kevin Harry.

I thank the entire staff at Sourcebooks for their enthusiastic support of this book, especially the detailed reading given by my editor Peter Lynch. A good editor makes you work, and Peter's comments and suggestions have increased the value and usability of this book on every page. I also thank Kelly Bale for her "hawk eye" copyediting. I look forward to promoting *Naturally Pain Free* guided by the expert support of Sourcebooks's publicity department headed by Liz Kelsch.

Index

About the Author

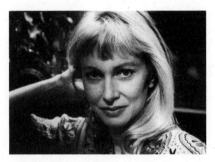

© Gad Cohen

"LETHA HADADY, D.AC., ONE OF THE nation's leading experts on natural Asian remedies, is leading a quiet ladylike revolution to bring herbal medicines from the Far East and elsewhere into everyday use in American homes." (*San Francisco Chronicle.*) *L.A. Times* Syndicate called her "the best-known blonde in Chinatown." Letha, a nationally certified acupuncturist (NCCAOM) has written four previous books on natural health and beauty. She is adjunct faculty for The Renfield Center for Nursing Education, Beth Israel Medical Center in New York, and teaches continuing education workshops through New York Open Center. Letha has led stress management workshops and acted as natural product consultant for Sony Entertainment Inc., Dreyfus, Ogilvy & Mather, and Consumer Eyes, Inc. in New York. She has been featured on many national television programs, including *The View*, NBC's *Today Show*, *Extra!*, and The Food Network, CNN, and ARTE (European television.) Her Ayurvedic health columns have appeared in *Heal India* magazine and *Healthy You!* published in India, Middle East, and Singapore. Letha is frequently a health expert on talk radio and podcasts in the U.S. and abroad. Her interactive website is www.asianhealthsecrets.com.